HERBAL DRUG INDUSTRY

From Cultivation to Innovation and Global Impact

HERBAL DRUG INDUSTRY

From Cultivation to Innovation and Global Impact

Abhishek Tiwari, PhD
Varsha Tiwari, PhD
Ajay Sharma, PhD
Editors

AAP APPLE ACADEMIC PRESS

First edition published 2026

Apple Academic Press Inc.
1265 Goldenrod Circle, NE,
Palm Bay, FL 32905 USA

760 Laurentian Drive, Unit 19,
Burlington, ON L7N 0A4, Canada

CRC Press
2385 NW Executive Center Drive,
Suite 320, Boca Raton FL 33431

4 Park Square, Milton Park,
Abingdon, Oxon, OX14 4RN, UK

Library and Archives Canada Cataloguing in Publication

CIP data on file with Canada Library and Archives

Library of Congress Cataloging-in-Publication Data

CIP data on file with US Library of Congress

ISBN: 978-1-779640-98-7 (hbk)
ISBN: 978-1-779640-99-4 (ebk)

DOI: 10.1201/9781779640994

About the Editors

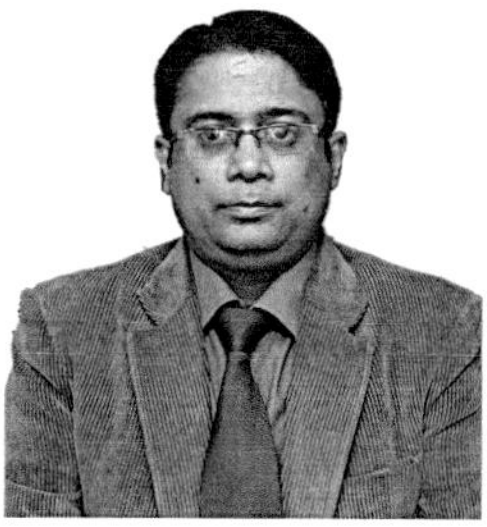

Abhishek Tiwari, PhD
Professor, Amity Institute of Pharmacy, Amity University Uttar Pradesh, Lucknow Campus, Lucknow, Uttar Pradesh, India

Abhishek Tiwari, PhD, is a Professor at the Amity Institute of Pharmacy, Lucknow, Amity University Uttar Pradesh, Noida, India. Dr. Tiwari has received more than the equivalent of nearly $108,000 USD in grants from various funding agencies including the Central Council for Research in Unani Medicine, New Delhi, India. Dr. Tiwari has been granted 35 patents and has filed nine patents for approval. He has published 76 papers in national and international journals. He has published more than 24 Indian and international books and 40 book chapters with Elsevier, Springer, Bentham, Wiley, and Astral International. He has guided two PhD and is currently guiding seven PhD students. Dr. Tiwari is an editorial member for various national and international journals. He received the best author award in 2019, best teacher award in 2019, and outstanding teacher awards in 2014 & 2015. He completed his BPharm at Jiwaji University, Gwalior, India, his MPharm at M.S. Ramaiah College of Pharmacy, Bangalore, and his PhD at Uttarakhand Technical University, Dehradun, India.

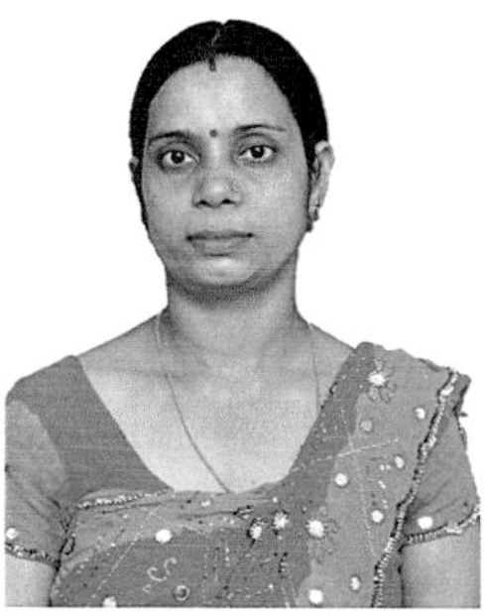

Varsha Tiwari, PhD
Professor, Amity Institute of Pharmacy of Amity University, Lucknow Campus, Uttar Pradesh, Lucknow, India

Varsha Tiwari, PhD, is a Professor with the Amity Institute of Pharmacy of Amity University, Lucknow, Uttar Pradesh, India. Dr. Tiwari has received more than nearly the equivalent of $1 million USD in grants from the Central Council for Research in Unani Medicine, New Delhi, India.

She has been granted 28 Indian, three South African, and three Australian patents. In addition, she has submitted a number of patents for approval. She has published 10 books and 28 book chapters with Elsevier, Springer, Bentham, Wiley, and Astral International. She has also published more than 65 research papers and has guided several doctoral, postgraduate, and graduate students. She has organized many conferences and also delivered many invited lectures at conferences. Dr. Varsha received Young Scientist, Young Author, and Pharmacy Recognition awards at the national level. She completed her doctorate at Uttarakhand Technical University and her MPharm at M. S. Ramaiah University, Bengaluru, India.

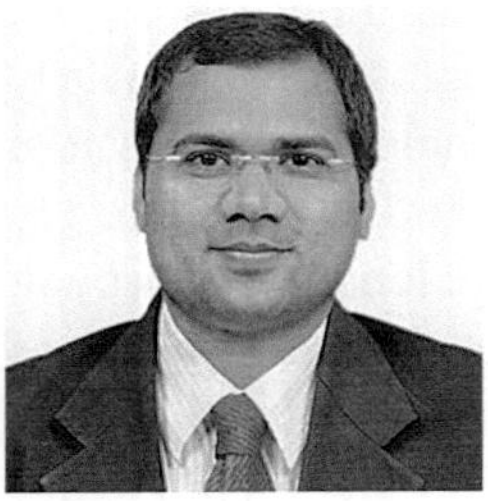

Ajay Sharma, PhD
Professor, Department of Pharmacognosy & Phytochemistry, School of Pharmaceutical Sciences, Delhi Pharmaceutical Sciences & Research University, New Delhi, Delhi, India

Ajay Sharma, PhD, is currently working as a Professor and Head of the Department of Pharmacognosy, School of Pharmaceutical Sciences, Delhi Pharmaceutical Sciences and Research University, New Delhi, India. He earned his PhD from the Poona College of Pharmacy, Bharati Vidyapeeth University, Pune, India. He has more than 15 years of teaching and research experience. His research area includes drug discovery and development from natural sources, ethnopharmacology, natural product chemistry, metabolomics, plant biotechnology, bioactivity-guided fractionation, and bioconversions. He has published more than 90 research articles in peer-review journals of national and international repute. He has presented more than 150 papers in national and international conferences. He has contributed four books and six book chapters and has published 10 Indian patents. He has been awarded a Postdoctoral Research Fellowship from Yeungnam University, Republic of Korea; Senior Research Fellowship from the Department of Biotechnology, New Delhi, India; and Junior Research Fellowship from the University Grants Commission, New Delhi, India during his studies. He has been awarded with research grants from the Central Council for Research in Unani Medicine (CCRUM), Ministry of Ayush (India), Department of Biotechnology (DBT) (India), All India Council for Technical Education (AICTE), and Madhya Pradesh

Council of Science and Technology (MPCOST). He has been awarded with Claude Leon Foundation Scholarship (2013) from the University of KwaZulu-Natal, Pietermaritzburg, Research Centre for Plant Growth and Development, South Africa; and a Postdoctoral Research Scholarship from the College of Pharmacy at International Islamic University, Pahang, Malaysia. He also received a Best Teacher Award during Eminent Teachers Award–2019 program organized by Amity University Madhya Pradesh in conjunction with Dainik Bhaskar, Gwalior; an APP Young Achiever Award during two-day international conference on Current Trends in Pharmaceutical Education Research, Edenburgh International College, Biratnagar, Nepal; an Innovation Award for Scientific Research—2018; and an AYUSH Award of CCRAS 2017 under the category Best Research Paper Award. He is a member of various national and international bodies. He been listed in the world's top 2% of scientists on the list of Stanford University consecutively for the last two years.

Contents

Contributors .... *xi*

Abbreviations .... *xvii*

Preface .... *xxi*

Introduction .... *xxiii*

1. **Herbal Drugs: Unveiling Nature's Pharmacopoeia for Modern Healthcare** **1**
Manish Kumar, Nidhi Arora, Priya, Sharad Visht, Shinu Pottathi, Manisha Bhatia, Abhishek Tiwari, Varsha Tiwari, Ajay Sharma, and Arya Lakshmi Marisetti

2. **Challenges in Upgrading and Modernizing Herbal Formulations** **29**
Pranay Wal, Ramkumar Pillappan, Rohini Karunakaran, Vishal Garg, Priyanka Gupta, Shweta Bhandari, Maninder Kaur, and Sourabh Kosey

3. **Plant Design, Layout, and Construction in Herbal Drug Production** **61**
Swapnali Patil, Pranali Pangam, and Poournima Sankpal

4. **Formulation and Production, and Management of Herbal Products** **77**
Akshay Kumar Lunawat, Tarun Sharma, Akshay Debanjan Mukherjee, Ankit Awasthi, Shubham Thakur, Manish Kumar, Abhishek Tiwari, Varsha Tiwari, and Arya Lakshmi Marisetti

5. **Regulatory Requirements for Herbal Drug Industries** **111**
Geetanjali Saini, Bhupendra Singh, Manish Vyas, Naresh Rangra, Prashant Kumar, and Sumit Durgapal

6. **Quality Standards and Monographs for Herbal Drugs** **141**
Arya Lakshmi Marisetti, Gana Manjusha K., Saurabh Dahiya, M. V. N. L. Chaitanya, D. S. N. B. K. Prasant, Venkateswara Rao Amara, and Ritu Karwasra

7. Testing of Natural Products and Drugs 181
Jaya Narhire, Ganesh Asabe, Nitin Wadate, Chantibabu Katta, Deepankar Bahuguna, Soham Loharkar, Gopal Bajad, Jitender Madan, Srinivas Nanduri, Samanthula Gananadhamu, Ashish Baldi, Snigdha Singh, Ramesh Chandra

8. Patents and Intellectual Property in Herbal Industry: The Outlook 219
Kavita Munjal, Arushi Sharma, Karan Sharma, Rohit Thakur, Ashish Baldi, and Vinod Kumar Gauttam

9. Patent Searches and Literature Review in Herbal Science 245
Gana Manjusha K., Arya Lakshmi Marisetti, and M. V. N. L. Chaitanya

10. Herbal Drug Licensing and Compliance 283
Ravikiran Vegada, Jankhana Baraiya, and Sourabh Jain

11. Future Trends and Conclusion 303
Ankita Wal, E. Selvakumari, C. S. Kandasamy, Himangi Vij, Biresh Kumar Sarkar, Arpan Kumar Tripathi, Samiksha Prashant Warke, and Mohd Masih Uzzaman Khan

Index 329

Contributors

Venkateswara Rao Amara
Department of Regulatory Toxicology, National institute of Pharmaceutical Education and Research (NIPER), Hajipur, Bihar, India

Nidhi Arora
Chandigarh Pharmacy College, Chandigarh Group of Colleges, Jhanjeri, Punjab, India

Ganesh Asabe
Department of Pharmaceutics, National Institute of Pharmaceutical Education and Research, Hyderabad, Telangana, India

Ankit Awasthi
Department of Pharmaceutics, ISF College of Pharmacy, Moga, Punjab, India

Deepankar Bahuguna
Department of Pharmaceutics, National Institute of Pharmaceutical Education and Research, Hyderabad, Telangana, India

Gopal Bajad
Department of Pharmaceutics, National Institute of Pharmaceutical Education and Research, Hyderabad, Telangana, India

Ashish Baldi
Department of Pharmaceutical Sciences and Technology, Maharaja Ranjit Singh Punjab Technical University, Punjab, India

Jankhana Baraiya
Assistant Professor, Department of Pharmacognosy, School of Pharmacy, RK University, Rajkot, Gujarat, India

Shweta Bhandari
Acropolis Institute of Pharmaceutical Education and Research, Indore, MP, India

Manisha Bhatia
M M College of Pharmacy, MM (DU), Mullana, Ambala, Haryana, India

M. V. N. L. Chaitanya
School of Pharmaceutical Sciences, Lovely Professional University, Punjab, India

Ramesh Chandra
Department of Chemistry, University of Delhi, Delhi, India; Dr B.R Ambedkar Centre for Biomedical Research, University of Delhi, Delhi, India; Institute of Nano Medical Sciences, University of Delhi, Delhi, India; Maharaja Surajmal Brij University, Bharatpur, Rajasthan, India

Saurabh Dahiya
Delhi Institute of Pharmaceutical Sciences and Research, Delhi Pharmaceutical Sciences & Research University, New Delhi, India

Sumit Durgapal
Department of Pharmaceutics, Uttaranchal University, Dehradun, Uttarakhand, India

Ankita Wal
PSIT-Pranveer Singh Institute of Technology (Pharmacy), Kanpur, Uttar Pradesh, India

Samanthula Gananadhamu
Department of Analytical Sciences, National Institute of Pharmaceutical Education and Research, Hyderabad, Telangana, India

Vishal Garg
Jaipur School of Pharmacy, Maharaj Vinayak Global University, Jaipur, Rajasthan, India

Vinod Kumar Gauttam
Professor & Dean, SGT College of Pharmacy, SGT University, Gurugram, India

Priyanka Gupta
Shivalik College of Engineering, Shimla Bypass Road Shiniwala, Dehradun, Uttarakhand, India

Sourabh Jain
Professor, Department of Pharmacognosy, Arihant School of Pharmacy & Bio-Research Institute, Gandhinagar, Gujarat, India

Gana Manjusha K.
Vignan Institute of Pharmaceutical Technology, Visakhapatnam, Adhara Pradesh, India

C. S. Kandasamy
Department of Pharmacognosy, Karpagam College of Pharmacy, Coimbatore, Tamil Nadu, India

Rohini Karunakaran
Unit of Biochemistry, Faculty of Medicine, AIMST University, Semeling, Kedah, Malaysia

Ritu Karwasra
Central Council for Research in Unani Medicine (CCRUM), Ministry of AYUSH, Government of India, New Delhi, India

Chantibabu Katta
Department of Pharmaceutics, National Institute of Pharmaceutical Education and Research, Hyderabad, Telangana, India

Maninder Kaur
G S R M Memorial College of Pharmacy, Lucknow, Uttar Pradesh, India

Mohd Masih Uzzaman Khan
Department of Pharmaceutical Chemistry & Pharmacognosy, Unaizah College of Pharmacy, Unaizah, Saudi Arabia

Sourabh Kosey
Department of Pharmacy Practice, ISF College of Pharmacy, Moga, Punjab, India

Manish Kumar
Department of Pharmaceutics, ISF College of Pharmacy, Moga, Punjab, India

Prashant Kumar
SRM Modinagar College of Pharmacy, SRM Institute of Science and Technology Delhi-NCR Campus, Delhi-Meerut Road, Modinagar, Ghaziabad, Uttar Pradesh, India

Soham Loharkar
Department of Pharmaceutics, National Institute of Pharmaceutical Education and Research, Hyderabad, Telangana, India

Akshay Kumar Lunawat
Department of Pharmaceutics, ISF College of Pharmacy, Moga, Punjab, India

Jitender Madan
Department of Pharmaceutics, National Institute of Pharmaceutical Education and Research, Hyderabad, Telangana, India

Arya Lakshmi Marisetti
Department of Pharmacognosy & Phytochemistry, School of Pharmaceutical Sciences, Delhi Pharmaceutical Sciences & Research University, New Delhi, Delhi, India

Akshay Debanjan Mukherjee
Department of Quality Assurance, ISF College of Pharmacy, Moga, Punjab, India

Kavita Munjal
Amity Institute of Pharmacy, Amity University, Noida, Uttar Pradesh, India

Srinivas Nanduri
Department of Chemical Sciences, National Institute of Pharmaceutical Education and Research, Hyderabad, Telangana, India

Jaya Narhire
Department of Pharmaceutics, National Institute of Pharmaceutical Education and Research, Hyderabad, Telangana, India

Pranali Pangam
Department of Pharmaceutical Quality Assurance, Vijayrao Naik College of Pharmacy, Shirval, Tal-Kankavli, Maharashtra, India

Swapnali Patil
Department of Pharmaceutics, Vijayrao Naik College of Pharmacy, Shirval, Tal-Kankavli, Maharashtra, India

Ramkumar Pillappan
Department of Pharmaceutics, NGSM Institute of Pharmaceutical Sciences, Mangalore, Karnataka, India

Shinu Pottathi
Department of Biomedical Sciences, College of Clinical Pharmacy, King Faisal University, Al-Ahsa, Saudi Arabia

D. S. N. B. K. Prasant
School of Pharmacy & Technology Management, SVKM's Narsee Monjee Institute of Management Studies (NMIMS), Polepally SEZ, TSIIC, Hyderabad, India

Priya
School of Pharmaceutical Sciences, CT University, Ludhiana, Punjab, India

Naresh Rangra
School of Pharmacy, Chitkara University, Baddi, Himachal Pradesh, India

Geetanjali Saini
NGI College of Pharmacy, Neelkanth Group of Institutions, Modipuram, Uttar Pradesh, India

Poournima Sankpal
Department of Pharmaceutical Chemistry, Bharati Vidyapeeth College of Pharmacy, Palus, Maharashtra, India

Biresh Kumar Sarkar
Department of Pharmacy, Central Ayurveda Research Institute, Central Council for Research in Ayurvedic Sciences, Kolkata, West Bengal, India

E. Selvakumari
Department of Pharmacognosy, College of Pharmacy, Mother Theresa Post Graduate and Research Institute of Health Sciences Puducherry, India

Ajay Sharma
Department of Pharmacognosy & Phytochemistry, School of Pharmaceutical Sciences, Delhi Pharmaceutical Sciences & Research University, New Delhi, Delhi, India

Tarun Sharma
Department of Pharmaceutics, ISF College of Pharmacy, Moga, Punjab, India

Arushi Sharma
Department of Pharmaceutics, Shiva Institute of Pharmacy, Bilaspur, Himachal Pradesh, India

Karan Sharma
Department of Pharmacology, Shiva Institute of Pharmacy, Bilaspur, Himachal Pradesh, India

Bhupendra Singh
NGI College of Pharmacy, Neelkanth Group of Institutions, Modipuram, Uttar Pradesh, India

Snigdha Singh
Department of Chemistry, University of Delhi, Delhi, India

Shubham Thakur
Department of Pharmaceutics, ISF College of Pharmacy, Moga, Punjab, India

Rohit Thakur
Department of Pharmaceutics, Shiva Institute of Pharmacy, Bilaspur, Himachal Pradesh, India

Abhishek Tiwari
Amity Institute of Pharmacy, Amity University Uttar Pradesh, Lucknow Campus, Lucknow, Uttar Pradesh, India

Varsha Tiwari
Amity Institute of Pharmacy, Amity University Uttar Pradesh, Lucknow Campus, Lucknow, Uttar Pradesh, India

Arpan Kumar Tripathi
KIPS, Shri Shankaracharya Professional University, Bhilai, Chhattisgarh, India

Ravikiran Vegada
Assistant Professor, Department of Pharmacognosy, Sharda School of Pharmacy, Pethapur, Gandhinagar, Gujarat, India

Himangi Vij
PSIT-Pranveer Singh Institute of Technology (Pharmacy), Kanpur, Uttar Pradesh, India

Sharad Visht
Faculty of Pharmacy, Tishk International University, Erbil, Kurdistan Region, Iraq

Manish Vyas
Research and development cell, Parul University, Vadodara, Gujarat, India

Nitin Wadate
Department of Pharmaceutics, National Institute of Pharmaceutical Education and Research, Hyderabad, Telangana, India

Pranay Wal
PSIT-Pranveer Singh Institute of Technology (Pharmacy), Kanpur, UP, India

Samiksha Prashant Warke
Department of Pharmaceutics, KYDSCT College of Pharmacy, Jalgaon, Maharashtra, India

Abbreviations

ABS	access and benefit-sharing
ADR	adverse drug reaction
AHP	American Herbal Pharmacopoeia
API	ayurvedic pharmacopoeia of India
ARTG	Australian Register for Therapeutic Goods
ASU	Ayurvedic, Siddha, and Unani
ATC	Anatomical Therapeutic Chemical
AYUSH	Ayurveda, Yoga & Naturopathy, Unani, Siddha, and Homoeopathy
BFAD	Bureau of Food and Drugs
BHP	British Herbal Pharmacopoeia
BP	British Pharmacopoeia
CAGR	compound annual growth rate
CBD	Convention on Biological Diversity
CE	capillary electrophoresis
CEC	capillary electrochromatography
CIP	cleaning-in-place
CMC	carboxymethylcellulose
CNS	central nervous system
DAD	diode array detectors
DCA	Drugs and Cosmetics Act
DRAs	Drug Regulatory Authorities
EAE	enzyme-assisted extraction
EMA	European Medicines Agency
EP	European Pharmacopoeia
EPO	European Patent Office
FDA	Food and Drug Administration
FTIR	Fourier transform-infrared spectroscopy
FTO	freedom to operate
GACP	Good Agricultural and Collection Practices
GC	gas chromatography
GC–MS	gas chromatography–mass spectrometry
GMPs	good manufacturing practices
HA	hyaluronic acid
HMPC	herbal medicinal products
HMs	herbal medicines

HNMs	herbal nanomedicines
HPI	Homoeopathic Pharmacopoeia of India
HPLC	high-performance liquid chromatography
HPTLC	high-performance thin-layer chromatography
HSCCC	high-speed counter-current chromatography
HVAC	heating, ventilation, and air conditioning
HWE	hot-water extraction
ICAR	Indian Council of Agricultural Research
ICBG	International Cooperative Biodiversity Groups
ICDRA	International Conference of Drug Regulatory Authorities
IP	intellectual property
IPC	Indian Pharmacopoeia Commission
IPC	International Patent Classification
IPR	intellectual property rights
IUCN	International Union for Conservation of Nature
JP	Japanese Pharmacopoeia
LM	language model
MA	marketing authorization
MAE	microwave-assisted extraction
MALDI	matrix-assisted laser desorption/ionization
MS	mass spectrometry
NAFDAC	National Agency for Food and Drug Administration and Control
NE	noise elimination
NHP	natural health products
NHPD	Natural Health Product Directorate
NLCs	nanostructured lipid carriers
NMPB	National Medicinal Plants Board
NMR	nuclear magnetic resonance spectroscopy
NPs	nanoparticles
OTC	over-the-counter
PAs	pyrrolizidine alkaloids
PEF	pulsed electric field
PLE	pressurized liquid extraction
prep-HPLC	preparative high-pressure liquid chromatography
RCT	randomized clinical trial
RH	relative humidity
RP	reverse-phase
RS	reference standards
SEP	sustainable entrepreneurship practices
SFE	supercritical fluid extraction
SMEs	small- and medium-sized enterprises

SPI	Siddha Pharmacopoeia of India
SRISTI	Society for Research and Initiatives for Sustainable Technology and Institutions)
SSC	Species Survival Commission
TCM	traditional Chinese medicine
THMPD	Traditional Herbal Medicinal Products Directive
TKDL	traditional knowledge digital library
TLC	thin-layer chromatography
TOF	time-of-flight
TRIPs	trade-related aspects of intellectual property rights
UAE	ultrasonic-assisted extraction
UPI	Unani Pharmacopoeia of India
USFDA	United States Food and Drug Administration
USP	US Pharmacopoeia
USPTO	United States Patent and Trademark Office
UV	ultraviolet
WHO	World Health Organization
WIPO	World Intellectual Property Organization
WTO	World Trade Organization

Preface

Herbal drugs have been used in healthcare systems all over the world for thousands of years. From ancient times, people have used plant-based remedies, and today, modern societies are rediscovering their benefits. This book, *Herbal Drug Industry*, explores the many aspects of herbal medicines, including their history, chemical makeup, uses, and the challenges they face today.

Chapter 1 introduces herbal drugs, tracing their rich history and cultural significance in various civilizations. It discusses the recent rise in the popularity of herbal medicines, highlighting their safety, natural origins, and benefits. It also explains the science behind these remedies and how they work in the body.

Chapter 2 covers the challenges in improving and modernizing herbal formulations. This chapter talks about quality issues like adulteration and misidentification and stresses the importance of good farming and manufacturing practices. It also highlights the role of green entrepreneurship in the cultivation and processing of medicinal plants.

Chapter 3 focuses on the design, layout, and construction of facilities for herbal drug production. It highlights the need for efficient workflows, minimizing contamination risks, and using advanced technologies to ensure safe and effective manufacturing processes that meet industry standards.

Chapter 4 delves into the formulation and production management of herbal products. It underscores the need for quality control, regulatory compliance, and sustainable sourcing practices. This chapter discusses the entire lifecycle of herbal products, ensuring their quality, safety, and effectiveness.

Chapter 5 explores the regulatory requirements for the herbal drug industry. It discusses different regulatory frameworks for herbal medicines and the challenges in ensuring their efficacy, safety, and quality. The chapter emphasizes the need for harmonized regulations to enhance the acceptance and credibility of herbal products worldwide.

Chapter 6 examines the quality standards and monographs for herbal drugs. It emphasizes the need for consistent high-quality standards in herbal medicine production and suggests revisions to ensure these standards adequately reflect the quality and effectiveness of herbal medicines.

Chapter 7 focuses on testing natural products and drugs. It details various analytical techniques and quality control tests required to ensure the safety and efficacy of herbal products, covering methods like chromatography and spectroscopy.

Chapter 8 addresses patents and intellectual property in the herbal industry. It discusses the increasing recognition of the value of herbal medicines and global trends in patenting these products. The chapter examines challenges and opportunities in patent laws and suggests reforms to encourage innovation and protect intellectual property rights.

Chapter 9 provides insights into patent searches and literature reviews. It outlines strategic methods for efficient information retrieval and emphasizes the importance of comprehensive literature reviews and using various tools for effective patent searches.

Chapter 10 discusses herbal drug licensing and compliance. It highlights the regulatory frameworks governing herbal products globally and stresses the importance of adhering to international standards to ensure their safety and quality.

Finally, chapter 11 looks toward the future, exploring emerging trends and concluding the book with a vision for the continued growth and integration of herbal medicines into modern healthcare systems. It highlights the potential of standardized protocols, cutting-edge research, and government initiatives in promoting the global acceptance and use of herbal remedies.

The authors will be please if this book activates the research and education lives of students, scientists and academic professionals along with create business potential. Information provided in this book will also serve the curiosity of general people about terpenoids and natural products.

This book would not have been possible without the assistance of Apple Academic Press, CRC Press, and Taylor & Francis publishers. The authors are especially grateful to Mrs. Sheetal Kumar and Mr. Rakesh Kumar for their scientific knowledge, helpful attitude, and encouragement.

Introduction

Herbal drugs, which come from various plant sources, have been used in healthcare for thousands of years. These natural remedies have been a cornerstone in many cultures around the world, providing relief and treatment for various ailments long before modern medicine was established. Herbal drugs are currently experiencing a resurgence in popularity due to their perceived safety, natural origins, and potential health benefits. This book aims to provide a comprehensive understanding of the herbal drug industry, from historical significance to modern applications, challenges, and future trends.

Herbal medicine has deep roots in the traditions of numerous cultures. Ancient civilizations, such as those in China, India, Egypt, and Greece, have long relied on plants for medicinal purposes. The enduring appeal of herbal remedies is tied to their cultural and traditional significance. Even today, many people prefer herbal drugs because they are considered more in tune with nature and less likely to cause side effects compared to synthetic medicines.

To appreciate the value of herbal drugs, it is essential to understand the science that supports their use. Plants contain a variety of chemical compounds, known as secondary metabolites, which include alkaloids, flavonoids, and terpenoids. These compounds are responsible for the medicinal properties of herbs. This book will explore how these substances interact with the human body to produce therapeutic effects. By understanding these interactions, we can better grasp why certain herbs are effective for specific health conditions.

Herbal drugs are used to treat a wide range of health issues. They can help with pain management, boost the immune system, support digestive health, and improve mental wellness, among other benefits. Through case studies and clinical evidence, this book will showcase the effectiveness of various herbal drugs in treating specific conditions. It will also highlight key herbs like ginseng, echinacea, and turmeric, explaining their historical use, chemical makeup, and current applications in healthcare.

One of the biggest challenges in the herbal drug industry is ensuring the quality and consistency of products. This book will discuss the importance of good agricultural and collection practices (GACP) and good manufacturing practices (GMP). It will also delve into the regulatory aspects and the need for rigorous clinical trials to establish the safety and efficacy of herbal drugs. Ensuring high standards in production and quality control is crucial for maintaining consumer trust and achieving therapeutic effectiveness.

Despite their benefits, herbal drugs face several challenges. Issues like adulteration, contamination, and variability in ingredient quality can impact their safety and efficacy. This book will examine these challenges and propose solutions, such as better agricultural practices and more stringent manufacturing standards. Additionally, the growing demand for herbal products presents opportunities for innovation and entrepreneurship in the industry.

The integration of advanced technologies, such as bioinformatics, genomics, and metabolomics, is revolutionizing herbal drug research. These technologies help identify potential new herbal drugs and understand their mechanisms of action at a molecular level. This book will explore how these advancements are shaping the future of the herbal drug industry, making it possible to develop more effective and targeted treatments.

Herbal drugs have been a vital part of human healthcare for centuries, and their relevance continues to grow in the modern world. This book provides a holistic view of the herbal drug industry, combining historical context, scientific understanding, practical applications, and insights into future trends. It serves as a valuable resource for healthcare professionals, researchers, and anyone interested in the potential of natural remedies to improve health and well-being. Through this exploration, we aim to highlight the enduring significance of nature's pharmacopoeia and its place in contemporary medicine.

—Editors

CHAPTER 1

Herbal Drugs: Unveiling Nature's Pharmacopoeia for Modern Healthcare

MANISH KUMAR[1*], NIDHI ARORA[2], PRIYA[3], SHARAD VISHT[4], SHINU POTTATHI[5], MANISHA BHATIA[6], ABHISHEK TIWARI[7], VARSHA TIWARI[7], AJAY SHARMA[8], and ARYA LAKSHMI MARISETTI[9]

[1]*Department of Pharmaceutics, ISF College of Pharmacy, Moga, Punjab, India*

[2]*Chandigarh Pharmacy College, Chandigarh Group of Colleges, Jhanjeri, Punjab, India*

[3]*School of Pharmaceutical Sciences, CT University, Ludhiana, Punjab, India*

[4]*Faculty of Pharmacy, Tishk International University, Erbil, Kurdistan Region, Iraq*

[5]*Department of Biomedical Sciences, College of Clinical Pharmacy, King Faisal University, Al-Ahsa, Saudi Arabia*

[6]*M. M. College of Pharmacy, MM (DU), Mullana, Ambala, Haryana, India*

[7]*Amity Institute of Pharmacy, Amity University Uttar Pradesh, Lucknow Campus, Lucknow, Uttar Pradesh, India*

[8]*Department of Pharmacognosy & Phytochemistry, School of Pharmaceutical Sciences, Delhi Pharmaceutical Sciences & Research University, New Delhi, Delhi, India*

[9]*Department of Pharmacognosy & Phytochemistry, School of Pharmaceutical Sciences, Delhi Pharmaceutical Sciences & Research University, New Delhi, Delhi, India*

*Corresponding author

Herbal Drug Industry: From Cultivation to Innovation and Global Impact.
Abhishek Tiwari, Varsha Tiwari, and Ajay Sharma (Eds.)

DOI: 10.1201/9781779640994-1

ABSTRACT

Herbal drugs, derived from diverse plant sources, have played a vital role in global healthcare systems for millennia. Their enduring appeal stems from cultural significance, natural origin, and perceived safety, making them increasingly relevant in modern medicine. This chapter offers a concise yet comprehensive overview of herbal drugs, emphasizing their historical roots, chemical constituents, mechanisms of action, therapeutic applications, and contemporary challenges. Key plant-derived compounds such as alkaloids, flavonoids, and terpenoids are highlighted for their pharmacological activities, including anti-inflammatory, antioxidant, and immunomodulatory effects. The therapeutic applications span multiple domains, including pain relief, digestive health, immune support, and mental well-being. Case studies and clinical evidence underscore their efficacy, while concerns about quality control, standardization, and regulatory oversight are addressed. Prominent herbal agents like ginseng, echinacea, and turmeric are explored for their established roles in modern therapeutic practice. The chapter also delves into emerging research trends, including the integration of bioinformatics, metabolomics, and genomics to enhance the discovery and understanding of herbal medicines.

1.1 INTRODUCTION TO THE HERBAL DRUG

1.1.1 OVERVIEW OF HERBAL DRUG

Herbal drugs, also known as botanical medicine or phytotherapy, utilize plants and plant extracts for therapeutic purposes. These remedies have been used for centuries across cultures worldwide and continue to be popular due to their perceived naturalness and potential health benefits. They encompass a wide range of substances, including leaves, roots, bark, flowers, and seeds [1].

Herbal drugs can be consumed in various forms, such as teas, capsules, tinctures, or applied topically as creams or poultices. They are believed to contain bioactive compounds that exert medicinal effects on the body, often targeting specific symptoms or conditions [2].

While many herbal remedies have anecdotal evidence supporting their efficacy, scientific research on their effectiveness varies. Some herbs have been extensively studied and validated for certain uses, while others lack robust clinical evidence. It is essential to approach herbal medicine with caution, considering potential interactions with medications and the variability in product quality and dosage [3].

Key points about herbal drugs include the following:

Natural origin: Herbal drugs derive from natural sources, primarily plants, and their constituents have been used for medicinal purposes throughout human history. These remedies harness the bioactive compounds found in various parts of plants, including leaves, roots, stems, flowers, and seeds, to promote health and treat ailments. The natural origin of herbal drugs underscores their perceived safety and efficacy, as they are often viewed as gentle alternatives to synthetic pharmaceuticals [4, 5].

Traditional use: Many herbal remedies have a long history of use in traditional medicine systems such as Ayurveda, traditional Chinese medicine (TCM), and Native American medicine. Traditional use of herbal drugs refers to the historical and cultural practices of using plants and plant-derived substances for medicinal purposes [6]. These remedies have been passed down through generations and often play a significant role in indigenous healing systems worldwide. Traditional herbal medicine relies on the knowledge and experience of local healers and has been integral to healthcare in many societies for centuries [7].

Bioactive compounds: Plants contain a diverse array of bioactive compounds, including alkaloids, flavonoids, terpenes, and essential oils, which contribute to their therapeutic effects.

Alkaloids: Nitrogen-containing compounds with diverse pharmacological activities. Examples include morphine from opium poppy and caffeine from coffee beans.

Flavonoids: Polyphenolic compounds with antioxidant, anti-inflammatory, and anticancer properties. Sources include green tea (catechins) and citrus fruits (hesperidin).

Terpenoids: Derived from the isoprene unit, terpenoids have various biological activities, including antimicrobial and anti-inflammatory effects. Examples include artemisinin from *Artemisia annua* (sweet wormwood) and menthol from mint plants [8].

Phenolic compounds: Known for their antioxidant properties, phenolic compounds also possess anti-inflammatory and anticancer activities. Resveratrol from grapes and curcumin from turmeric are examples.

Glycosides: Sugar-bound compounds found in plants with diverse medicinal properties. Cardiac glycosides like digoxin from *Digitalis purpurea* are used in heart conditions [9].

Saponins: Compounds with foaming properties and various pharmacological effects, including antimicrobial and anticancer activities. Ginsenosides from ginseng are well-known saponins.

Essential oils: Volatile compounds with aromatic properties and therapeutic effects. Lavender oil and tea tree oil are examples with antimicrobial and soothing properties.

These compounds often work synergistically within the plant, contributing to its overall medicinal properties. However, the efficacy and safety of herbal drugs depend on factors such as dosage, formulation, and interactions with other compounds [10].

Holistic approach: Herbal medicine often takes a holistic approach to health, considering the balance and interaction of physical, mental, and spiritual aspects of well-being. Instead of merely treating symptoms, it focuses on addressing the root causes of illness and promoting balance within the individual [11].

Herbal medicine within a holistic framework often integrates various modalities, including nutrition, lifestyle modifications, stress management techniques, and mind-body practices like yoga or meditation. The goal is to support the body's innate healing abilities and restore harmony between different aspects of a person's being [18].

This approach recognizes that health is influenced by multiple factors, including physical, emotional, social, and environmental elements. By incorporating herbal remedies into a broader framework of holistic health, individuals can strive for comprehensive well-being and resilience [12].

Cultural significance: Herbal remedies are often deeply rooted in cultural practices and are passed down through generations.

Cultural heritage: Herbal remedies have been passed down through generations within cultures, forming an integral part of traditional medicine systems such as TCM, Ayurveda, and Native American healing practices [13].

Spiritual and ritualistic use: Many cultures incorporate herbs into spiritual rituals and ceremonies, believing in their ability to heal not just the body but also the spirit. For example, smudging ceremonies using sage or other herbs are common in indigenous cultures [14].

Connection to nature and the land: Herbal medicine emphasizes the connection between humans and the natural world. Indigenous cultures often have deep-rooted relationships with local plants, considering them sacred and respecting their harvesting and usage practices [15].

Community and identity: Herbal remedies foster community bonds and are often shared among family members and within communities. They play a role in preserving cultural identity and traditional knowledge [16].

Adaptation and innovation: While traditional herbal knowledge is ancient, it continues to evolve as cultures adapt to changing environments and incorporate new understandings. Modern herbalists blend traditional practices with contemporary knowledge and scientific research [17].

Regulatory considerations: Regulatory frameworks for herbal drugs vary globally. Some countries have established regulations to ensure the safety, quality, and efficacy of herbal products. In general, these products may fall under dietary supplement regulations, traditional medicine regulations, or a combination of both, depending on the jurisdiction [19].

United States: In the United States, herbal drugs are often regulated as dietary supplements under the Dietary Supplement Health and Education Act of 1994. The Food and Drug Administration (FDA) oversees the regulation of dietary supplements, ensuring they are safe and labeled accurately. However, manufacturers are not required to demonstrate efficacy before marketing, unlike prescription drugs [20].

European Union: Herbal drugs are regulated under the Traditional Herbal Medicinal Products Directive (THMPD) in the European Union (EU). This directive establishes standards for the registration and marketing of traditional herbal medicines. To be approved, herbal drugs must demonstrate their safety, quality, and traditional use.

Canada: Health Canada regulates herbal drugs as natural health products (NHPs). NHPs must undergo premarket assessment for safety, efficacy, and quality before they can be legally sold in Canada. The Natural and Nonprescription Health Products Directorate oversees this process [21].

China: Herbal drugs are an integral part of TCM. The China Food and Drug Administration regulates TCM products, including herbal drugs, to ensure their safety, quality, and efficacy [22].

India: In India, herbal drugs are regulated as Ayurvedic, Siddha, and Unani (ASU) medicines under the Ministry of AYUSH (Ayurveda, Yoga & Naturopathy, Unani, Siddha, and Homoeopathy). The regulatory framework includes standards for the manufacture, sale, and distribution of ASU medicines [23].

These are just a few examples, and regulatory frameworks can differ significantly in other countries and regions. It is essential for manufacturers and consumers to understand and comply with the specific regulations governing herbal drugs in their respective areas.

Potential benefits: Herbal drugs are studied for their potential benefits in treating various health conditions, including but not limited to pain, inflammation, digestive issues, and respiratory problems [24].

Anti-inflammatory effects: Certain herbs like turmeric, ginger, and boswellia possess anti-inflammatory properties, which may help alleviate symptoms of conditions like arthritis and inflammatory bowel disease.

Antioxidant activity: Many herbs contain antioxidants such as flavonoids and polyphenols, which can help neutralize harmful free radicals in the body, potentially reducing the risk of chronic diseases like cancer and cardiovascular disease [25].

Digestive health: Herbs like peppermint, ginger, and chamomile are known for their digestive benefits, including alleviating symptoms of indigestion, bloating, and nausea.

Stress reduction: Adaptogenic herbs like Ashwagandha and rhodiola are believed to help the body adapt to stress and promote relaxation, potentially reducing symptoms of anxiety and improving overall well-being [26].

Immune support: Some herbs, including echinacea, elderberry, and garlic, are thought to enhance immune function, potentially reducing the frequency and severity of colds and other infections [37].

Cognitive enhancement: Certain herbs like *Ginkgo biloba* and *Bacopa monnieri* are believed to improve cognitive function and memory, though more research is needed to confirm their efficacy [36].

It is important to note that while herbal drugs offer potential benefits, individual responses can vary, and not all claims are supported by robust scientific evidence. It is advisable to consult with a healthcare professional before incorporating herbal remedies into your healthcare regimen, especially if you have underlying health conditions or are taking medications [27].

Challenges: Standardization of herbal products, understanding interactions with conventional medicines, and ensuring consistent quality are challenges associated with herbal medicine.

It is important to note that while some herbal drugs have demonstrated therapeutic effects, not all herbal remedies are supported by rigorous scientific evidence. As with any form of medicine, it is advisable to consult with healthcare professionals before using herbal drugs, especially in conjunction with conventional treatments [28].

Quality control and standardization: Ensuring consistent quality and potency of herbal products can be challenging due to variability in plant sources, growing conditions, harvesting methods, and manufacturing processes. Lack of standardization may lead to variability in the concentration of active ingredients, affecting the efficacy and safety of herbal drugs [42].

Safety concerns: While herbal drugs are often perceived as natural and safe, they can still pose risks, including adverse reactions, herb–drug interactions, and contamination with pesticides, heavy metals, or microbial pathogens. Some herbs may also have toxic effects if consumed in high doses or for prolonged periods [35].

Limited scientific evidence: Despite their widespread use, many herbal remedies lack rigorous scientific research to support their safety and efficacy. Conducting clinical trials on herbal drugs presents challenges, including funding, ethical considerations, and the complexity of studying multicomponent plant extracts [29].

Regulatory issues: Herbal drugs are subject to less stringent regulation compared to pharmaceutical drugs in many countries. This can result in inconsistent oversight of manufacturing practices, labeling accuracy, and product quality, leading to potential risks for consumers [30].

Cultural and traditional knowledge: Traditional herbal medicine often relies on empirical knowledge passed down through generations. While this knowledge can offer valuable insights, it may also perpetuate misconceptions or unsupported claims about the efficacy of certain herbs [38].

1.1.2 INFRASTRUCTURE FOR HERBAL DRUGS

The infrastructure for herbal drugs involves various components that contribute to the cultivation, processing, research, development, regulation, and distribution of herbal medicines. It encompasses various stakeholders, including farmers, manufacturers, regulators, and healthcare practitioners, who play crucial roles in ensuring the quality, safety, and efficacy of herbal medicines [39].

***Cultivation and harvesting*:** Herbal medicines often rely on the sustainable cultivation and harvesting of medicinal plants. This involves selecting appropriate growing conditions, planting, nurturing, and harvesting plants at the right time to preserve their therapeutic properties.

Farming practices: Herbal drugs often begin with the cultivation of medicinal plants using sustainable and standardized farming practices [34].

Cultivation: Herbal drugs are often cultivated in specific environments that mimic their natural habitat. Factors such as soil type, sunlight exposure, and water availability are crucial for successful cultivation. Some herbs can be grown in home gardens, while others require specialized farming practices [33].

Harvesting: Timing is critical for harvesting herbal drugs to ensure optimal potency and efficacy. Different plant parts, such as leaves, flowers, roots, or seeds, may need to be harvested at specific stages of growth. Harvesting methods vary depending on the plant species and the desired medicinal compounds [32].

Processing: After harvesting, herbal drugs may undergo processing steps such as drying, grinding, or extraction to preserve their therapeutic properties. Proper processing techniques help maintain the quality and stability of herbal products [31].

Quality control: Quality control measures are essential to ensure the safety and efficacy of herbal drugs. This includes testing for contaminants, verifying the identity of plant species, and assessing the concentration of active compounds [42].

Processing and extraction: After harvesting, medicinal plants undergo processing to extract active compounds or prepare them into various forms such as powders, extracts, tinctures, or capsules. Manufacturing facilities must adhere to good manufacturing practices (GMPs) to ensure product quality and safety [40].

Quality assurance: Stringent quality control measures during processing to ensure consistency and purity of herbal extracts [41].

Facilities: Processing and extraction facilities need to be designed and maintained to meet GMP standards. This includes appropriate layout, sanitation, ventilation, and equipment to prevent contamination and ensure product integrity [39].

Equipment: Specialized equipment such as extraction machines, distillation units, drying chambers, and milling machines are essential for processing herbal raw materials into standardized extracts or formulations [43].

Quality control: Infrastructure for quality control involves laboratories equipped with instruments for chemical analysis, microbiological testing, and other assays to verify the identity, purity, and potency of herbal products [42].

Storage: Adequate storage facilities with controlled temperature and humidity are necessary to preserve the stability and shelf-life of herbal raw materials and finished products [45].

Research and development: Continuous research is essential to validate the efficacy of herbal medicines, identify active compounds, elucidate mechanisms of action, and explore potential drug interactions. Research also contributes to the development of standardized herbal extracts and formulations [44].

Botanical research: Scientific studies on the bioactive compounds, pharmacological properties, and potential therapeutic effects of medicinal plants [47].

Formulation development: Research into developing standardized herbal formulations for specific health conditions [46].

Research institutions: Academic institutions, government research agencies, and private organizations play vital roles in conducting basic and clinical research on herbal drugs. These institutions provide funding, expertise, and facilities for studying the pharmacology, toxicology, and clinical applications of herbal remedies [49].

Botanical gardens and herbaria: These facilities preserve and study plant species, providing researchers with access to diverse botanical resources for drug discovery and development. They contribute to the identification, authentication, and sustainable cultivation of medicinal plants [7].

Analytical laboratories: High-quality analytical facilities equipped with advanced instrumentation are essential for assessing the chemical composition, purity, and quality of herbal drugs. These labs employ techniques such as chromatography, spectroscopy, and mass spectrometry (MS) to analyze active constituents and detect contaminants [53].

Regulatory agencies: Government regulatory bodies establish guidelines and standards for the quality, safety, and efficacy of herbal drugs. They oversee product registration, labeling, and manufacturing practices to ensure consumer protection and public health [56].

Clinical trial infrastructure: Infrastructure for conducting clinical trials is necessary to evaluate the therapeutic effects and safety profiles of herbal medicines. This includes research hospitals, clinics, and specialized centers capable of recruiting participants, administering interventions, and collecting data in controlled settings [54].

Traditional knowledge documentation: Efforts to document and preserve traditional knowledge about medicinal plants are essential for integrating traditional herbal practices with modern scientific research. Collaborative initiatives with indigenous communities promote cultural preservation and facilitate the sustainable use of herbal resources [48].

Industry collaboration: Collaboration between pharmaceutical companies, herbal product manufacturers, and research institutions accelerates the development and commercialization of herbal drugs. Partnerships enable access to funding, expertise, and distribution channels, fostering innovation in product development and marketing strategies [50].

Regulatory compliance: The regulatory landscape for herbal drugs involves ensuring their safety, quality, and efficacy through infrastructure and compliance measures. Regulatory bodies establish guidelines for manufacturing, labeling, and marketing herbal products to protect public health and promote consumer confidence [52].

Regulatory agencies: Government agencies overseeing the safety, efficacy, and quality of herbal drugs [56].

Quality standards: Establishment of monographs and quality standards for herbal products [55].

Quality control and testing: Robust quality control measures are essential to verify the identity, purity, and strength of herbal ingredients. Analytical techniques such as chromatography, spectroscopy, and microbiological assays are used to assess the composition and quality of herbal products [51].

Product labeling and claims: Regulatory agencies require accurate labeling of herbal drugs, including ingredient lists, dosage instructions, and warnings about potential side effects or interactions. Claims regarding the therapeutic properties of herbal products must be supported by scientific evidence and comply with advertising regulations [58].

Safety monitoring: Herbal drugs should undergo safety assessments to identify and mitigate potential risks to consumers. This includes monitoring adverse reactions, conducting toxicity studies, and evaluating the safety of long-term use or interactions with other medications [57].

Registration and licensing: Herbal drugs may need to be registered or licensed by regulatory authorities before they can be marketed and sold to consumers. This process typically involves submitting documentation on product formulation, manufacturing processes, safety data, and clinical evidence supporting efficacy [59].

Manufacturing facilities: The manufacturing facilities for herbal drugs encompass a diverse range of processes, from sourcing raw materials to production, quality control, and packaging. These facilities must adhere to stringent regulatory standards to ensure the safety, efficacy, and consistency of herbal products [60].

GMPs: Manufacturing facilities must comply with GMP regulations specific to herbal products. These guidelines ensure that manufacturing processes are well-controlled and consistently produce herbal drugs of high quality [61].

Quality control laboratories: These laboratories play a crucial role in testing raw materials, in-process samples, and finished products for identity, purity, potency, and safety. They employ various analytical techniques, such as high-performance liquid chromatography, gas chromatography, and MS, to assess the quality of herbal drugs [63].

Cultivation and sourcing: Manufacturing facilities may have partnerships or their cultivation sites to ensure a consistent and sustainable supply of herbal raw materials. They may also establish relationships with reputable suppliers to source high-quality botanicals [62].

Extraction and processing equipment: Manufacturing facilities require specialized equipment for extracting bioactive compounds from botanical raw materials. This may include techniques such as solvent extraction, supercritical fluid extraction, or steam distillation. Processing equipment is also necessary for drying, milling, and granulating herbal materials [64].

Packaging and labeling: Herbal drugs must be packaged and labeled accurately to meet regulatory requirements and ensure consumer safety. Packaging materials should be selected carefully to preserve the stability and potency of the product, while labeling should provide clear information on dosage, usage instructions, and potential allergens [65].

Education and training: Healthcare practitioners require education and training in herbal medicine to safely and effectively recommend herbal remedies to patients. This includes understanding herb–drug interactions, dosing guidelines, and evidence-based uses of herbal therapies [107].

Training programs: Educational initiatives for farmers, herbalists, and professionals involved in the herbal industry.

Research collaboration: Partnerships between academia and industry for advancing herbal medicine research.

Academic programs: Universities and colleges offer academic programs ranging from certificates to advanced degrees in herbal medicine. These programs cover disciplines such as pharmacognosy, phytochemistry, herbal pharmacology, and traditional herbal medicine practices. Students learn about plant identification, cultivation techniques, extraction methods, quality control, and clinical applications [90].

Continuing education: Professionals in healthcare, including pharmacists, physicians, nurses, and herbalists, pursue continuing education programs to enhance their knowledge and skills in herbal medicine. These programs provide updates on research findings, regulatory requirements, and clinical practices [66].

Research initiatives: Academic institutions, research organizations, and government agencies conduct research on herbal medicines to evaluate their safety, efficacy, mechanisms of action, and potential interactions. This research contributes to evidence-based practice and informs educational curricula [67].

Regulatory framework: Governments establish regulations and standards for the education, training, and practice of herbal medicine practitioners to ensure public safety and quality assurance. Regulatory bodies may accredited educational programs, license practitioners, and monitor product quality [70].

Public awareness and consumer education: Public health agencies, nonprofit organizations, and professional associations promote awareness of herbal medicine safety, efficacy, and responsible use through educational campaigns, workshops, and informational resources.

Distribution and marketing: The infrastructure, distribution, and marketing of herbal drugs involve various elements, including cultivation, processing, distribution channels, and promotional activities [73].

Supply chain management: Efficient distribution networks to ensure timely availability of herbal products [74].

Marketing strategies: Promoting herbal medicines through various channels, including traditional and digital platforms [72].

Cultural acceptance and demand: Cultural attitudes toward herbal medicine greatly influence its distribution and marketing. In regions where traditional medicine is deeply rooted in culture, there tends to be higher demand for herbal drugs. For example, TCM and Ayurveda in India have established markets and distribution networks based on centuries-old practices [69].

Regulatory frameworks: Regulatory policies play a crucial role in shaping the distribution and marketing of herbal drugs. Different countries have varying regulations governing the production, sale, and advertising of herbal products. These regulations often dictate quality control standards, labeling requirements, and permissible health claims. For example, the EU is THMPD sets out specific requirements for the registration and marketing of herbal medicines [70].

Quality control and standardization: Ensuring the quality and safety of herbal drugs is essential for consumer confidence and regulatory compliance. Infrastructure for quality control involves standardized cultivation practices, harvesting methods, and manufacturing processes. Organizations such as the United States Pharmacopeia and the Pharmacopoeia of the People's Republic of China provide standards for herbal product quality [68].

Distribution channels: Herbal drugs are distributed through various channels, including pharmacies, health food stores, online retailers, and traditional medicine practitioners. The choice of distribution channel often depends on factors such as target market, product type, and regulatory requirements. In recent years, e-commerce platforms have emerged as significant distribution channels for herbal products, offering a wide reach and convenience for consumers.

Marketing strategies: Marketing herbal drugs involves communicating their benefits, addressing consumer concerns, and complying with regulatory restrictions on health claims. Marketing strategies may include educational campaigns, endorsements by healthcare professionals, and advertising through various media channels. Social media platforms have become increasingly important for reaching consumers interested in NHPs [72].

Pharmacovigilance: Pharmacovigilance for herbal drugs involves monitoring and assessing the safety of these products throughout their lifecycle, from premarket approval to postmarket surveillance. It aims to identify, evaluate, and prevent adverse effects or other safety concerns associated with herbal medicines [77].

Regulatory framework: Governments and regulatory agencies established frameworks to oversee the safety of herbal drugs. This includes guidelines for product registration, labeling requirements, and adverse event reporting mechanisms [76].

Adverse event reporting systems: These systems allow healthcare professionals and consumers to report any adverse effects or reactions associated with herbal products. These reports are crucial for identifying potential safety concerns and taking appropriate regulatory actions [79].

Monitoring programs: Continuous monitoring of herbal drugs in the market helps identify emerging safety issues. This can involve postmarketing surveillance studies, pharmacovigilance databases, and collaboration with healthcare providers and researchers [6].

Quality control: Ensuring the quality and consistency of herbal products is essential for their safety and efficacy. Quality control measures include testing for contaminants, standardization of active ingredients, and adherence to GMPs [75].

Research and evaluation: Conducting research on the safety and efficacy of herbal medicines contributes to evidence-based decision-making. This includes clinical trials, systematic reviews, and pharmacological studies to understand their mechanisms of action and potential risks [78].

International collaboration: International collaboration in the infrastructure of herbal drugs involves cooperation among countries, researchers, and institutions to enhance the research, development, regulation, and promotion of herbal medicines globally. This collaboration aims to leverage diverse expertise, resources, and perspectives to address common challenges and opportunities in the field of herbal medicine [84].

Global standards: Collaboration with international organizations to align standards and facilitate the global trade of herbal drugs.

Research exchange: Sharing research findings and knowledge across borders [80].

Research and development: Collaborative research initiatives facilitate the investigation of the efficacy, safety, and mechanisms of action of herbal medicines. By pooling resources and expertise, researchers can conduct multicenter clinical trials, explore traditional knowledge, and develop standardized methods for quality control and product evaluation [71].

Regulatory harmonization: Harmonizing regulatory frameworks across countries streamlines the registration, quality control, and market access of herbal drugs. International collaboration enables the exchange of regulatory practices, guidelines, and data to ensure the safety, efficacy, and quality of herbal products while facilitating their global trade [83].

Capacity building: Collaborative efforts support capacity building in herbal medicine research, education, and manufacturing. Training programs, workshops, and knowledge-sharing initiatives strengthen the skills of researchers, healthcare professionals, regulators, and industry stakeholders, fostering innovation and sustainability in the herbal medicine sector [81].

Cultural and ethical considerations: Recognizing the cultural diversity and traditional knowledge associated with herbal medicine, international collaboration promotes respectful engagement with local communities and indigenous practices. Ethical guidelines and frameworks safeguard intellectual property rights, biodiversity, and the equitable sharing of benefits derived from herbal resources [82].

Public awareness and education: Collaborative campaigns and educational programs raise public awareness about the potential benefits and risks of herbal medicines. By disseminating evidence-based information and promoting responsible use, international collaboration fosters informed decision-making among consumers, healthcare providers, and policymakers [85].

Consumer awareness: Consumers need access to accurate information about herbal medicines to make informed decisions about their use. This includes understanding potential benefits, risks, and limitations, as well as consulting qualified healthcare professionals when necessary [88].

Regulatory bodies: Government agencies, such as the FDA in the United States or the European Medicines Agency in Europe, regulate herbal drugs to ensure their safety, quality, and efficacy. These agencies provide guidelines and regulations for the manufacturing, labeling, and marketing of herbal products, contributing to consumer confidence [89].

Healthcare professionals: Physicians, pharmacists, and other healthcare providers play a crucial role in educating consumers about herbal drugs. They can provide evidence-based information, discuss potential interactions with prescription medications, and offer guidance on incorporating herbal remedies into overall healthcare plans [87].

Educational initiatives: Academic institutions, healthcare organizations, and nonprofit groups conduct educational programs and workshops to enhance consumer awareness of herbal drugs. These initiatives may include seminars, online courses, and informational materials that cover topics such as herbal safety, efficacy, and proper usage [86].

Consumer information sources: Reliable sources of information, including reputable websites, books, and pamphlets, offer guidance on selecting and using herbal drugs. Government health agencies, universities, and health-care organizations often provide evidence-based resources that empower consumers to make informed decisions about herbal remedies [90, 91].

1.2 VARIOUS DOSAGE FORMS IN HERBAL MEDICINES

Herbal medicines are available in various dosage forms, providing flexibility in administration and catering to different patient preferences. The choice of dosage form often depends on the properties of the herbal remedy, intended therapeutic effect, and practical considerations. Here are some common dosage forms in herbal medicine.

1.2.1 HERBAL TEAS (INFUSIONS AND DECOCTIONS)

Preparation: Made by steeping plant material (leaves, flowers, or roots) in hot water.

Examples: Chamomile tea, peppermint tea, ginger tea.
Benefits: Easy preparation, mild taste, and suitable for various herbs [98].

1.2.2 TINCTURES

Preparation: Extracts of herbs using alcohol or a combination of alcohol and water.

Examples: Echinacea tincture, ginseng tincture.

Benefits: Concentrated form, long shelf life, and easy to dose [99].

1.2.3 CAPSULES AND TABLETS

Preparation: Dried herbal extracts or powders encapsulated or compressed into tablet form.

Examples: Garlic capsules, *G. biloba* tablets.

Benefits: Convenient, precise dosing, and often standardized for consistent potency [100].

1.2.4 POWDERS

Preparation: Finely ground herbal material.

Examples: Ashwagandha powder, turmeric powder.

Benefits: Versatile, can be mixed into liquids or foods, and customizable dosing [101].

1.2.5 TOPICAL PREPARATIONS

Preparation: Creams, ointments, or balms containing herbal extracts for external application.

Examples: Arnica cream, calendula ointment.

Benefits: Targeted application for skin conditions or localized pain relief [102].

1.2.6 SYRUPS

Preparation: Herbal extracts combined with a sweet syrup base.

Examples: Elderberry syrup, cough syrups.

Benefits: Palatable, especially for children, and can be soothing for respiratory issues [103].

1.2.7 ESSENTIAL OILS

Preparation: Concentrated volatile oils extracted from aromatic plants.

Examples: Lavender oil, tea tree oil.

Benefits: Aromatherapy, topical application, or diffusion for various therapeutic effects [104].

1.2.8 LOZENGES AND PASTILLES

Preparation: Solid dosage forms designed to dissolve slowly in the mouth.

Examples: Licorice lozenges, throat pastilles.

Benefits: Convenient for throat and respiratory issues, pleasant taste [105].

1.2.9 HERBAL EXTRACT SPRAYS

Preparation: Liquid herbal extracts in a spray form.

Examples: Propolis throat spray, echinacea spray.

Benefits: Convenient for oral application, easy to carry.

1.2.10 POULTICES AND COMPRESSES

Preparation: Herbal materials applied directly to the skin, often with the help of a cloth or bandage.

Examples: Comfrey poultice, chamomile compress.

Benefits: Localized treatment for inflammation or injuries [106].

It is important for individuals to follow recommended dosage instructions and consult with healthcare professionals, especially when combining herbal medicines with conventional treatments. Additionally, the choice of dosage form may depend on individual preferences, health conditions, and specific therapeutic goals.

1.3 CLINICAL DATA ON HERBAL DRUGS (FIGURES 1.1 AND 1.2)

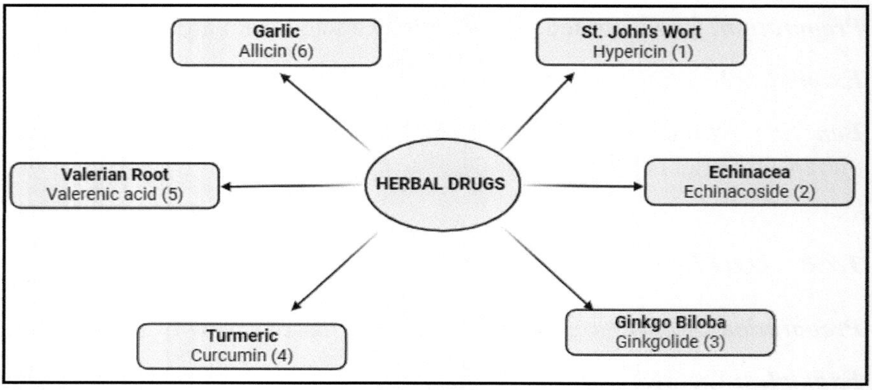

FIGURE 1.1 Pictorial representation of the herbal drugs used in clinical trials.

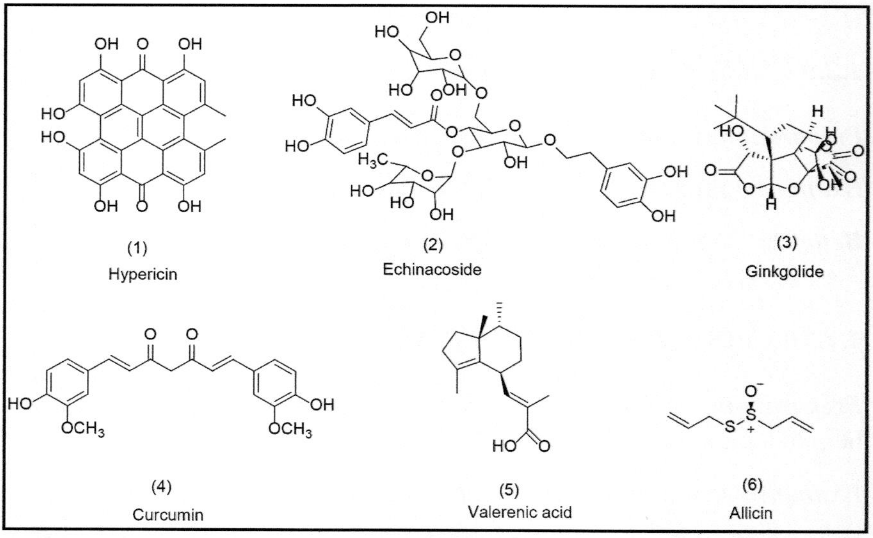

FIGURE 1.2 The chemical structure data of herbal drugs used in clinical trials.

Table 1.1 allows for easy comparison of different herbal drugs, their respective conditions treated, study types, sample sizes, and key findings or results from clinical studies (Table 1.1). Keep in mind that the specific details and formatting may vary depending on the exact information available for each herbal drug [92–97].

TABLE 1.1 Clinical Trials Data of Herbal Drugs

Herbal Drug	Condition Treated	Study Type	Sample Size	Results
St. John's Wort/ Klamath Weed	Depression	Randomized controlled trial	200 participants	Significant reduction in depressive symptoms compared to placebo ($p < 0.05$)
Echinacea	Common cold	Meta-analysis	1000 participants	Shortened duration and severity of cold symptoms compared to placebo ($p < 0.01$)
Ginkgo biloba	Cognitive decline	Longitudinal study	500 elderly participants	Slowed progression of cognitive decline over 2-year period compared to control group ($p < 0.001$)
Turmeric	Inflammation	Systematic review	Various studies included	Demonstrated anti-inflammatory effects comparable to NSAIDs in multiple trials
Valerian root	Insomnia	Double-blind RCT	300 participants	Improved sleep quality and reduced sleep latency compared to placebo ($p < 0.05$)
Garlic	Hypertension	Cohort study	1000 hypertensive patients	Modest reduction in blood pressure observed over 6-month period compared to baseline ($p < 0.01$)

KEYWORDS

- **herbal drugs**
- **case studies**
- **clinical evidence**

REFERENCES

1. World Health Organization. *WHO Traditional Medicine Strategy: 2014–2023*. World Health Organization, 2013.
2. Snyder, M., Lindquist, R., Tracy, M. F., & Chen, K.-M. Evolution and use of complementary therapies and integrative health approaches. *Complementary Therapies in Nursing: Promoting Integrative Care*, 2022, pp. 3–20.
3. Bent, S. Herbal medicine in the United States: Review of efficacy, safety, and regulation: Grand rounds at University of California, San Francisco Medical Center. *J Gen Int Med* 2008, 23, 854–859.
4. Harvey, A. L. Natural products in drug discovery. *Drug Discov Today* 2008, 13(19–20), 894–901.
5. Newman, D. J., & Cragg, G. M. Natural products as sources of new drugs over the nearly four decades from 01/1981 to 09/2019. *J Nat Prod* 2020, 83(3), 770–803.
6. Ekor, M. The growing use of herbal medicines: Issues relating to adverse reactions and challenges in monitoring safety. *Front Pharmacol* 2014, 4, 177.
7. Fabricant, D. S., & Farnsworth, N. R. The value of plants used in traditional medicine for drug discovery. *Environ Health Perspect* 2001, 109(suppl 1), 69–75.
8. Rahimi, R., & Abdollahi, M. Herbal medicines for the management of irritable bowel syndrome: A comprehensive review. *World J Gastroenterol* 2017, 23(30), 509–525.
9. Newman, D. J., & Cragg, G. M. Natural products as sources of new drugs from 1981 to 2014. *J Nat Prod* 2016, 79(3), 629–661.
10. Atanasov, A. G., et al., Discovery and resupply of pharmacologically active plant-derived natural products: A review. *Biotechnol Adv* 2015, 33(8), 1582–1614.
11. Kligler, B., & Lee, R. Integrative medicine and holistic approaches to health and well-being. *Primary Care Clinics* 2004, 31(4), 1075–1086.
12. Boon, H., Verhoef, M., O'Hara, D., Findlay, B., & Majid, N. Integrative health care: Arriving at a working definition. *Altern Ther Health Med* 2004, 10(5), 48–56.
13. Bodeker, G., Ong, C. K., & Grundy, C. WHO Global Atlas of Traditional, Complementary and Alternative Medicine. 2005.
14. Cunningham, A. B. Applied ethnobotany: People, Wild Plant Use and Conservation. 2001.
15. Farnsworth, N. R., & Soejarto, D. D. Global Importance of medicinal plants. In: Akerele, A., Heywood, V., & Synge, H., (Eds.), *The Conservation of Medicinal Plants*, 1991.

16. Moerman, D. E. Native American ethnobotany. 1998.
17. Pieroni, A., & Vandebroek, I. Travelling cultures and plants: The ethnobiology and ethnopharmacy of human migrations. 2007.
18. US Department of Health and Human Services. Complementary, alternative, or integrative health: What's in a name. *National Center for Complementary and Integrative Health* (2021).
19. Young, A. L., & Scott Bass, I. The Dietary Supplement Health and Education Act. *Food & Drug LJ* 1995, 50, 285.
20. Grupstra, R. J., Goedecke, T., Scheffers, J., Strassmann, V., & Gardarsdottir, H. Review of studies evaluating effectiveness of risk minimization measures assessed by the European Medicines Agency between 2016 and 2021. *Clin Pharmacol Ther* 2023, 114(6), 1285–1292.
21. Ng, J. Y., & Luong, M. Evaluation of the Canadian natural health product regulatory framework in academic research: A scoping review. *Eur J Integr Med* 2020, 37, 101159.
22. Liang, Z., Lai, Y., Li, M., Shi, J., Lei, C. I., Hu, H., & Oi Lam Ung, C. Applying regulatory science in traditional Chinese medicines for improving public safety and facilitating innovation in China: A scoping review and regulatory implications. *Chin Med* 2021, 16, 1–16.
23. Katiyar, C. K., Chakrabarty, A. K., Dubey, S. K., Pandey, P. K., Tumulu, M., & Narwaria, A. Enhancing quality of Ayush products—Strategies and efforts of the ministry of Ayush and Ayush industry. *J Res Ayurvedic Sci* 2023, 7(Suppl 1), S73–S81.
24. Pan, S. Y., et al., New perspectives on Chinese herbal medicine (Zhong-Yao) research and development. *Evid-Based Complement Alternat Med* 2013, 2013, 269625.
25. Ghasemzadeh, A., et al. Antioxidant Potential and Its Relationship with Polyphenol and Flavonoid Content in Plants. *Oxidative Med Cell Longev* 2016, 2016, 905–987.
26. Kennedy, D. O., & Wightman, E. L. Herbal extracts and phytochemicals: Plant secondary metabolites and the enhancement of human brain function. *Adv Nutrit* 2011, 2(1), 32–50.
27. Patel, S. Adaptogenic herbs in aging-related disorders. *Evid-Based Complement Alternat Med* 2015, 2015, 1–11.
28. Ernst, E. The risk-benefit profile of commonly used herbal therapies: Ginkgo, St. John's Wort, Ginseng, Echinacea, Saw Palmetto, and Kava. *Ann Intern Med* 2002, 136(1), 42–53.
29. Zhou, S., et al., Challenges in herbal medicine research: A journal overview. *Evid-Based Complement Alternat Med* 2003, 1(1), 3–7.
30. World Health Organization. *Quality Control Methods for Medicinal Plant Materials*. World Health Organization, 1998.
31. Júnior, J. O. C. S., Costa, R. M. R., Teixeira, F. M., & Barbosa, W. L. R.. Processing and quality control of herbal drugs and their derivatives. *Quality Control of Herbal Medicines and Related Areas*, Intech: Rijeka, Croatia, 2011, pp. 195–222.
32. Tanko, H., Carrier, D. J., Duan, L., & Clausen, E. Pre- and post-harvest processing of medicinal plants. *Plant Genet Resour* 2005, 3(2), 304–313.
33. Board, N. I. I. R. *Herbs Cultivation & Their Utilisation*. Asia Pacific Business Press Inc., 2003.

34. Mwale, M., Bhebhe, E., Chimonyo, M., & Halimani, T. E. Use of herbal plants in poultry health management in the Mushagashe small-scale commercial farming area in Zimbabwe. *Int J Appl Res Vet Med* 2005, 3(2), 163–170.
35. Ara, I., Maqbool, M., Bukhari, B., Ara, N., & Hajam, T. A. Present status, standardisation and safety issues with herbal drugs. *Int J Res Pharm Sci Technol* 2020, 1(3), 95–101.
36. Goel, B., & Maurya, N. K. Memory booster herb (natural cognitive enhancers): An overview. *Int J Physiol Nutrit Phys Educ* 2019, 4(1), 975–979.
37. Naik, S. R., Thakare, V. N., & Joshi, F. P. Functional foods and herbs as potential immune adjuvants and medicines in maintaining a healthy immune system: A commentary. *J Complement Integr Med* 2010, 7(1).
38. Teschke, R., Larrey, D., Melchart, D., & Danan, G. Traditional Chinese medicine (TCM) and herbal hepatotoxicity: RUCAM and the role of novel diagnostic biomarkers such as microRNAs. *Medicines* 2016, 3(3), 18.
39. Zhang, M., Wang, C., Zhang, R., Chen, Y., Zhang, C., Heidi, H., & Li, M. Comparison of the guidelines on good agricultural and collection practices in herbal medicine of the European Union, China, the WHO, and the United States of America. *Pharm Res* 2021, 167, 105533.
40. Qu, L., Li, X., Xiong, Y., Wang, Z., Zhou, Y., Zou, W., Tang, J., & Wang, M. Opportunities and hurdles to European market access for multi-herbal traditional Chinese medicine products: An analysis of EU regulations for combination herbal medicinal products. *Pharm Res* 2022, 186, 106528.
41. Mykhailenko, O., Desenko, V., Ivanauskas, L., & Georgiyants, V. Standard operating procedure of Ukrainian saffron cultivation according to good agricultural and collection practices to assure quality and traceability. *Ind Crops Prod* 2020, 151, 112376.
42. Choi, D. W., Kim, J. H., Cho, S. Y., Kim, D. H., & Chang, S. Y. Regulation and quality control of herbal drugs in Korea. *Toxicology* 2002, 181, 581–586.
43. Tambare, P., Tamboli, F. A., & More, H. N. Standardisation of herbal drugs: An overview. *Int Res J Pharm* 2011, 2(12), 56–60.
44. World Health Organization. *World Health Organization Traditional Medicine Strategy 2014–2023*. World Health Organization: Geneva, 2013.
45. Son, J.-Y., Shin, J.-W., & Son, C.-G. Stability study for herbal drugs according to storage conditions and periods. *J Korean Med* 2009, 30(2), 127–132.
46. Ahmed, H. M., Nabavi, S., & Behzad, S. Herbal drugs and natural products in the light of nanotechnology and nanomedicine for developing drug formulations. *Mini Rev Med Chem* 2021, 21(3), 302–313.
47. Li, W. Botanical drugs: A future for herbal medicines. *J Contemp Health L. & Policy* 2002, 19, 117.
48. Gurib-Fakim, A. Medicinal plants: Traditions of yesterday and drugs of tomorrow. *Mol Asp Med* 2006, 27(1), 1–93.
49. Kim, H. K., & Verpoorte, R. Sample preparation for plant metabolomics. *Phytochem Anal* 2010, 21(1), 4–13.
50. Scossa, F., Benina, M., Alseekh, S., Zhang, Y., & Fernie, A. R. The integration of metabolomics and next-generation sequencing data to elucidate the pathways of

natural product metabolism in medicinal plants. *Planta Med* 2018, 84(12/13), 855–873.
51. Kaack, K. V., Knudsen, B. F., & Rosenberg, L. Guidelines for good agricultural and collection practice for sambucusnigra flowers and berries as active ingredients in traditional herbal medicine and dietary supplements. In: *I International Symposium on Elderberry 1061*, 2013, pp. 225–235.
52. Govindaraghavan, S., & Sucher, N. J. Quality assessment of medicinal herbs and their extracts: Criteria and prerequisites for consistent safety and efficacy of herbal medicines. *Epilepsy Behav* 2015, 52, 363–371.
53. Farooqui, N. A., Dey, A., Singh, G. N., Easwari, T. S., & Pandey, M. K. Analytical techniques in quality evaluation of herbal drugs. *Asian J Pharm Res* 2014, 4(3), 112–117.
54. Willcox, M., Siegfried, N., & Johnson, Q. Capacity for clinical research on herbal medicines in Africa. *J Alternat Complement Med* 2012, 18(6), 622–628.
55. Länger, R., Stöger, E., Kubelka, W., & Helliwell, K. Quality standards for herbal drugs and herbal drug preparations—appropriate or improvements necessary. *Planta Med* 2018, 84(06/07), 350–360.
56. Rousseaux, C. G., & Schachter, H. Regulatory issues concerning the safety, efficacy and quality of herbal remedies. *Birth Defects Res Part B: Dev Reprod Toxicol* 2003, 68(6), 505–510.
57. Chan, T. Y. K. Monitoring the safety of herbal medicines. *Drug Saf* 1997, 17(4), 209–215.
58. Kušar, A. N. I. T. A., & Pravst, I. Quality and safety of botanical food products and their labelling. *Agro Food Ind Hi Tech* 2014, 25, 33–35.
59. Verma, N. Current regulatory challenges and approaches in the registration of herbal drugs in Europe. *Clin Res Regul Affairs* 2016, 33(1), 9–24.
60. Han, J.-E., Park, M., Park, J.-H., Oh, D., Kim, K. H., & Sung, S.-H. Quality control of pharmacopuncture: A comparative study of good manufacturing practice and external herbal dispensary standards. *J Pharmacopunct* 2021, 24(2), 59.
61. He, T.-T., Ung, C. O. L., Hu, H., & Wang, Y.-T. Good manufacturing practice (GMP) regulation of herbal medicine in comparative research: China GMP, cGMP, WHO-GMP, PIC/S and EU-GMP. *Eur J Integr Med* 2015, 7(1), 55–66.
62. Muriuki, J., Franzel, S., Mowo, J., Kariuki, P., & Jamnadass, R. Formalisation of local herbal product markets has potential to stimulate cultivation of medicinal plants by smallholder farmers in Kenya. *Forests, Trees and Livelihoods* 2012, 21(2),, 114–127.
63. Muyumba, N. W., Mutombo, S. C., Sheridan, H., Nachtergael, A., & Duez, P.. Quality control of herbal drugs and preparations: The methods of analysis, their relevance and applications. *Talanta Open* 2021, 4, 100070.
64. Mohammad A., Huda, S. N., Manan, Z. A., Alwi, S. R. W., Chua, L. S., Mustaffa, A. A., & Yunus, N. A. Herbal processing and extraction technologies. *Sep Purif Rev* 2016, 45(4), 305–320.
65. Amekyeh, H., Kumadoh, D., Adongo, D. W., Orman, E., Abubakar, S., Dwamena, A., & OkweesiAggrey, M. Evaluation of packaging, labels, and some physicochemical properties of herbal antimalarial products on the Ghanaian market. *Heliyon* 2024, 10(5), e27032.

66. Strohecker, J. L., & Athens, W. Design of an online continuing education module: Herbal and dietary supplements impact warfarin safety and efficacy. In: *Adult and Continuing Education: Concepts, Methodologies, Tools, and Applications*, IGI Global, 2014, pp. 580–589.
67. Inamdar, N., Edalat, S., Kotwal, V. B., & Pawar, S. Herbal drugs in the milieu of modern drugs. *Int J Green Pharm (IJGP)* 2008, 2(1).
68. Alamgir, A. N. M., & Alamgir, A. N. M. Herbal drugs: Their collection, preservation, and preparation; evaluation, quality control, and standardisation of herbal drugs. *Therapeutic Use of Medicinal Plants and Their Extracts: Volume 1: Pharmacognosy*, 2017, pp. 453–495.
69. Rana, K. K., & Rana, S. Review on present status and future of herbal medicine. *Beats Nat Sci* 2014, 1(2), 1–8.
70. Sahoo, N., Manchikanti, P., & Dey, S. Herbal drugs: Standards and regulation. *Fitoterapia* 2010, 81(6), 462–471.
71. Lee, K.-H. Research and future trends in the pharmaceutical development of medicinal herbs from Chinese medicine. *Public Health Nutr* 2000, 3(4a), 515–522.
72. Gunjan, M., Naing, T. W., Saini, R. S., Ahmad, A., Naidu, J. R., & Kumar, I. Marketing trends & future prospects of herbal medicine in the treatment of various diseases. *World J Pharm Res* 2015, 4(9), 132–155.
73. Calixto, J. B. Efficacy, safety, quality control, marketing and regulatory guidelines for herbal medicines (phytotherapeutic agents). *Brazil J Med Biol Res* 2000, 33, 179–189.
74. Octavia, A., Sriayudha, Y., & Ali, H. Innovation capability and supply chain management: Empirical study of Indonesian traditional herbal medicine products. *Int J Supply Chain Manag* 2020, 9(1), 601–608.
75. Shinde, V. M., Dhalwal, K., Potdar, M., & Mahadik, K. R. Application of quality control principles to herbal drugs. *Int J Phytomed* 2009, 1(1), 4–8.
76. Okumu, M. O., Ochola, F. O., Onyango, A. O., Mbaria, J. M., Gakuya, D. W., Kanja, L. W., Kiama, S. G., & Onyango, M. A. The legislative and regulatory framework governing herbal medicine use and practice in Kenya: A review. *Pan Afr Med J* 2017, 28(1), 232.
77. Barnes, J. Pharmacovigilance of herbal medicines: A UK perspective. *Drug Saf* 2003, 26, 829–851.
78. Abd, W., Shahezwan, M., Sakthong, P., & Winit-Watjana, W. Development and validation of novel scales to determine pharmacist's care for herbal and dietary supplement users. *Res Soc Admin Pharm* 2020, 16(4), 475–487.
79. Posadzki, P., Watson, L. K., & Ernst, E. Adverse effects of herbal medicines: An overview of systematic reviews. *Clin Med* 2013, 13(1), 7.
80. Booker, A., Johnston, D., & Heinrich, M.. Value chains of herbal medicines—Research needs and key challenges in the context of ethnopharmacology. *J Ethnopharmacol* 2012, 140(3), 624–633.
81. Kala, C. P., & Sajwan, B. S. Revitalising Indian systems of herbal medicine by the National Medicinal Plants Board through institutional networking and capacity building. *Curr Sci* 2007, 93(6), 797–806.
82. Chatfield, K., Salehi, B., Sharifi-Rad, J., & Afshar, L. Applying an ethical framework to herbal medicine. *Evid-Based Complement Alternat Med* 2018, 2018, 1903629.

83. Al-Safi, S. A., Ayoub, N. M., Ayoub, A. M., Al-Momany, E., Al-Doghim, I., Al-Balas, Mosa'B., Alkofahi, A. S., Aboul-Enein, F. H., & Aboul-Enein, B. H. Public awareness of the abuse of herbs and drugs to decrease body weight: A novel national survey in Jordan. *J Public Health* 2008, 16, 205–213.
84. Abraham, J. International conference on harmonisation of technical requirements for registration of pharmaceuticals for human use. In: *Handbook of Transnational Economic Governance Regimes*, Brill Nijhoff, 2010, pp. 1041–1053.
85. Bodeker, G. *WHO Global Atlas of Traditional, Complementary, and Alternative Medicine*, World Health Organization, 2005, Vol. 1.
86. Weber, W. J., & Hopp, D. C. National centre for complementary and integrative health perspectives on clinical research involving natural products. *Drug Metab Dispos* 2020, 48(10), 963–965.
87. Barnes, J., Anderson, L. A., & Phillipson, J. D. *Herbal medicines*, No. 3rd Edn, Pharmaceutical Press, 2007.
88. Chinou, I., Knoess, W., & Calapai, G. Regulation of herbal medicinal products in the EU: An up-to-date scientific review. *Phytochem Rev* 2014, 13, 539–545.
89. Vlietinck, A., Pieters, L., & Apers, S. Legal requirements for the quality of herbal substances and herbal preparations for the manufacturing of herbal medicinal products in the European Union. *Planta Med* 2009, 75(07), 683–688.
90. Lee, E. L., Richards, N., Harrison, J., & Barnes, J. Prevalence of use of traditional, complementary and alternative medicine by the general population: A systematic review of national studies published from 2010 to 2019. *Drug Saf* 2022, 45(7), 713–735.
91. Lee, E. L., Harrison, J., & Barnes, J. Mapping prevalence and patterns of use of, and expenditure on, traditional, complementary and alternative medicine in New Zealand: A scoping review of qualitative and quantitative studies. *N Z Med J* 2021, 134(1541), 57–74.
92. Barrett, B., Brown, R., Rakel, D., Mundt, M., Bone, K., Barlow, S., & Ewers, T. Echinacea for treating the common cold: A randomised trial. *Ann Intern Med* 2010, 153(12), 769–777.
93. Daily, J. W., Yang, M., & Park, S. Efficacy of turmeric extracts and curcumin for alleviating the symptoms of joint arthritis: A systematic review and meta-analysis of randomised clinical trials. *J Med Food* 2016, 19(8), 717–729.
94. Snitz, B. E., O'Meara, E. S., Carlson, M. C., Arnold, A. M., Ives, D. G., Rapp, S. R., Saxton, J., et al., Ginkgo biloba for preventing cognitive decline in older adults: A randomised trial. *JAMA* 2009, 302(24), 2663–2670.
95. Pittler, M. H., & Ernst, E. Clinical effectiveness of garlic (Allium sativum). *Mol Nutr Food Res* 2007, 51(11), 1382–1385.
96. Linde, K., Berner, M. M., & Kriston, L. St John's wort for major depression. *Cochrane Database Syst Rev* 2008, 2008(4), CD000448.
97. Taavoni, S., Ekbatani, N., Kashaniyan, M., & Haghani, H. Effect of valerian on sleep quality in postmenopausal women: A randomised placebo-controlled clinical trial. *Menopause* 2011, 18(9), 951–955.
98. Özcan, M. M., Ünver, A., Uçar, T., & Arslan, D. Mineral content of some herbs and herbal teas by infusion and decoction. *Food Chem* 2008, 106(3), 1120–1127.

99. Hudz, N., Makowicz, E., Shanaida, M., Białoń, M., Jasicka-Misiak, I., Yezerska, O., Svydenko, L., & Wieczorek, P. P. Phytochemical evaluation of tinctures and essential oil obtained from Saturejamontana herb. *Molecules* 2020, 25(20), 4763.
100. Mudrić, J., Arsenijević, J., Maksimović, Z., Ibrić, S., Gopčević, K., & Đuriš, J. Tablet and capsule formulations incorporating high doses of a dry optimised herbal extract: The case of Satureja kitaibelii. *J Drug Deliv Sci Technol* 2021, 66, 102776.
101. Etti, C. J., Yusof, Y. A., Chin, N. L., & Tahir, S. M. Effects of formulation on flowability of selected herbal powders using compendial methods and powder flow analyser. *Int Food Res J* 2016, 23, S225.
102. Aiyalu, R., Govindarajan, A., & Ramasamy, A. Formulation and evaluation of topical herbal gel for the treatment of arthritis in animal model. *Brazil J Pharm Sci* 2016, 52, 493–507.
103. Jadhao, A. G., Sanap, M. J., & Patil, P. A. Formulation and Evaluation of Herbal Syrup. *Asian J Pharm Res Dev* 2021, 9(3), 16–22.
104. Kowalski, R., Baj, T., Kowalska, G., & Pankiewicz, U. Estimation of potential availability of essential oil in some brands of herbal teas and herbal dietary supplements. *PLoS One* 2015, 10(6), e0130714.
105. Ramya, S. *Formulation and Standardization of Antiemetic Herbal Lozenges as per Ayush and Pharmacopoeial Standards*. PhD dissertation., Periyar College of Pharmaceutical Sciences, Tiruchirappalli, 2021.
106. Chatawatee, B., Chokpaisarn, J., Yusuf, M., Waehama, F., Kunworarath, N., Kongsuwan, C., & Mae, M. S. Effectiveness of knee acupressure along with herbal knee poultice for knee osteoarthritis treatment: A pilot pre-post clinical study. *J Herb Med* 2022, 32, 100498.
107. Zhang, A. L., Changli Xue, C., Fong, H. H. S. Integration of herbal medicine into evidence-based clinical practice: Current status and issues. In: Benzie, I. F. F., Wachtel-Galor, S. (Eds.), *Herbal Medicine: Biomolecular and Clinical Aspects*, 2nd edn., CRC Press/Taylor & Francis: Boca Raton, FL, USA: 2011.

CHAPTER 2

Challenges in Upgrading and Modernizing Herbal Formulations

PRANAY WAL[1*], RAMKUMAR PILLAPPAN[2], ROHINI KARUNAKARAN[3], VISHAL GARG[4], PRIYANKA GUPTA[5], SHWETA BHANDARI[6], MANINDER KAUR[7], and SOURABH KOSEY[8]

[1]PSIT-Pranveer Singh Institute of Technology (Pharmacy), Kanpur, Uttar Pradesh, India

[2]Department of Pharmaceutics, NGSM Institute of Pharmaceutical Sciences, Mangalore, Karnataka, India

[3]Unit of Biochemistry, Faculty of Medicine, AIMST University, Semeling, Kedah, Malaysia

[4]Jaipur School of Pharmacy, Maharaj Vinayak Global University, Jaipur, Rajasthan, India

[5]Shivalik College of Engineering, Dehradun, Uttarakhand, India

[6]Acropolis Institute of Pharmaceutical Education & Research, Indore, Madhya Pradesh, India

[7]G.S.R.M. Memorial College of Pharmacy, Lucknow, Uttar Pradesh, India

[8]Department of Pharmacy Practice, ISF College of Pharmacy, Moga, Punjab, India

*Corresponding author

Herbal Drug Industry: From Cultivation to Innovation and Global Impact.
Abhishek Tiwari, Varsha Tiwari, and Ajay Sharma (Eds.)

DOI: 10.1201/9781779640994-2

ABSTRACT

Herbal formulations are increasingly in demand for primary healthcare due to their affordability, cultural acceptance, physiological compatibility, and fewer side effects. However, their use is not without limitations. Compared to conventional medicines, herbal formulations often face challenges related to pharmacognosy and standardization. Quality issues can be categorized into external problems—such as adulteration, misidentification, and contamination—and internal issues related to ingredient complexity and variability. Strict adherence to Good Agricultural and Collection Practices (GACP) and Good Manufacturing Practices (GMP) can help minimize external risks. A major challenge in the industry is the consistent supply of high-quality medicinal and aromatic plants. Promoting green entrepreneurship through the development of agri-clinics, testing facilities, and training programs can address this issue. Encouraging the next generation to take risks, manage resources, and innovate in medicinal plant cultivation supports both sustainability and employment. Green entrepreneurship encompasses all stages from production and processing to marketing and transport and offers low entry barriers, making it especially appealing to youth. By creating a supportive ecosystem that rewards green initiatives, India can overcome current obstacles and build a robust, sustainable herbal medicine industry.

2.1 INTRODUCTION

The world's largest provider of medicinal herbs is India. Only 7000–7500 of the 20,000 or so known medicinal herbs in India are used by traditional healers to treat various illnesses. Within the many Indian medical systems, the percentage of plants used is as follows: Ayurveda 2000, Siddha 1300, Unani 1000, and homoeopathy 800. Approximately 25,000 potent plant-based remedies are employed in conventional and indigenous medicine in India. In India, the conventional medical system is utilized by around 1.5 million professionals for medical reasons. In India, the commercialization of conventional herbal formulations and natural medical goods is projected to involve around 7800 manufacturing operations, requiring over 2000 t of raw medicinal material from plants annually [1]. Throughout time immemorial, traditional medicine and herbal remedies have been widely used for medicinal purposes to maintain health through a variety of methods.

Biochemical and pharmacological analyses have been conducted on numerous plant extracts over the past century to determine their chemical makeup and validate their medicinal value.

Many different types of natural resources, including vegetation microbes, fungal organisms, and aquatic organisms, are the source of a vast array of natural goods. Of them, plants constitute an essential source of molecules with pharmacological activity, namely, many popular drugs produced from plants. Presently, more than 100 potent phytochemicals are employed in medicine, and plant-derived preparations provide primary healthcare to about 80% of the global population. By purifying procedures, phytochemicals with a range of molecular sizes, chemical types, and molecular structure have been gathered as extracts, fractions, or bioactive molecules [2]. Herbal medicine merchandise has been around for centuries and has shown promise in treating a variety of illnesses, including cancer. However, several significant issues have hindered their widespread adoption in the biological and pharmaceutical communities, such as the toxicology and effectiveness of most natural recipes, unclear chemical constituents in herbals, unidentified ingredients, and molecular pathways [3]. While conventional medicine has strong methods for demonstrating effectiveness, guaranteeing quality, standardizing good manufacturing practices, testing for safety, and monitoring side effects after a product is marketed, there are no comparable regulations for herbal products. This is true even though conventional herbal remedies have been accepted by many cultures and geographical areas. Yet, it must be noted that several guidelines' documents on security and toxicology [4]. Notwithstanding the long tradition of the use of herbal goods and their encouraging results on illness treatment, recent reports indicated that investigation on herbal medications and herbal medicines has reduced some of the negative aspects about medical care, product growth, market expansion, and molecular applications. Herbal formulations might be difficult to upgrade and modernize for a variety of reasons. Although herbal remedies have been widely used for ages and are frequently connected to traditional medicine, there are certain obstacles that must be overcome to incorporate them into contemporary healthcare procedures. Cultivating herbal crops offers a sustainable way to obtain high-value commercial raw materials for the food, drugs, agrochemical, and cosmetics industries. It also creates new opportunities for farmers to make more money and significantly advances the rural economy [5]. Despite a growing trend in the cultivation of medicinal herbs, a persistent issue is the reluctance of many farmers to produce these plants as their primary source of revenue. The reason for this is that the market is unclear since the production of this herbal remedy is still classified as a "gray area." Farmers that grow therapeutic plants still do not know who will buy their products or what their price requirements are. There currently exists a discrepancy among the demand for medicinal plant production—needed by the herbal medicine industry—and the supply—produced by farmers.

There is a distinction between both demand and supply, particularly when it comes to demand, which is higher than supply. This is an entrepreneurial chance that needs to be taken advantage of to strengthen the economics of the people [6]. Developing medicinal herb entrepreneurship is just one of the initiatives aimed at advancing the production of medicinal plants. More work needs to be put into the development of medicinal plant entrepreneurship to shorten the trade chain for medicinal plant cultivation, which should increase the selling price that producers earn.

To create advantageous cooperation for medicinal herb farmers, businessmen, and the herbal medicine businesses, the Agency for the Assessment and Application of Technology is currently carrying out an investigation on the growth of medicinal plant entrepreneurial activity as an example to be executed. An essential prerequisite for businesses and other organizations that deal with Ayurveda and herbal goods is the quality assessment of herbal preparations. As a method of quality control (QC), standardization establishes a set of guidelines that convey these ideas. All procedures used in the production of herbal medications are included in the method of standardization. QC, which depends on procedures both before and after harvesting, guarantees performance that is safe, reliable, and consistent. Good manufacturing procedures (GMPs) and good agricultural practices are included in these [6].

The World Health Organization (WHO) has promoted the creation of national guidelines and standards for assessing the efficacy of conventional medications. It additionally underlined the significance of protecting biodiversity and creating national pharmacopeia and monographs on therapeutic plants. Stringent restrictions are required for the herbal business, and they are essential. Regulations pertaining to herbal pharmaceuticals in India have been documented, along with a summary of the regulatory landscape of herbal medicine in the Brazil, China, USA, Canada, Australia, and Germany. For being introduced into the marketplace, an herbal remedy must undergo safety standardization, as per WHO rules [7].

The herbal remedies that community members and indigenous cultures have found to be useful have been the basis for much of the development of the current pharmaceutical sector. Despite this, businesses continue to profit from the sale of these drugs without giving credit or acknowledgment to the individuals who initially discovered those plants. Protection of intellectual property can take the shape of ideas, knowledge, data, or other "matters of the mind" that are not readily apparent or known to others in their lack of revelation or access. A specific piece of proprietary information may be claimed solely or jointly by one person, by a group of people, by a company or organization, or by the government. A sole owner of a certain piece of intellectual property has several options, including selling it to other parties, bartering or trading it with others, giving it away, using it themselves, or doing nothing with it [8]. As we continue to unearth the medicinal capabilities of herbs, a future in which herbal remedies actively make contributions to the diverse terrain of medical treatment will be made possible by a harmonious blending of traditional wisdom with contemporary scientific inquiry. Exploring herbal formulations and learning about the wide range of nature's pharmacy supports a holistic approach to well-being that respects the intricate interaction between humans and plants.

2.2 HERBAL FORMULATIONS

For ages, herbal remedies, which come from the complex realm of plants, have been a crucial component of medical care for humans. Herbal medicine has been used since the dawn of civilization, when local knowledge and experience established the basis for the creation of various herbal remedies. Herbal remedies have seen a resurgence in popularity recently, drawing the attention of people looking for alternatives to traditional treatment as the popularity of holistic and organic approaches to healthcare has increased. Plant compositions, or parts of them, had been used extensively in herbal remedies for antiquity; today, most people on the earth still utilize botanical medicines [9]. Herbal remedies have roots in ancient societies all over the world. Plants have long been used in traditional medicine systems, including Ayurveda in India, traditional Chinese medicine (TCM) in China, and indigenous traditions around the world. The wisdom handed down throughout the ages emphasizes the effectiveness of herbs in treating a range of medical issues. Herbs were more than just food; they were also valued for their medicinal qualities, which led to the creation of mixtures that attempted to bring the body's equilibrium and harmony back. Herbal formulations come in a variety of forms, each designed to meet a particular need related to health. One calming and simple approach to absorb the health benefits of plants is through herbal teas, which are arguably the oldest type of herbal therapy [10]. Herbal extracts can be conveniently consumed as tinctures, capsules, or pills, or used topically as ointments and lotions. Herbs are combined in Ayurvedic and TCM formulations, which have their roots in ancient philosophies, to support overall well-being. Throughout the past century, numerous plant extracts have been the focus of chemical and pharmacological studies aimed at ascertaining their chemical makeup and substantiating the applications of traditional medicinal practices.

The public is beginning to turn more and more toward herbal medicines since they are perceived as "alternative remedies" that are less harmful and more benign than synthetic ones. Furthermore, a substantial body of scientific research backs the medical application of herbal remedies for a variety of illnesses. In recent years, scientists have made significant investments in the investigation and creation of innovative methods for delivering herbal drugs [11].

The organic chemicals used in herbal treatments are sourced from an herb that has been the foundation of traditional medicinal methods since ancient times. In the field of drug formulation creativity, science, and technology have progressed to the point where phyto-forms of administration have evolved from basic mixes and tablets to extremely sophisticated tech-based pharmaceutical delivery mechanisms [12]. In addition to lowering presystemic metabolic rates and possible harm from the placement of drugs in nontargeted areas, the application of sophisticated equipment in the application of herbal remedies or plant-based goods additionally enhanced active drugs stability and increased adherence among patients due to ease of administration and adequate dosage [13]. It is especially difficult to design unique medicine methods of administration for herbal products because of the wide range of active components. Therefore, to protect the molecule from various physiological stressors including acidic pH, the reticuloendothelial route, and metabolism, innovative drug delivery strategies are required to optimize drug bioavailability. Therefore, for improved treatment results, herbal remedies or natural substances should be incorporated into cutting-edge drug delivery systems [14].

Innovative herbal medicine delivery systems are developed to get over the limitations of the herbal dose forms that are now available because of the many advantages that herbal medicines bring to humanity. New herbal medicine delivery technologies can help attain site specificity. By increasing the medication's surface area, the novel drug delivery technique not only makes drugs more soluble and active, but it also makes nanoparticles more permeable via the blood–brain barrier [15]. Pharmaceutical science, medicinal chemistry, polymer chemistry, and molecular genetics are all combined to create modern drug delivery methods, which have unique physicochemical properties including huge surface area to mass ratio, high sensitivity, regulated and ultrasmall dimensions, and functional structure. There are obstacles even though herbal remedies provide a natural and comprehensive approach to wellness. It is crucial to use herbal goods responsibly and with knowledge due to the possibility of herb–drug interactions, QC, and standardization of herbal products. To fully realize the benefits of herbal formulations while maintaining their safety and effectiveness, it is imperative to combine traditional wisdom with contemporary scientific rigor [16].

2.2.1 CURRENT TRENDS IN HERBAL FORMULATIONS

These days, herbal medicine is becoming more and more significant and helpful, particularly considering the difficulties we have in treating a broad variety of medical conditions. More pleasant and efficient medication dosage forms are needed in the modern era. The present development in herbal form of administration is to improve the solubility, bioavailability, pharmacologic behavior, stability, minimize toxicity, raise compliance, and so on. Several of these are listed in Table 2.1 [17]. Herbal treatments in the form of gathers, enriched parts, or biomarker components are known as herbal nanomedicines (HNMs). Given their lower toxicities and enhanced bioavailability, HNMs offer certain benefits [18]. The application of nanomedicines to enhance the bioavailability of several chemical and botanical bioactive substances has demonstrated encouraging outcomes. Regarded as a nanomedicine, nanogels provide remarkable stability, drug loading capability, biologic consistency, robust penetrating ability, and environmental stimulus response. Nanogels have gained prominence in several fields, such as organ aiming for, diagnostics, chemotherapy drug delivery, delivery of genes, and herbal remedies. Recently, biotechnology has made extensive use of nanogels, primarily in the areas of genetics, protein production, and enzyme immobilization. They are a benefit to cutting-edge medical treatment plans. Additionally, amphiphilic nanogels are used because to their substantial drug-carrying capacity, which is achieved through aggregates and sedimentation. The primary goals of next-generation nanogels are to deliver drugs to targets more safely and effectively; they may even be able to show promising results in tissue engineering [19]. Herbal and conventional pharmaceutical products are quite sophisticated and unique, supporting our everyday health-conscious lifestyle. The widespread usage of herbal goods in our daily lives has led to a current trend toward the adoption of herbal and traditional items. There is a great need for several conventional and herbal products to address their shortcomings. Many conventional and herbal pharmacies are currently creating new information and fashions to produce the necessary dosage forms.

TABLE 2.1 Current Trends in Herbal Formulations

S. No.	Category	Type	Subtype
1.	Oral dosage forms	Granules	Effervescent granules
			Rapid release granules
		Tablets	FDT
			RDT
		Capsules	
		Suspension	
		Contemporary syrup	
		Linctus	
		Emulsions	
		Microemulsion	
		SEDDs	
2.	Novel drug dosage form (oral/parenteral)	Nanogel	
		Liposomes	
3.	Topical dosage forms	Dentifrices	
		Toothpastes	
		Hair dye	
		Face pack	
		Hand wash	
		Shampoo	
		Gel	
		Sprays	
		Hydrogel	
4.	Ophthalmic dosage forms	Eye drops	

Notes: FDT: fast dissolving tablet, RDT: rapid disintegrating tablets, SEDDs: self-emulsifying drug delivery systems

2.2.2 DRAWBACKS OF HERBAL FORMULATIONS

When technology and science have grown in the field of pharmaceutical formulation innovation, herbal dosage forms have evolved from straightforward mixtures and tablets to extremely sophisticated technology-based drug delivery systems [12]. Utilizing cutting-edge technology to deliver medicinal herbs or plant-based products enhanced the stability of active pharmaceutical ingredients, decreased presystemic metabolic activity and potential toxicity from drug deposition in nontargeted areas, and increased patient compliance due to medication adequacy and ease of administration [13]. It is especially difficult to design unique medicine delivery strategies for herbal medicines because of the wide range of active components. Therefore, to increase medication bioavailability by shielding the molecule from additional physiological distractions including acidic pH, the reticuloendothelial pathway, and metabolic activities, innovative drug delivery strategies are required [14].

Innovative herbal preparations such as liposomes, phytotomies, microspheres, nanocapsules, polymeric nanoparticles, nanoemulsions, transferosomes, and ethosomes have been made possible by the utilization of plant bioactive components [20]. The stomach's extremely acidic pH will break down many of the chemicals in herbal medicines before they even reach the bloodstream, and other ingredients may be susceptible to first-pass metabolism, which would reduce the bioavailability of herbal medications. Small size, drug-delivering nanocarriers added to herbal remedies will deliver the right amount of medication to the active site, bypassing all barriers including the stomach's acidic pH and the liver's metabolism, thus the drug will have a long-lasting effect and start working sooner [21].

Nonetheless, this resolved the issue with the physio-chemical characteristics and composition of the herbal dosage forms. A few of the significant disadvantages of herbal formulations, aside from this, are covered below.

2.2.2.1 HERBAL DRUG TOXICITY

The broad range of toxicological issues linked to the consumption of herbal medicines has been repeatedly linked to serious detrimental deaths, including cardiovascular issues, psychiatric issues, neurological implications, liver damage or failure, hematologic as well as kidney toxic effects, and neurological consequences [22].

Herbal toxicity is typically diagnosed by ruling out other possible causes and considering the time interval between the negative outcome and the herb's consumption. However, in many instances, the application of suitable methodologies for determining herbal poison in causation evaluation has failed to demonstrate any causative effect or has only suggested a weak causal association [23]. Furthermore, an array of investigations has documented the possible harmful properties of herbal medications, even though little or no causation of herb toxicology could be proven in numerous cases. According to Jones and Lawson [24], there is a significant correlation between the usage of blue cohosh herbal therapy and severe congestive heart failure in neonates. Both the existence of vasoactive glycosides and an alkaloid recognized to have adverse impacts on the myocardium may be responsible for the result. Moreover, blue cohosh has acute cardiotoxic and sympathomimetic actions that can constrict coronary blood vessels and reduce heart oxygenation, which can result in morbidity and death in the fetus or in infants subjected by mother consumption. In the same way, cardiac glycosides were connected to hyperkalemia, an adverse reaction that was seen in a patient who was taking numerous herbal remedies [25]. Even with a variety of assays to assess cause and effect, diagnosing hepatotoxicity caused by herbal drugs remains difficult. Despite the reality that HMPs have been widely used for millennia, there are very few clinical investigations including them that have appeared in the scientific literature. Consequently, postmarked drug surveillance is an invaluable source of safety data, and causality analysis shows a connection among a putative HMP and a side effect that has been detected [26]. While there is not a single, widely acknowledged technique for determining causality, the approaches that are currently in use rely on expert, computational, and probability-based studies in addition to the caliber of adverse event reports. Anecdotal accounts of any negative effects from herbs are less believable unless causation is shown.

Human cases of acute intoxication following ingestion of thujone-rich essential oils have also been documented. It has been shown that thujone or items comprising thujone can produce disruptions to the central nervous system, which can result in convulsions, unconsciousness, and even death [27]. Likewise, it has been revealed that *Glycyrrhiza glabra*, which is frequently utilized for treating upper respiratory tract inflammation as well as ulcers in the duodenum and stomach, suppresses the renin–aldosterone mechanism. Long-term consumption of liquorice may result in these side effects, including high blood pressure, low potassium levels, myopathy, and irregular heartbeats [28]. Overall, it is evident that although the adverse consequences of herbs have been well documented in industrialized nations, developing nations have not given the same level of attention to the subject.

Herbs can also be harmful if they cause the body to produce reactive intermediates because of the stimulation of metabolism of their contents through phases I and II reactions. The ensuing reactive intermediates can adhere covalent to proteins and DNA, which can cause mutation, carcinogenicity, and toxicity to organs [29]. Herbs collected from contaminated areas or unsound agricultural techniques, medicinal plant products tainted with pesticides and microbiological pollutants, heavy metals, hazardous materials, and adulterants that may be harmful to consumers are additional concerns that could jeopardize safety.

2.2.2.2 HERBAL FORMULATIONS INTERACTIONS

The usage of herbal medicine in modern times is common, but one problem that modern society has is getting patients to tell their doctors that they also take conventional medications in addition to herbal goods. Although potentially herb–drug interactions might be equally favorable or neutral, several empirical investigations have demonstrated the adverse or contradictory interactions between medications and herbs [30].

Numerous pharmacologically biologically active elements are typically present in herbal medications, which significantly raises the likelihood of interactions. The possibility of interactions between herbs and drugs may often be greater than that of drug–drug interactions. Herb–drug interactions may either boost or reduce the pharmacological or toxicological impacts through the pharmacokinetic parameters herb–drug communication, which occurs when one medication interferes with the other's ability to be eliminated, metabolized, or absorbed, and the pharmacodynamic herb–drug communication, which occurs when two distinct drugs act in opposing ways and ultimately impacts the dose reaction and the processes of therapeutic or toxic effects [31]. Herb–drug interactions are frequently observed when cardiovascular drugs with a narrow therapeutic index, like warfarin and digoxin, are taken together with herbs. For example, taking warfarin and St. John's Wort together lowers prothrombin time, which may lead to a decrease in the anticoagulant action and a requirement for a higher dose of warfarin [32].

The available data supporting the possibility of interactions between herbal medicine and conventional medications primarily comes from case series, patient reports, and a small number of clinical trials. The evaluation of drug-herbal interactions is challenging due to the unreliability of the herbal products' composition. However, there are several potential interactions, including those involving enzymes that metabolize drugs and drug transport structures, in addition to pharmacodynamic effects.

Possible interactions, nevertheless, cannot be foreseen because most herbal medicines and supplements lack a thorough understanding of their pharmacokinetic and pharmacodynamic properties. This explains why *in vitro* complementary-drug interactions require confirmation and evaluation in clinical trials to determine their therapeutic significance [33].

2.2.2.3 CLINICAL TRIALS OF HERBAL FORMULATIONS

Herbal medicinal goods are sold as nutritional supplements and are governed by the Dietary Supplement Health and Education Act, which avoids the strict quality standards of the Drugs and Cosmetics Act 1940 by not requiring evidence of safety or efficacy. Lead poisoning has been documented in relation to the administration of Ayurvedic HMPs lately and this could result in diseases such as status epilepticus, fatal baby encephalopathy, fetal paralysis, sensory neural hearing loss, and fetal retardation in development [34]. Several factors make carrying out clinical trials involving conventional and herbal treatments problematic. For example, it can be difficult, impractical, or even impossible to establish active and control groups that are the same color, smell, and taste. Similarly, using a placebo presents challenges because the herbal study medicine may have a distinct flavor and potent perfume that are difficult to replicate when creating a placebo [35].

Comparative placebo research on herbal medications also presents ethical problems since it is unacceptable to provide uninformed people a placebo rather than a treatment that is already available and effective for their ailment. When formulating products with multiple plant extracts, the issues frequently become more numerous. Additionally, employing bioactive markers to standardize the chemicals needs special care [36].

In the first phase of medication research, pharmacokinetic investigations provide challenges in estimating the number of "active" molecules in bodily fluids, particularly in Ayurvedic formulations.

Large-scale clinical trials involving medicinal plants are plagued by the fact that storage environments can also affect the bioavailability of herbal medicines, potentially causing loss of action or fungus or microbial contamination that results in batch-to-batch fluctuation. When producing Ayurvedic medicines, the significance of GMPs is typically overlooked; as a result, when working with commercial formulations, it is important to monitor adulteration and substitution. The choice of dosing schedule could potentially cause issues. Whether a crude medication or an extract is used, the dosage must be determined, and the extract's dosage is determined using its extractive value [34].

In addition to oral therapy, the medical system frequently recommends other treatments that may or might not be standardized. Additionally, as they exist in contemporary medical science, there is no typical benchmark composition, particularly when a single medicinal therapy is involved for multiple therapeutic domains [37].

Another problem is the wide range of variability in the crude raw herb material due to factors including climate, harvesting techniques, collecting protocols, environmental dangers, and geographic regions. This makes it challenging to standardize the result for an acceptable standard that can be replicated. Several herbal systems' combined strategy fails to distinguish between the patient and the disease, which is one of the other causes. The clinical trial's inclusion and exclusion criteria are made more challenging by this method [38].

Moreover, Ayurveda suggests several treatments for the same patient at different phases of the disease, adding yet another challenging to control variable in a scientific experiment. In clinical trials, the treatment result can be additionally influenced by dietary factors [39].

Most herbal remedies used in conventional systems are administered to humans with the need for toxicity testing, hence it is possible that their carcinogenic, embryotoxic, and embryotoxic consequences will go unnoticed in traditional medicine. It is challenging to organize double-blind randomized clinical studies with Ayurvedic medications. Particularly in the case of herbal remedies, the placebo-controlled, double-blind randomized trial may be regarded as the gold standard for scientific proof of safety and effectiveness. Randomized clinical studies with herbal medicine, nevertheless, may prove challenging to carry out due to the necessity for sizable volunteer groups, extended study periods, and high costs associated with medical treatment [40].

Furthermore, a significant issue is that funding for these trials is typically not easily accessible. Hazardous herbs, toxic metals, microbiological, and other contaminants (including pesticides), along with intentional adulteration with pharmaceutical products, are among the problems pertaining to the security and efficacy of herbal remedies [41].

Another issue with alternative medicine investigation is that professionals of complementary medicine frequently doubt the validity of randomized clinical trials in the context of complementary medication due to the comprehensive approach—which treats the soul, body, and mind simultaneously—that is necessary and since complementary medicine is typically customized for each patient. Experts argue that it is improper to administer a single treatment to every participant in a randomized clinical trial in an identical way and in the exact same dose [42].

2.2.2.4 ABSENCE OF REGULATORY CONTROL

There is a dearth of research supporting the security and efficacy of herbal products, but over 30,000 nutritional supplements are available for purchase in the United States, and more than 1000 are added every year. Most patients think that the government regulates CAM security, but the FDA in the United States simply needs a copy of the good's label sent by the manufacturer. Even though an innovative nutritional supplement or composition contains novel, experimental, and uncontrolled herbal components, it can be released and sold quickly and with little to no restriction. Although there is limited regulation, the Dietary Complement Health and Education Act of 1994 permits the sale of unproven herbal items [43]. Regrettably, a lot of supplements include impurities or substances that can interact negatively with other medications. Many of these substances would undoubtedly be prohibited if premarket security checks were conducted on them. It is not very beneficial to restrict a certain substance or collection of compounds because producers can easily release new formulations. The FDA was notified of hundreds of cases of ephedra poisoning between 1995 and 1997, which resulted in cardiac arrhythmia deaths, myocardial infarctions, strokes, and seizures. Young people in otherwise healthy states who utilized ephedra for loss of weight and vitality boost had side effects [44]. Consequently, the FDA ultimately outlawed ephedra. However, other chemically comparable sympathomimetic amines replaced ephedra in weight-loss and energy-boosting supplements. Synephrine, for example, has become the most widely used substitute for ephedra. Its pharmacology and structure are comparable. Herbal items are regarded as natural by the public. Consequently, the misconception that natural goods are safe is pervasive [43].

2.2.2.5 INSUFFICIENT QUALITY ASSURANCE

The FDA and other regulatory agencies need to take immediate action in response to the significant differences in low-to-lot variability, storage practices, and manufacturing processes used to produce herbal supplements. Although the US Pharmacopeia has been creating QC standards, supplement producers are not obligated to abide by them.

This kind of freedom permits the unrestricted sale of inexpensively produced and even outdated herbal remedies. The main issues are still the variety of sources of herbs and the uneven ingredient labeling. According to the Harris Poll from 2008, over 40% of all herbal goods either do not contain as much of the active component as stated on the label or use less expensive compounds in place of more costly ones [45]. Herbal goods are frequently contaminated with heavy metals, adulterated with medications, and include forbidden animal and plant substances [46]. Adulteration using antibiotics, nonsteroidal anti-inflammatory medications, hormones, and heavy metals—both deliberate and accidental—occurs often. The public, including children, is marketed steroids that have not been tested or controlled. Testing revealed unrecorded prescription medicines in 13 types of dietary supplements, prompting the FDA to publish nine alerts about safety in 2007 advising customers to discontinue using them [47]. Subsequent health testing or treatment can reveal the implications of utilizing herbal products. Producers are required by FDA rules to refrain from tainting goods with heavy metals, insecticides, other plants, or prescription medications. However, there have been numerous reports of adulterant chemicals found in products, putting unaware customers at risk for adverse reactions and interactions with drugs [43].

2.2.2.6 SOCIAL MISINFORMATION

Compared to any previous period, deceptive marketing strategies have allowed erroneous claims regarding the safety and effectiveness of herbs to reach the public. Herbal items are advertised on television, radio, on the web, and in periodicals, newspapers, and novels. Untested, oral traditions are the foundation for the use of herbs as medicine. Certain advertisements even state that the substance being promoted is the most potent in the entire globe, patented, doctor advised, or available now without a doctor's prescription. Herbal supplement sales may only be discontinued upon demonstration of product hazard and submission of supporting documentation to the Secretary of the Department of Health and Human Services. But the FDA fails to regularly test nutritional supplements, and prior to it can limit dietary supplements use or remove it entirely from the market, it must prove that the dietary supplement is "unsafe" (Guidance for Industry, 2009). Protection of consumers' regulations must be implemented, and manufacturers should have the weight of evidence when proving the safety of a supplement, not government agencies or customers [43].

2.2.3 MODERNIZATION OF HERBAL FORMULATIONS

Today's technologies for QC of herbal medicines include capillary electrophoresis, chromatographic techniques for fingerprint analyzing thin-layer chromatography, liquid chromatography, high-performance liquid chromatography, and gas chromatography, microscopic analyses, DNA polymorphism techniques that evaluate sequences of DNA and determine connections among genomic DNA split sequences and proportions of active elements, and biologicals. Modernizing herbal medicine technically is essential to establishing QC and promoting standardization by both quantitative and qualitative investigation of active ingredients and biological activity. Furthermore, rather than relying solely on personal experience, effort ought to be taken to assure efficacy through medical research, including double-blind clinical trials, and to guarantee safe through examination of toxicology and adverse reactions. Dietary supplements also need to adhere to strict QC guidelines.

The qualities of herbal formulations—including their pharmacological effect and quantitative composition—are being studied and documented using contemporary analytical and pharmacological methodologies in relation to their constituent parts.

The following three strategies are proposed for the creation of novel, secure, and efficient world-class medication scans. Three approaches are available: active principals (bioactive substances), active fractions, and active formulations. Both now and in the future, research must be done on bioactive fraction and active compositions in addition to bioactive principles (lead compounds or leads) to carry on the tradition of herbal medicine and the applications of additional medicinal herbs for the development of drugs in the 21st century [43].

2.3 ENTREPRENEURSHIP DEVELOPMENT IN THE HERBAL INDUSTRY

A strategy for building human capital and preparing the next generation of risk-takers and resource managers is the cultivation of entrepreneurship among medicinal and aromatic plants. The study's goal is to comprehend the situation, current developments, and prospective uses of aromatic and medicinal herbs for the growth of entrepreneurship. The production, manufacturing, sales, commerce, and transportation of raw materials, as well as the provision of inputs and offerings, are all included in the entrepreneurial activities related to herbal formulations. The pharmaceutical and herb businesses are in demand for herbal formulations. The pharmaceutical business has been facing supply issues due to the rising demand for drugs. Among the biggest challenges the industry is facing is finding enough aromatic and medicinal plants to make high-quality medicines. Developing laboratories and Agri-clinics, as well as offering farmers technical advice and consulting from skilled entrepreneurs, represent a few of the significant areas of new prospects in this industry [48]. These days, running a small- or medium-sized business is not only difficult, but full with obstacles. One of the primary issues raised by the shift to sustainable entrepreneurship practices (SEP) is how to maintain competitiveness. Businesses of all sizes encountered this conundrum, which made small- and medium-sized enterprises (SMEs) more susceptible to outside economic shocks than larger companies in this cutthroat, sustainability-focused corporate environment, ultimately leading to their demise.

The embrace of sustainable practices by SMEs having a substantial annual revenue has been effectively evaluated by earlier investigators; nonetheless, the degree of engagement amongst SMEs is still low, particularly in the herbal business. In part because there is a lack of understanding and awareness of desirable sustainable antecedent and procedures that could result in excellent performance from manufacturers; in addition, there is a lack of market demand as well as awareness of environmentally friendly goods [49].

The World Bank has started initiatives to aid in the cultivation and preservation of herbal remedies. In addition, the Indian government has been encouraging the growing of therapeutic plants via several initiatives and plans. To foster cooperation amongst many stakeholders and advance the Indian medicinal plant industry, the National Medicinal Plants Board (NMPB) was established in 2000 [50]. Given the enormous potential for entrepreneurship in the herbals sector, the goal of the next section is to examine and talk about the approaches and issues related to herbs-based firm development. There are numerous challenges and strategies to build an herbal business, such as raw material accessibility, collection, and farming, managing the supply chain, herbal manufacturing, advertising, standardization, quality assurance, security, efficacy, customer satisfaction, and business viability. This could help businesses create profitable business plans for the herbal industry [51].

2.3.1 POVERTY DECLINE

The majority of the impoverished reside in isolated rural areas which are full of assets like such forests. These regions experience varying combinations of issues, such as inadequate administration, market mechanisms, and resource endowment. About 275 million individuals (or 27% of the country's population) are estimated to reside on India's forest fringes, primarily reliant on the country's woods for their livelihood. In isolated places and among chronically impoverished populations, migration is rather high as a means of risk management and as a means of raising quality of life and the well-being of households [52]. The long-term effects of being away from home and family, coupled with the potential for increased risk of illness and being exposed to toxic substances, can make migration's ultimate effects less advantageous. It is critical that development plans and policies give forest more consideration. Furthermore, innovations and value improvements made to forest resources, particularly herbals, may assist to lessen poverty and its related issues. More than 270 million individuals throughout India alone rely either completely or in part on nontimber forest generate, such as herbs, to sustain their employment; the growing need for herbal-based environmentally friendly products contributes to the improvement of income as well as the growth of rural nations. This enormous asset of herbals offers countless opportunities for starting plant-based skincare products and pharmaceutical businesses [50].

2.3.2 MANAGEMENT OF RESOURCES

The Indian government is always working to set up and modernize conventional medical systems, including homoeopathy, natural remedies, Unani, Ayurveda, and Siddha. In 1964, a chapter pertaining to the licensing and manufacturing of Ayurvedic, Siddha, and Unani medications for trade was added to the medications and Cosmetics Act 1940. According to the Indian Medicine Central Council Act, 1970, the Central Council of Indian Medicine was founded in 1971 with the goal of establishing minimal requirements for study in the three Indian systems of medicine—Ayurveda, Siddha, and Unani [53]. The NMPB was established in 2000 with the goal of developing the herbal medicine industry. As a result, each state and union territory in India established the State Medicinal Plants Board. In accordance with the Biological Diversity Act of 2002, State Biodiversity Boards were also established. Through Biodiversity Management Committees, they prepare People's Biodiversity Registers, aiding in the documentation and administration of herbals. The Biological Diversity Act of 2002 addresses biodiversity conservation as well as providing an environment for business or scientific users to utilize natural assets in India and share profits [51].

Given the wide range of parties involved in the herbal industry—including growers, herbalists, manufacturers, universities, research centers, state forest departments, and nongovernmental organizations—the NMPB has been tasked with coordinating with every of the organizations on all pertinent matters pertaining to the growth of medicinal herbs industry. To meet the growing need for herbals and close the gaps between demand as well as supply, businesses must augment their resources. Selective herb growing on private land, in waste areas, along with outside of forested areas may increase the availability of herbal resources. If the various methods for gathering herbs sustainably are adhered to, they could aid in resource management [54].

2.3.3 CERTIFICATION

A tool to assess the long-term viability of medicinal plants along with the caliber of herbal medications is the WHO's 2003 guidance on acceptable agronomic and gathering methods for medicinal plants. Regulations unique to each nation have been devised for the collection and production of medicinal plants, especially, India. Herbal certification benefits the business by lowering the possibility of recall and disapproval, boosting customer confidence, and guaranteeing legal compliance. The business's and herbals' viability may both benefit from the accreditation. The entire procedure of growing and gathering medicinal plants for business purposes needs to be closely watched since the produce that is proclaimed and registered needs to meet certification requirements [55].

2.3.4 MARKETING

The marketplace for herbs is primarily divided into four categories: herbal raw materials; nutraceuticals (foods containing health dietary habits for preventing illnesses and therapy); phyto-pharmaceuticals (medicinal plants items featuring isolated pure active ingredients for treating diseases); and cosmeceuticals (cosmetic goods having therapeutic features). The global market is shifting toward organic products for beauty and medicinal purposes, which presents huge possibilities for the development of herb-based businesses [56]. Notwithstanding the enormous demand for herbs, producers, collectors, processors, and merchants have difficulty locating favorable markets because they lack precise data on the costs, quality, and number of herbs. A stable marketplace and an elevated percentage of loyal clients are two metrics that help define the success of a company. Herbal-based organization must implement new growth strategies and processes in response to the swift advancements in technologies. The manufacturing process is enhanced by the introduction of novel innovations, leading to market expansion. The significance of botanical products as an element of international trade is contingent upon their application as ingredients in the pharmaceutical sector. Because of the worth addition, herbal medications made by extracting purified active ingredients are typically more costly than those sold on the global market [54]. A stable marketplace and an elevated percentage of loyal clients are two metrics that help define the success of a company. Herbal-based organization must implement new growth strategies and processes in response to the swift advancements in technologies. The manufacturing process is enhanced by the introduction of novel innovations, leading to market expansion. The significance of botanical products as an element of international trade is contingent upon their application as ingredients in the pharmaceutical sector. Because of the worth of addition, herbal medications made by extracting purified active ingredients are typically more costly than those sold on the global market [51].

2.3.5 LAW AND POLICY

The unlawful use of herbal formulations is regulated or outlawed by country-specific regulations and acts. Obtaining raw materials for a business must adhere to worldwide agreements and country-specific regulations, so it is critical for entrepreneurs to comprehend government regulations and regulatory structures. Globally, the problems surrounding natural formulas research and bio-prospecting improve certain conflicts due to biopiracy as well as the rights of benefit exchange. An entrepreneur aiming to create a novel herbal medication ought to be cognizant of these crucial matters regarding the utilization of genetic resources [54]. In addition to protecting innovation and bringing in money, patenting goods or processes can be leveraged to forge strategic business partnerships that will support an organization's expansion. Patent rights can encourage invention, generate money for study, and aid in the creation of new markets and understanding holders and knowledge [51].

2.4 ENTREPRENEURSHIP STARTUP

An agri-enterprise incubator, Medi-Hub TBI examines all facets of technological leadership, business, and incubator in the field of aromatic and therapeutic plants. The incubator, which is the initial one of its sorts to serve the requirements of start-ups in the medicinal and aromatic plant industries, was put into operation in 2020 with funding assistance from the Indian Council of Agricultural Research (ICAR) and the Department of Agricultural Research and Education (DARE) of the Ministry of Agriculture and Farmers Welfare, Government of India. The ICAR-Directorate of Medicinal and Aromatic Plants Research (DMAPR), located in Anand, Gujarat, India, is the host institution for Medi-Hub TBI. Under the auspices of ICAR, ICAR-DMAPR is a national organization dedicated to studying the medicinal and aromatic plants of India [57].

The following goods made from medicinal plants can be the basis of small-scale businesses that are mentioned in Figure 2.1 [58].

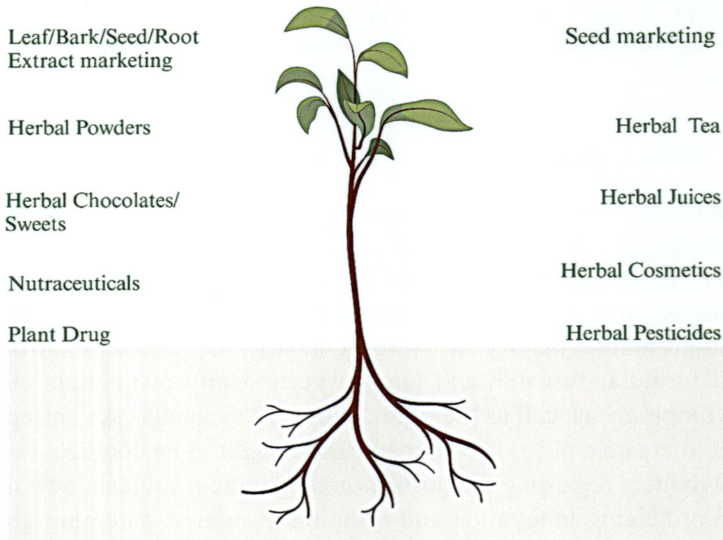

FIGURE 2.1 Small-scale business ideas related to herbs.

Research priorities ought to initially focus on creating appropriate plant material including a package of related procedures for the growth of such species prior starting a start-up. Based on the predominant soil, water, and environmental variables at a given site, organized cultivation of herbal plants requires cultural procedures that are specific to species and locations. Therefore, to obtain the right kind of medicinal and aromatic plants, efforts must be taken to standardize growing methods and harvesting periods. Research and development initiatives as well as methods for cultivating must be designed with these considerations in mind. In the process of creating cultivated variations, attempts must be made to genetically improve a minimum of some of those species in comparison to species that exist in natural settings by a variety of breeding techniques, such as conventional genetic modification and the application of biotechnology.

Farmers' acceptance of such crops is significantly hampered by the lack of timely and appropriate planting materials. More nurseries must be built around the state to provide farmers with easy access to planting material. Considering the growing market for organic goods—particularly for aromatic and medicinal plants—efforts ought to be focused on developing species that can be grown in organic agricultural environments.

The production of herbal plants in greenhouses and as intercrops can potentially be made more common if suitable cultivation techniques are established and crop finances are favorable. Improvements in regional value addition, evaluation, harvesting, and storing techniques, as well as other basic interventions, can significantly boost returns to the community. Realizing the advantages has been significantly hampered by a lack of understanding of these challenges. To increase agricultural yields, farmers and extension agents must be given more training and support.

Additionally, postharvest marketing processes, such as harvesting, grading, and standardization, system of certification, packing, and shipping, need to be enhanced to fulfill domestic as well as global quality requirements. To comply with international requirements, International Organization of Standards (ISO) certification systems might also be required [59].

2.5 PROJECT SELECTION AND PROJECT REPORTS

Farmers and business owners who want to grow herbals or launch an herbal-based business are encouraged to carefully evaluate the following factors, such as

- Determine whether the location is appropriate for growing herbals: tests on the water and soil are preferred.
- Assemble comprehensive data regarding the herbals that are going to be grown: farmers and government agencies at the federal and state levels supply the information that is needed.
- Talk about the plan to start a farming business or create value with all the partners.
- Examine the market and ensure that you are satisfied with the marketing prospects and the demand going forward.

- Make financial arrangements including loans, incentives, self-investment, and so on.
- Establish drying and irrigation services.
- Cultivate as organically, get certified organic status from reputable organizations.
- Obtain quality planting material from reliable vendors.
- To prevent planting delays, plant the crop during the appropriate season and time.

Make sure there is regular labor force monitoring in the event of missing landlordism, especially when applying inputs (fertilizers, manures, and additional chemicals), while many workers are being engaged in tasks like harvesting, weeding, and so on [59].

Ayurvedic pharmacopeia released by the Central Government includes quality criteria for 645 single Ayurvedic medicines and 202 compound compositions; Unani pharmacopeia includes quality norms for 298 single pharmaceuticals and 150 compound compositions; and Siddha pharmacopeia includes quality standards for 139 individual drugs. The Central Council for Research in Ayurvedic Sciences, Ministry of Ayurvedic Sciences, Government of India, New Delhi, has issued broad standards for the development of Ayurvedic formulations of drugs, summarized in Figure 2.2 [60].

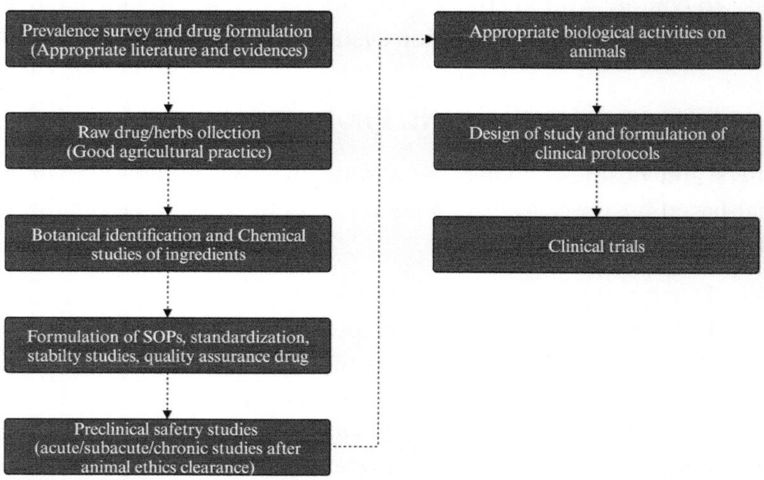

FIGURE 2.2 Parameters for Ayurvedic formulations established by the Central Council for Research in Ayurvedic Sciences

2.6 QUALITY AND REGULATORY CONCERNS

Even though herbal medicines are frequently used for illness management, evaluation, therapy, and prevention, efficient oversight and QC remain major concerns on a global scale challenge. The increasing and widespread use of botanicals has led to a safety, efficacy, and quality issue for world health. The subsequent development of traditional medicine depends on scientific verification and technological standardization of herbal medicine. Using products of guaranteed quality appropriately could also significantly lower the hazards connected to using herbal medication. Yet, very few nations have passed laws regulating the use of herbal remedies; most do not have enough laws governing botanicals, and the efficacy of herbal items offered is typically not assured. The Medicines Control Agency and the Medical Device Agency merged to establish the Medicines and Healthcare Products Regulatory Agency (MHRA) in April 2003. MHRA oversees ensuring the security and caliber of all medications [61].

Since many other nations, mainly in Africa and some regions of Asia, lack such regulations, it is imperative that these be developed globally. Herbal product studies are similarly lacking; while natural product research is extensively conducted, relatively few studies yield meaningful outcomes that are incorporated into the healthcare system. As a result, it may come as no surprise to learn that there have only been a tiny number of poorly controlled clinical studies for isolated bioactive phytoconstituents.

In general, evaluating herbal remedies can be challenging; the main obstacles are accurately identifying plants and isolating their active constituents concerning this. The latter is more complicated and requires extra care since a single medical plant might have hundreds of naturally occurring elements, and the atmosphere, time of collection, or plant origin all affect the qualities of medicinal plants. Thus, policies pertaining to several topics are desperately needed, such as financial and other allocation of resources; training, education, and provider licensing; legislation and regulation for herbal goods and therapeutic practices; and development and research [62].

To guarantee the superior quality of herbal medications, GMP is desperately needed. Well-designed, randomized, double-blind, placebo-controlled clinical trials are required to determine the safety and efficacy of herbal medicines in addition to allopathic medications to allow for a pharmaceutical regulatory body to fulfill the high standards of the public.

Study on herbal items and Indian Ayurvedic medicines will have new avenues for fundamental and practical study thanks to systematic clinical trials. The year 2000 marked the implementation of GMP for Ayurvedic, Siddha, and Unani medicine. The Indian Pharmacopoeia of 2007 contained 59 monographs on herbs and herbal products, but the Indian Pharmacopoeia of 2010 featured 89 (Indian Pharmacopoeia, 2010) [63].

2.7 SUMMARY AND CONCLUSION

Numerous natural resources, such as fungi, aquatic organisms, and bacteria found in vegetation, are the source of an enormous variety of natural commodities. Among these, plants are a vital source of molecules having pharmacological activity—that is, a sizable number of widely used medications are derived from plants. More than 100 powerful phytochemicals are currently used in medicine, and plant-derived treatments supply the world's population with primary healthcare. The wide spectrum of toxicological problems associated with using herbal remedies has been frequently connected to gravely harmful fatalities.

Herbal toxicity is usually diagnosed by excluding other potential causes and accounting for time that has passed between the adverse event and the ingestion of the herb. Herbal medicines usually contain a multitude of pharmacologically biologically active ingredients, which greatly increases the possibility of interactions. Herbal and pharmacological interactions can frequently occur more frequently than drug–drug interactions. Through the pharmacokinetic parameters herb–drug communication—which happens when one medication interferes with the other's ability to be eliminated, metabolized, or absorbed—and the pharmacodynamic herb–drug communication, herb–drug interactions can either increase or decrease the pharmacological or toxicological impacts. Double-blind randomized clinical trials with Ayurvedic remedies are difficult to arrange. The placebo-controlled, double-blind randomized experiment is considered the gold standard for scientific evidence of safety and efficacy, especially when it comes to herbal medicines.

The fact that financing for these clinical trials is usually difficult to come by is another big problem. Problems with the safety and effectiveness of herbal treatments include poisonous plants, heavy metals, microbial, and other pollutants (such as pesticides) as well as deliberate adulteration with pharmaceuticals. In addition to failing to do routine testing on nutritional supplements, the FDA must demonstrate that a supplement is "unsafe" before it may restrict its usage or take it off the market completely. Regulations for the protection of consumers must be put into place, and when it comes to demonstrating the safety of a supplement, manufacturers—rather than governmental organizations or consumers in the case of herbal formulations—should bear the burden of proof. The Indian government is always attempting to establish and update traditional medicinal systems, such as Siddha, Ayurveda, Unani, homoeopathy, and natural medicines. Herbal certification helps the company by increasing customer confidence, ensuring legal compliance, and reducing the likelihood of recall and dissatisfaction. The accreditation could be beneficial to the business's and herbals' viability.

An ongoing problem is that many farmers are reluctant to grow these plants as their main source of income. Even if there is an increasing trend in the production of therapeutic herbs, cultivate medicinal plants are still unsure about their target market and what their acceptable price range is.

Demand and supply are not the same things, especially when it comes to demand being greater than supply. One of the programs aiming at increasing the output of medicinal plants is the development of medicinal herb entrepreneurship. To reduce the trade chain for medicinal plant cultivation and raise the selling price that producers receive, more effort must be made into the development of medicinal plant entrepreneurship. The entire process of cultivating and harvesting medicinal plants for commercial use must be constantly monitored because the declared and registered produce must adhere to certification standards. Initiatives for research and development and cultivation techniques need to be planned with these factors in mind. To produce cultivated variations, at least some of those species must be genetically improved compared to species found in the wild using a range of breeding methods, including traditional genetic modification and the use of biotechnology. Development of species suitable for organic agricultural settings should be the main priority, given the expanding market for organic products, especially aromatic and medicinal plants. Furthermore, to meet both domestic and international quality standards, postharvest marketing procedures like harvesting, grading, and standardization, as well as the certification system, packing, and shipping, must be improved. ISO certification systems may also be necessary to meet international criteria. It is also advised to abide by a few regulations to guarantee excellent agricultural practices. A future in which herbal remedies actively contribute to the vast field of medical treatment will be made possible by the harmonic fusion of ancient wisdom with modern scientific investigation as we continue to uncover the therapeutic properties of herbs. Investigating herbal remedies and discovering the vast array of natural remedies can promote a comprehensive approach to health that honors the complex relationship between people and plants.

KEYWORDS

- **herbal formulations**
- **good agricultural**
- **collection practices**
- **green entrepreneurship**
- **Ayurvedic formulations**

REFERENCES

1. Pandey, M. M., Rastogi, S., & Rawat, A. K. Indian herbal drug for general healthcare: An overview. *Int J Alternat Med* 2008, 6, 3.
2. Han, H. S., Koo, S. Y., & Choi, K. Y. Emerging nanoformulation strategies for phytocompounds and applications from drug delivery to phototherapy to imaging. *Bioact Mater* 2022, 14, 182–205.
3. Atanasov, A. G., Zotchev, S. B., Dirsch, V. M., & Supuran, C. T. Natural products in drug discovery: Advances and opportunities. *Nat Rev Drug Discov* 2021, 20, 200–216.
4. Neergheen-Bhujun, V. S. Underestimating the toxicological challenges associated with the use of herbal medicinal products in developing countries. *Biomed Res Int* 2013, 2013, 804086.
5. Mulyono, D., Pinardi, D., & Jufri, A. Development of medicinal plant culture through empowerment of entrepreneur. In: *International Seminar on Promoting Local Resources for Sustainable Agriculture and Development (ISPLRSAD 2020). Atlantis Press 2021*. Atlantis Press, pp. 420–426.
6. Siahaan, S., & Aryastami, N. K. Studi kebijakan pengembangan tanaman obat di Indonesia. *Media Penelitian dan Pengembangan Kesehatan* 2018, 28, 157–166.
7. Chege, I. N., Okalebo, F. A., Guantai, A. N., Karanja, S., & Derese, S. Herbal product processig practices of traditional medicine practitioners in Kenya—Key information interviews. *JHMN* 2018, 16, 1–23.

8. Kartal, M. Intellectual property protection in the natural product drug discovery, traditional herbal medicine and herbal medicinal products. *Phytother Res* 2007, 21, 113–119.
9. Jain, N., Gupta, B. P., Thakur, N., Jain, R., Banweer, J., Jain, D. K., & Jain, S. (2010). Phytosome: A novel drug delivery system for herbal medicine. *Int J Pharm Sci Drug Res* 2010, 2, 224–228.
10. SAME AS 1
11. Mandal, S. C., & Mandal, M. Current status and future prospects of new drug delivery system. *Pharm Times* 2010, 42(4), 13–16.
12. Chakrobarty, K., Shivakumar, A., & Ramachandran, S. Nanotechnology in herbal medicine. *Int J Herb Med* 2016, 4, 21–27.
13. Devi, V. K., Jain, N., & Valli, K. S. (2010). Importance of novel drug delivery systems in herbal medicines. *Pharmacogn Rev* 2010, 4, 27.
14. Nalini, T., Kumari, S., & Basha, K. Novel nanosystems for herbal drug delivery. *World J Pharm Pharm Sci* 2017, 6(5), 1447–1463.
15. Bonifacio, B. V., da Silva, P. B., Ramos, M. A. D. S., Negri, K. M. S., Bauab, T. M., & Chorilli, M. Nanotechnology-based drug delivery systems and herbal medicines: A review. *Int J Nanomed* 2014, 9, 1–15.
16. Balekundri, A., & Mannur, V. Quality control of the traditional herbs and herbal products: A review. *Futur J Pharm Sci* 2020, 6, 1–9.
17. Zaigham, H., Tauheed, A., & Ali, A. Recent trend in traditional medicine dosage form and present status of Unani and Ayurvedic medicine. *Int J Pharm Sci & Res* 2019, 10, 1640–1649.
18. Teja, P. K., Mithiya, J., Kate, A. S., Bairwa, K., & Chauthe, S. K. Herbal nanomedicines: Recent advancements, challenges, opportunities and regulatory overview. *Phytomed* 2022, 96, 153890.
19. Sindhu, R. K., Gupta, R., Wadhera, G., & Kumar, P. Modern herbal nanogels: Formulation, delivery methods, and applications. *Gels* 2022, *8*, 97.
20. Semalty, A., Semalty, M., & Rawat, M. S. M. The phyto-phospholipid complexes-phytosomes: A potential therapeutic approach for herbal hepatoprotective drug delivery. *Pharmacog Rev* 2007, 1(2), 369–374.
21. Khogta, S., Patel, J., Barve, K., & Londhe, V. Herbal nano-formulations for topical delivery. *J Herb Med* 2020, 20, 100300.
22. Ernst, E. Cardiovascular adverse effects of herbal medicines: A systematic review of the recent literature. *Can J Cardiol* 2003, 19, 818–827.
23. Teschke, R., Schmidt-Taenzer, W., & Wolff, A. Spontaneous reports of assumed herbal hepatotoxicity by black cohosh: Is the liver-unspecific Naranjo scale precise enough to ascertain causality. *Pharmacoepidemiol Drug Saf* 2011, 20, 567–582.
24. Jones, T. K., & Lawson, B. M. Profound neonatal congestive heart failure caused by maternal consumption of blue cohosh herbal medication. *J Pediatr* 1998, 132, 550–552.
25. Haden, M., Marshall, D. A. S., & Murphy, B. (2011). Toxic levels of glycosides in herbal medication: A potential cause of hyperkalaemia. *Scott Med J* 2011, 56, 1–3.
26. Jordan, S. A., Cunningham, D. G., & Marles, R. J. Assessment of herbal medicinal products: Challenges, and opportunities to increase the knowledge base for safety assessment. *Toxicol Appl Pharmacol* 2010, 243, 198–216.

27. Pelkonen, O., Abass, K., & Wiesner, J. Thujone and thujone-containing herbal medicinal and botanical products: Toxicological assessment. *Regul Toxicol Pharmacol* 2013, 65, 100–107.
28. Russo, S., Mastropasqua, M., Mosetti, M. A., Persegani, C., & Paggi, A. Low doses of liquorice can induce hypertension encephalopathy. *Am J Nephrol* 2000, 20, 145–148.
29. Padiyara, R. S., & Khan, S. F. A review of commonly used herbal medicines. *ICHP* 2006, 9, 22–36.
30. Cheng, C. W., Fan, W., Ko, S. G., Song, L., & Bian, Z. X. Evidence-based management of herb-drug interaction in cancer chemotherapy. *Explore* 2010, 6, 324–329.
31. Cohen, P. A., & Ernst, E. Safety of herbal supplements: A guide for cardiologists. *Cardiovasc. Ther* 2010, 28, 246–253.
32. Henderson, L., Yue, Q. Y., Bergquist, C., Gerden, B., & Arlett, P. St John's wort (Hypericum perforatum): Drug interactions and clinical outcomes. *Br J Clin Pharmacol* 2002, 54, 349–356.
33. Goey, A. K., Mooiman, K. D., Beijnen, J. H., Schellens, J. H., & Meijerman, I. Relevance of in vitro and clinical data for predicting CYP3A4-mediated herb–drug interactions in cancer patients. *Cancer Treat Rev* 2013, 39, 773–783.
34. Sharma, A. K., Kumar, R., Mishra, A., & Gupta, R. Problems associated with clinical trials of Ayurvedic medicines. *Rev Bras Farmacogn* 2010, *20,* 276–281.
35. Saper, R. B., Kales, S. N., Paquin, J., Burns, M. J., Eisenberg, D. M., Davis, R. B., & Phillips, R. S. Heavy metal content of ayurvedic herbal medicine products. *JAMA* 2004, 292, 2868–2873.
36. Rothman, K. J., & Michels, K. B. The continuing unethical use of placebo controls. *N Engl J Med* 1994, 331, 394–398.
37. Ramandeep, K., Vikas, G., Francis, C. A., & Parveen, B. Scope and bottlenecks in clinical trials of herbal drugs-present scenario. *J Pharm Res* 2015, 14, 26–32.
38. Bauer, R., & Tittel, G. Quality assessment of herbal preparations as a precondition of pharmacological and clinical studies. *Phytomed* 1996, 2, 193–198.
39. Chaudhury, M. R., Chandrasekaran, R., & Mishra, S. Embryotoxicity and teratogenicity studies of an ayurvedic contraceptive—pippaliyadi vati. *J Ethnopharmacol* 2001, 74, 189–193.
40. Chan, K. Some aspects of toxic contaminants in herb medicines. *Chemosphere* 2003, 52, 1361–1371.
41. Moore, C., & Adler, R. Herbal vitamins: Lead toxicity and developmental delay. *Pediatrics* 2000, 106, 600–602.
42. Fugh-Berman, A. Herb-drug interactions. *Lancet* 2000, 355, 134–138.
43. Abdel-Aziz, S. M., Aeron, A., & Kahil, T. A. Health benefits and possible risks of herbal medicine. In: *Microbes in Food and Health*, 2016, pp. 97–116.
44. Laakmann, G., Schüle, C., Baghai, T., & Kieser, M. St. John's wort in mild to moderate depression: The relevance of hyperforin for the clinical efficacy. *Pharmacopsychiatry* 1998, 31, 54–59.
45. Brody, J. E. *Americans Gamble on Herbs as Medicine*. The New York Times, 2009. Available from: http: //query.nytimes.com/gst/fullpage.html?res_9B0D EFDA123B F93AA35751C0A96F958260. Accessed 2023.

46. Saper, R. B., Phillips, R. S., Sehgal, A., Khouri, N., Davis, R. B., Paquin, J., Thuppil, V., & Kales, S. N. Lead, mercury, and arsenic in US- and Indian manufactured ayurvedic medicines sold via the Internet. *JAMA* 2008, 300, 915–23.
47. Corns, C. M. Herbal remedies and clinical biochemistry. *Ann Clin Biochem* 2003, 40, 489–507.
48. Rathore, R., & Mathur, A. Entrepreneurship development in medicinal and aromatic plants: Prospects and challenges. *Int J Econ Plants* 2018, 5, 32–35.
49. Muhammad Auwal, A., Mohamed, Z., Nasir Shamsudin, M., Sharifuddin, J., & Ali, F. External pressure influence on entrepreneurship performance of SMEs: A case study of Malaysian herbal industry. *J Small Bus Entrep* 2020, 32, 149–171.
50. Kala, C. P., & Sajwan, B. S. Revitalizing Indian systems of herbal medicine by the National Medicinal Plants Board through institutional networking and capacity building. *Curr Sci* 2007, 93, 797–806.
51. Kala, C. P. Medicinal and aromatic plants: Boon for enterprise development. *J Appl Res Med Aromat Plants* 2015, 2, 134–139.
52. Deshingkar, P. *Migration, Remote Rural Areas and Chronic Poverty in India.* Overseas Development Institute: London, 2010, p. 31.
53. Kala, C. P. Programme zur Revitalisierung von Naturheilverfahren mitArzneipflanzen in Indien. *Zeitschrift fur Arznei- & Gewurzpflanzen* 2008, 13, 138–139.
54. Kala, C. P. Medicinal plants conservation and enterprise development. *Med Plants* 2009, 1, 79–95.
55. Humphries, S. S., & Kainer, K. A. Local perceptions of forest certification for community-based enterprises. *Forest Ecol Manag* 2006, 235, 30–43.
56. Garrity, D. P. Agroforestry and the achievement of the Millennium Development Goals. *Agrofor Syst* 2004, 6, 5–17.
57. dmapr.icar.gov.in/Medi_hub/home.html
58. Rajeswara, R., Rajput, D. K., Nagaraju, G., & Adinarayana, G. Scope and potential of medicinal and aromatic plants products for small and medium enterprises. *J Pharmacogn* 2012, 3, 112–114.
59. Das, S., Reddy, I. S., Kumar, P., Kumar, R., Bhushan, S., & Singh, S. B. *Agri-entrepreneurship Development in Medicinal andAromatic Plants*. Parmar Publication, 2022, pp. 118–120.
60. Government Set Up Validations and Quality Control Regulations of Herbal Medicines| Ayush Next https://ayushnext.ayush.gov.in/detail/writeUps/government-set-up-validations-and-quality-control-regulations-of-herbal-medicines
61. Sen, S., Chakraborty, R., & De, B. Challenges and opportunities in the advancement of herbal medicine: India's position and role in a global context. *J Herb Med* 2011, 1, 67–75.
62. World Health Organization. *WHO Traditional Medicine Strategy 2002–2005*. World Health Organization: Geneva, 2002.
63. Warude, D., & Patwardhan, B. Botanicals: Quality and regulatory issues. *J Sci Indus Res* 2005, 64, 83–92.

CHAPTER 3

Plant Design, Layout, and Construction in Herbal Drug Production

SWAPNALI PATIL[1*], PRANALI PANGAM[2], and POOURNIMA SANKPAL[3]

[1]*Department of Pharmaceutics, Vijayrao Naik College of Pharmacy, Shirval, Tal-Kankavli, Maharashtra, India*

[2]*Department of Pharmaceutical Quality Assurance, Vijayrao Naik College of Pharmacy, Shirval, Tal-Kankavli, Maharashtra, India*

[3]*Department of Pharmaceutical Chemistry, Bharati Vidyapeeth College of Pharmacy, Palus, Maharashtra, India*

*Corresponding author

ABSTRACT

The design, layout, and construction of herbal drug production facilities play a pivotal role in ensuring the efficient and safe manufacturing of herbal pharmaceuticals. Effective plant design begins with a comprehensive analysis of the specific requirements of herbal drug production, considering factors such as raw material storage, processing equipment, quality control, and regulatory compliance. The layout must optimize workflow, minimize contamination risks, and facilitate easy cleaning and maintenance. Construction materials and techniques must adhere to industry standards to meet good manufacturing practices and ensure product quality. Sustainability and energy efficiency are increasingly important considerations in modern plant design. Moreover, integration of automation and digital technologies is critical for precision and consistency in herbal drug production. These technologies enhance process control, data monitoring, and traceability, thereby improving product quality

Herbal Drug Industry: From Cultivation to Innovation and Global Impact.
Abhishek Tiwari, Varsha Tiwari, and Ajay Sharma (Eds.)

DOI: 10.1201/9781779640994-3

and regulatory compliance. In conclusion, a well-planned and executed design, layout, and construction process in herbal drug production facilities are essential for achieving high-quality products, ensuring regulatory compliance, and promoting sustainability in the rapidly growing herbal pharmaceutical industry.

3.1 INTRODUCTION

The herbal drug industry has undergone a remarkable transformation, evolving into a dynamic sector at the intersection of traditional wisdom and modern pharmaceutical innovation. In response to a global shift toward natural and sustainable healthcare alternatives, herbal drugs, derived from plant sources, have garnered widespread recognition for their perceived efficacy and lower incidence of side effects compared to synthetic pharmaceuticals. The demand for herbal remedies has surged, driven by a burgeoning consumer base seeking holistic healthcare solutions rooted in nature's pharmacopeia. As this demand continues to grow, the establishment of state-of-the-art herbal drug production facilities becomes paramount, demanding a comprehensive understanding of plant design, layout, and construction. This guide aims to provide an exhaustive exploration of the multifaceted considerations involved in setting up such facilities, catering not only to compliance requirements but also to strategic imperatives for success in this rapidly evolving pharmaceutical landscape [1, 2].

In this context, the journey commences with the strategic selection of an appropriate site, transcending geographical considerations to encompass a thorough evaluation of regulatory compliance and environmental impact. This initial phase sets the stage for the facility's adherence to stringent good manufacturing practices (GMPs) and other regulatory standards, ensuring that the herbal drugs produced meet the highest levels of quality and safety. The chosen site must withstand comprehensive risk assessments, considering potential natural disasters, proximity to pollution sources, and other factors that could compromise the integrity of the manufacturing process. Zoning regulations come under close scrutiny to confirm not only the present suitability of the site for pharmaceutical manufacturing but also its potential for accommodating future expansions [3, 4].

Following the meticulous selection of a site, the facility design becomes a key player in the operational success of herbal drug production. Beyond the logistical aspects, the layout design is an intricate process aimed at optimizing workflow, minimizing material movement, and ensuring a seamless progression from raw material intake to the packaging of the finished product. Cleanroom design principles are integral to controlling variables such as airborne particles, temperature, and humidity all critical factors in meeting the stringent standards of GMP for herbal drug production. A flexible and modular design is recommended to allow for easy adaptation to evolving production needs and the assimilation of emerging technologies, thereby ensuring the long-term resilience and sustainability of the facility [5].

Equipment selection, the next crucial phase, demands a nuanced understanding of the various processes involved in herbal drug manufacturing. From extraction methods such as steam distillation, solvent extraction, to supercritical fluid extraction, the chosen equipment must align seamlessly with these processes. Material compatibility is non-negotiable, necessitating equipment constructed from materials that are inert, corrosion-resistant, and easy to clean. Automation integration takes precedence to enhance precision, reduce manual handling, and elevate overall production efficiency to meet the growing demand for herbal drugs [4, 6].

Layout considerations within the facility further contribute to the overall success of herbal drug production. The systematic handling of raw materials, from intake and inspection to storage, demands a meticulous approach. A robust quality control system for incoming raw materials is imperative, involving identity testing, purity assessments, and checks for contaminants. Storage conditions must be optimized to preserve the integrity of herbal ingredients and prevent degradation. Extraction and processing areas should be strategically designed with adequate ventilation and temperature control to optimize the quality of herbal drugs. Segregation of different processing stages, such as extraction and formulation, is crucial to prevent cross-contamination and maintain the purity of the final product [7, 8].

In the formulation and mixing stages, layouts must prevent cross-contamination, and equipment should facilitate thorough cleaning. Stringent cleaning protocols should be established, and equipment design should allow for easy disassembly and access for cleaning-in-place (CIP) systems [9]. Quality control and assurance play a central role in herbal drug production, necessitating the integration of a quality control laboratory equipped with advanced analytical tools. Real-time monitoring systems should be implemented to detect deviations from quality standards promptly, allowing for immediate corrective actions [10].

Construction guidelines for herbal drug production facilities require careful consideration of materials, hygiene, utilities, and regulatory compliance. Construction materials must comply with industry standards and be chemically resistant to substances used in herbal drug production [11, 12]. Hygienic design principles, including smooth surfaces, effective seals, proper drainage, and cleaning-friendly layouts, are essential to minimize areas where contaminants can accumulate. Utility systems, including power, water, and HVAC (heating, ventilation, and air conditioning), should be designed for efficiency and equipped with redundancy to ensure continuous production in case of system failures. Early engagement with regulatory authorities is crucial to expedite approvals, and comprehensive documentation throughout the construction process is necessary to demonstrate compliance with regulatory requirements. In conclusion, as the demand for herbal drugs continues to rise, the importance of plant design, layout, and construction cannot be overstated. Establishing a successful herbal drug production facility requires a holistic approach that encompasses site selection, facility design, equipment selection, layout considerations, construction guidelines, and strict adherence to regulatory standards. This comprehensive guide seeks to empower industry professionals and stakeholders with the knowledge needed to navigate the complexities of establishing and operating herbal drug production facilities, ultimately contributing to the delivery of high-quality herbal pharmaceuticals in an increasingly competitive and dynamic market. As the herbal drug industry stands at the nexus of tradition and innovation, the meticulous design and construction of production facilities are fundamental to meeting the evolving healthcare needs of a discerning global consumer base [11, 13].

3.2 RISING SIGNIFICANCE OF HERBAL DRUG PRODUCTION

The resurgence of interest in herbal medicines stems from a growing awareness of the limitations and side effects associated with conventional pharmaceuticals. Herbal drugs, derived from natural sources, offer a compelling alternative, often presenting fewer adverse effects and a broader spectrum of therapeutic benefits. The inherent complexity of plant-derived compounds provides a diverse range of bioactive molecules, each with unique healing properties. This diversity allows for a nuanced and personalized approach to healthcare, catering to individual needs and preferences [14, 15].

The global shift toward herbal drug usage is not merely a trend; it reflects a fundamental change in consumer attitudes and preferences. Patients are increasingly seeking treatment options that align with their holistic well-being, and herbal drugs, with their roots deeply embedded in traditional medicine, offer a promising avenue. This shift has prompted pharmaceutical companies to invest significantly in herbal drug research, development, and production, giving rise to a burgeoning need for advanced and efficient manufacturing facilities [16].

3.3 PLANT DESIGN

3.3.1 SITE SELECTION

In the intricate process of site selection for an herbal drug production facility, a comprehensive approach is essential to ensure the alignment of the chosen site with regulatory standards and environmental requirements. This begins with a thorough evaluation of both local and international regulations governing pharmaceutical manufacturing. Early engagement with regulatory authorities is crucial to gain insights into specific requirements and streamlining approval processes. An indispensable component of site selection is the conduct of an Environmental Impact Assessment, which delves into potential ecological consequences. This assessment encompasses an in-depth analysis of air and water quality, soil conditions, and overall impact on local ecosystems [17]. Moreover, sustainability practices are integral to the site-selection process, emphasizing the incorporation of energy-efficient technologies and waste management strategies to minimize the ecological footprint of the facility. Proximity to raw material sources holds paramount significance, with an emphasis on choosing a location in close proximity to reliable sources to ensure a stable and efficient supply chain. Transportation infrastructure, including roads, ports, and airports, is meticulously assessed to facilitate the smooth movement of raw materials and finished products. Furthermore, the accessibility of utilities such as water, electricity, and gas is considered to support manufacturing operations effectively. The chosen site should not only comply with zoning regulations specific to pharmaceutical manufacturing but also allow for future expansion, considering both physical space and regulatory constraints. In essence, a judiciously selected site forms the cornerstone of a successful herbal drug production facility, laying the groundwork for compliance, efficiency, and long-term sustainability [18].

3.3.2 FACILITY DESIGN

In the realm of herbal drug production, facility design plays a pivotal role in shaping the operational efficiency and overall success of the manufacturing process. A meticulous approach to facility design begins with a focus on workflow optimization, ensuring a smooth and logical progression from raw material intake to the packaging of the finished product. This involves conducting a detailed analysis of the entire production process, mapping out each stage to identify potential bottlenecks and streamline operations. The layout is crafted with precision, adhering to lean manufacturing principles to minimize waste, reduce lead times, and enhance productivity [19].

The allocation of separate areas for various production stages is a critical aspect of facility design. Distinct zones are designated for herbal extraction processes, processing activities such as grinding and mixing, and formulation and packaging stages [20]. This ensures not only a logical and sequential arrangement of equipment but also prevents cross-contamination between different stages of production. Adherence to GMP is paramount in facility design, guiding the implementation of cleanroom design principles. This involves controlling variables such as airborne particles, temperature, and humidity to meet pharmaceutical industry standards. Additionally, hygienic practices, including the use of easily cleanable materials and rigorous sanitation procedures, are integrated into the design. The establishment of robust documentation and record-keeping systems is a key element, ensuring comprehensive tracking of processes and compliance with GMP requirements. Ultimately, a well-designed facility sets the stage for efficient and compliant herbal drug production, meeting both industry standards and consumer expectations [21] (Table 3.1).

TABLE 3.1 List of Machinery, Equipment, and Minimum Manufacturing Premises Required for the Manufacturing of Herbal Medicine

Sr. No.	Category of Medicine	Minimum Manufacturing Space Required	Machinery/Equipment Recommended
		1200 ft^2 covered area with separate cabins partitions for each activity. If Unani medicine is manufactured in same premises an additional area of 400 ft^2 will be required	
1.	Churna/Nasya/ Manjan/Lepa Kwath Chum	200 ft^2	Grinder/disintegrator/pulverizer/ powder mixer/sieves/shifter
2.	Pills/Vatti/Gutika matirai	100 ft^2	Ball mill, mass mixer/power mixer, pill/vati cutting machine, stainless steel trays/containers for storage. Driers/mechanized chatee (for mixing guggul) where required
3.	Tablets	100 ft^2	Ball mill, mass mixer/powder mixer, granulator drier, tablet compressing machine and sugarcoating, mechanized chatte
4.	Kajal	100 ft^2	Karthen lamps for collection of kajal, tipple roller mill, sieves, filling/packing manufacturing room should be provided with exhaust fan and ultraviolet lamps
5.	Capsules	100 ft^2	Air-conditioner, dehumidifier, hygrometer, thermometer, capsule filling machine, and chemical balance
6.	Ointment/Marham pasai	100 ft^2	Tube filling machine, crimping medicine/ointment mixer, end runner/mill (where required)
7.	Asava/Aristha	100 ft^2	
8.	Sufoof (powder)	200 ft^2	Grinder/pulverizer, seiver, trays, scoups, powder mixer, (where required)
9.	Raughan (oils) (crushing and boiling)	100 ft^2	Oil expeller, patilas, oil filter bottle filling machine, bottle drier, bhatti

3.3.3 EQUIPMENT SELECTION

Choosing the right equipment is a critical aspect of herbal drug production, directly impacting the quality and efficiency of the manufacturing process. The selection process begins by considering the specific needs of herbal drug processing, taking into account factors such as extraction methods, drying techniques, and formulation processes. Equipment is tailored to the unique characteristics of the herbal materials, ensuring optimal yield efficiency and preservation of potency [22].

Material compatibility is a central consideration in equipment selection. It involves prioritizing machinery constructed from materials that resist corrosion, as herbal extracts may contain acidic or corrosive compounds. This not only extends the lifespan of the equipment but also prevents contamination and maintains the integrity of the final product. Equipment is chosen with an emphasis on designs that facilitate easy cleaning and sterilization, crucial aspects in maintaining product quality and meeting regulatory standards [11].

Validation processes are instituted to ensure that each piece of machinery operates within specified parameters, guaranteeing reliability and consistency in the manufacturing process. Regular calibration programs further contribute to equipment accuracy and precision. The integration of advanced technologies, automation where applicable, and a commitment to ongoing maintenance ensures that the selected equipment aligns seamlessly with the goals of producing high-quality herbal drugs in an efficient and sustainable manner. In essence, equipment selection is a strategic and nuanced process that forms the backbone of a successful herbal drug production operation [23].

Strategic layout planning: Efficient layout considerations are instrumental in ensuring the seamless and compliant operation of an herbal drug production facility. Divided into key segments, each aspect of layout considerations contributes to the overall success of the manufacturing process [24].

3.3.3.1 ZONING

The layout of an herbal drug production plant plays a pivotal role in optimizing efficiency and ensuring a seamless workflow. Zoning, or the division of the plant into distinct functional areas, is a key aspect of strategic layout planning. These zones may include spaces dedicated to raw material storage, extraction and processing, quality control, packaging, and administrative functions. Each zone serves a specific purpose, contributing to the overall coherence and effectiveness of the herbal drug production process [25].

3.3.1.2 RAW MATERIAL HANDLING

Raw material handling is a critical phase in the herbal drug production process, demanding a systematic and well-designed approach. The facility layout is structured to accommodate the intake, inspection, and storage of raw materials. To maintain the highest standards of quality, a robust quality-control system is implemented, involving identity testing, purity assessments, and checks for contaminants. Storage conditions are optimized to preserve the integrity of herbal ingredients and prevent degradation. An emphasis on efficient logistical workflows minimizes material movement and enhances the overall efficiency of the raw material handling process [25].

3.3.1.3 EXTRACTION AND PROCESSING AREAS

Designing optimal extraction and processing areas is essential to extract and process herbal materials efficiently while maintaining product quality. The layout includes dedicated spaces for extraction processes, such as maceration, percolation, or supercritical fluid extraction. Adequate ventilation and temperature control are integrated to optimize the quality of herbal drugs. Process segregation is carefully implemented, creating distinct areas for different stages of production. This segregation prevents cross-contamination and ensures the purity of the extracted materials. The strategic layout also accounts for the sequential progression of processes, contributing to the overall efficiency and compliance of the facility [26].

3.3.1.4 FORMULATION AND MIXING

Layout considerations for formulation and mixing areas focus on preventing cross-contamination and ensuring precise and controlled processes. Separate areas are allocated for formulation and mixing stages to prevent interference between different herbal formulations. The design emphasizes equipment that facilitates thorough cleaning and sanitation, preventing any residue from affecting subsequent formulations. Stringent cleaning protocols are established, and equipment design incorporates features that enable easy disassembly and access for CIP systems. By maintaining strict controls and cleanliness in these areas, the layout ensures the integrity of herbal formulations and the prevention of any potential quality issues [20, 27].

3.3.1.5 QUALITY CONTROL AND ASSURANCE

Quality control and assurance are integral components of herbal drug production, demanding specialized layouts to meet stringent standards. The facility integrates a dedicated quality control laboratory equipped with advanced analytical tools such as high-performance liquid chromatography and mass spectrometry. This laboratory is strategically placed to allow for real-time monitoring and immediate intervention if deviations from quality standards are detected. Real-time monitoring systems are implemented at various stages of production to identify and address potential issues promptly. The layout ensures a seamless integration of quality control measures at every step, contributing to the production of high-quality herbal drugs that meet regulatory requirements and consumer expectations.

3.3.1.6 SAFETY PROTOCOLS

The safety of personnel and the integrity of the herbal drug production process are non-negotiable priorities. Layout planning must incorporate stringent safety protocols, including emergency exits, fire suppression systems, and adequate ventilation. Compliance with occupational health and safety regulations is paramount, ensuring that the working environment is secure and conducive to the well-being of all involved [28].

3.3.1.7 FLEXIBILITY FOR EXPANSION

Anticipating future growth and expansion is a hallmark of strategic layout planning. The herbal drug industry is dynamic, with innovations and market demands evolving rapidly. A well-designed layout should incorporate flexibility, allowing for the seamless integration of additional equipment, storage capacity, or even entire production lines. This forward-thinking approach ensures that the herbal drug production plant remains adaptable to the evolving landscape of the pharmaceutical industry [29].

3.3.2 CONSTRUCTION CHALLENGES AND CONSIDERATIONS

3.3.2.1 MATERIAL SELECTION

The materials chosen for construction play a pivotal role in ensuring the longevity, safety, and compliance of the herbal drug production facility. Complying with industry standards, materials must be selected based on their compatibility with pharmaceutical manufacturing and herbal drug production. Prioritizing corrosion-resistant materials is essential, especially considering potential exposure to acidic or corrosive substances during the production process. These materials should also be easy to clean and sterilize to prevent contamination and maintain product quality. The selection process extends to equipment, surfaces, and structural elements, all of which contribute to creating a facility that meets the stringent requirements of a pharmaceutical manufacturing environment [30].

3.3.2.2 HYGIENIC DESIGN

Hygienic design principles are paramount in preventing microbial contamination and maintaining the highest standards of cleanliness throughout the facility. The layout and construction should incorporate smooth surfaces and effective seals to minimize areas where contaminants can accumulate. Proper drainage systems are essential to facilitate easy cleaning and prevent standing water, reducing the risk of microbial growth. The design should also consider the use of impermeable and easy-to-clean materials to maintain a sterile environment. These hygienic design practices extend to equipment selection, ensuring that machinery and surfaces are easily accessible for thorough cleaning, sterilization, and sanitation [31].

3.3.2.3 UTILITIES AND SUPPORT SYSTEMS

Efficient utility and support systems are integral to the construction guidelines of a herbal drug production facility. Consideration for water, electricity, and HVAC systems is crucial. Utilities should be designed to support the specific needs of herbal drug production, ensuring a reliable and consistent supply. Backup systems for critical utilities, such as power and water, should be in place to guarantee continuity of production in the event of utility failures. Embracing energy-efficient technologies and considering renewable energy sources contribute not only to sustainability but also to the operational efficiency of the facility. Robust systems for waste management and disposal should also be integrated into the construction guidelines, aligning with environmental sustainability practices [32].

3.3.2.4 COMPLIANCE WITH REGULATORY STANDARDS

Construction guidelines for a herbal drug production facility must align with stringent compliance and regulatory requirements. Engaging with regulatory authorities early in the planning and construction phases is essential to identify specific requirements and streamline approval processes. Documentation throughout the construction process is critical, demonstrating adherence to regulatory standards and facilitating the regulatory approval process. Compliance with GMP is non-negotiable, and the facility design and construction should reflect this commitment to quality and safety. Ensuring that the facility complies with local and international regulations, including zoning laws, environmental regulations, and building codes, is imperative. Continuous monitoring and updates to construction practices based on evolving regulatory standards contribute to the long-term success and compliance of the herbal drug production facility [9, 32].

3.3.2.5 PROJECT MANAGEMENT

Efficient project management is instrumental in bringing the herbal drug production plant from blueprint to reality. Coordinating with architects, engineers, contractors, and regulatory authorities requires a comprehensive and well-executed plan. Timely completion is essential not only for meeting market demands but also for minimizing costs and ensuring that the plant is operational within the anticipated timeframe.

3.3.2.6 VALIDATION AND QUALIFICATION

Validation and qualification are essential processes in the lifecycle of herbal drug production plants, ensuring that the facility is designed, constructed, and operates in compliance with regulatory standards and industry best practices. These processes are crucial to guarantee the safety, efficacy, and quality of herbal drugs produced within the facility. Post-construction, the plant undergoes a thorough validation and qualification process. This involves a meticulous examination to verify that the plant meets the specified design criteria and operates in accordance with regulatory guidelines. Validation and qualification are integral steps in ensuring the safety, efficacy, and quality of the herbal drugs produced within the facility [33].

3.4 CONCLUSION

In conclusion, the design, layout, and construction of herbal drug production plants represent a multifaceted journey that requires a harmonious blend of scientific precision, engineering acumen, and regulatory diligence. The rising prominence of herbal drugs in the pharmaceutical landscape underscores the importance of establishing cutting-edge facilities that can meet the demands of a dynamic and evolving industry. By integrating efficient design principles, strategic layout planning, and strict adherence to regulatory standards during construction, pharmaceutical companies can pave the way for the sustainable growth of herbal drug production. The journey from plant conception to operation is not merely about constructing physical structures; it is a commitment to providing healthcare solutions that resonate with the natural rhythms of healing. As the herbal drug industry continues to flourish, the design and construction of advanced production plants will play a pivotal role in shaping the future of pharmaceuticals.

KEYWORDS

- **herbal drug production**
- **good manufacturing practices**
- **facility layout**
- **sustainability**
- **automation**
- **quality control**
- **regulatory compliance**

REFERENCES

1. Bowonder, B., et al., The global pharmaceutical industry: Changing competitive landscape. *Int J Technol Manage* 2003, 25(3–4), 201–226.
2. Petrova, E. Innovation in the pharmaceutical industry: The process of drug discovery and development. In: *Innovation and Marketing in the Pharmaceutical Industry: Emerging Practices, Research, and Policies*. Springer, 2013, pp. 19–81.
3. Zhou, L. G., & Wu, J. Y. Development and application of medicinal plant tissue cultures for production of drugs and herbal medicinals in China. *Nat Prod Rep* 2006, 23(5), 789–810.
4. Alamgir, A., & Alamgir, A. Cultivation of herbal drugs, biotechnology, and in vitro production of secondary metabolites, high-value medicinal plants, herbal wealth, and herbal trade. In: *Therapeutic Use of Medicinal Plants and Their Extracts: Volume 1: Pharmacognosy*, 2017, pp. 379–452.
5. He, T.-T., et al., Good manufacturing practice (GMP) regulation of herbal medicine in comparative research: China GMP, cGMP, WHO-GMP, PIC/S and EU-GMP. *Eur J Integr Med* 2015, 7(1), 55–66.
6. Ahad, B., et al., Medicinal plants and herbal drugs: An overview. In: *Medicinal and Aromatic Plants: Healthcare and Industrial Applications*, 2021, pp. 1–40.
7. Wichtl, M. *Herbal Drugs and Phytopharmaceuticals: A Handbook for Practice on a Scientific Basis*. CRC Press, 2004.
8. Lu, D.-Y., et al., Natural drug cancer treatments, strategies from herbal medicine to chemical or biological drugs. *Stud Nat Prod Chem* 2020, 66, 91–115.
9. Bandaranayake, W. M. Quality control, screening, toxicity, and regulation of herbal drugs. In: *Modern Phytomedicine: Turning Medicinal Plants into Drugs*, 2006, pp. 25–57.
10. Balekundri, A., & Mannur, V. Quality control of the traditional herbs and herbal products: A review. *Future J Pharm Sci* 2020, 6, 1–9.
11. Mukherjee, P. K. *Quality Control and Evaluation of Herbal Drugs: Evaluating Natural Products and Traditional Medicine*. Elsevier, 2019.
12. Organization, W. H. *WHO Guidelines on Good Agricultural and Collection Practices [GACP] for Medicinal Plants*. World Health Organization, 2003.
13. Organization, W. H. Quality assurance of pharmaceuticals: A compendium of guidelines and related materials. In: *Good Manufacturing Practices and Inspection*. World Health Organization, 2007, Vol. 2.
14. Dubey, N., Kumar, R., & Tripathi, P. Global promotion of herbal medicine: India's opportunity. *Curr Sci* 2004, 86(1), 37–41.
15. Verma, S., & Singh, S. Current and future status of herbal medicines. *Vet World* 2008, 1(11), 347.
16. Pan, S.-Y., et al., New perspectives on how to discover drugs from herbal medicines: CAM's outstanding contribution to modern therapeutics. *Evid-Based Complement Altern Med* 2013, 2013, 627375.
17. McPherson, E. M. *Plant Location Selection Techniques*. Elsevier, 1995.
18. Rediske, G., et al., Wind power plant site selection: A systematic review. *Renew Sustain Energy Rev* 2021, 148, 111293.

19. Sbárbaro, D., & Del Villar, R. *Advanced Control and Supervision of Mineral Processing Plants*. Springer Science & Business Media, 2010.
20. Alamgir, A., & Alamgir, A. Herbal drugs: Their collection, preservation, and preparation; evaluation, quality control, and standardization of herbal drugs. In: *Therapeutic Use of Medicinal Plants and Their Extracts: Volume 1: Pharmacognosy*, 2017, pp. 453–495.
21. Sahoo, N., & Manchikanti, P. Herbal drug regulation and commercialization: An Indian industry perspective. *J Alternat Complement Med* 2013, 19(12), 957–963.
22. Muyumba, N., et al., Quality control of herbal drugs and preparations: The methods of analysis, their relevance and applications. *Talanta Open* 2021, 4, 100070.
23. Indrayanto, G. The importance of method validation in herbal drug research. *J Pharm Biomed Anal* 2022, 214, 114735.
24. Mutua, K. J. *Operational Challenges in the Growth of Small & Medium Enterprises in Kisumu County, Kenya*. University of Nairobi, 2013.
25. Seider, W. D., et al., *Product and Process Design Principles: Synthesis, Analysis, and Evaluation*. John Wiley & Sons, 2017.
26. Prado, J., & Rostagno, M. *Natural Product Extraction: Principles and Applications*. Royal Society of Chemistry, 2022.
27. Byeon, J. C., et al., Recent formulation approaches to oral delivery of herbal medicines. *J Pharm Investig* 2019, 49, 17–26.
28. Zamawe, C., et al., Effectiveness and safety of herbal medicines for induction of labour: A systematic review and meta-analysis. *BMJ Open* 2018, 8(10), e022499.
29. Wachtel-Galor, S., & Benzie, I. F. *Herbal Medicine*. Lester Packer, PhD, 2011, p. 1.
30. Hoffmann, D. *Medical Herbalism: The Science and Practice of Herbal Medicine*. Simon and Schuster, 2003.
31. Yang, L., & Tsai, T.-H. Neuroprotective effect and herbal-drug pharmacokinetic interaction of Gastrodia elata extract on valproic acid. *Biomed Pharmacother* 2022, 156, 113938.
32. Parveen, A., et al., Challenges and guidelines for clinical trial of herbal drugs. *J Pharm Bioallied Sci* 2015, 7(4), 329.
33. Mukherjee, P. K. *Evidence-based Validation of Herbal Medicine*. Elsevier, 2015.

CHAPTER 4

Formulation and Production, and Management of Herbal Products

AKSHAY KUMAR LUNAWAT[1], TARUN SHARMA[1], AKSHAY DEBANJAN MUKHERJEE[2], ANKIT AWASTHI[1], SHUBHAM THAKUR[1], MANISH KUMAR[1*], ABHISHEK TIWARI[3], VARSHA TIWARI[3], and ARYA LAKSHMI MARISETTI[4]

[1]*Department of Pharmaceutics, ISF College of Pharmacy, Moga, Punjab, India*

[2]*Department of Quality Assurance, ISF College of Pharmacy, Moga, Punjab, India*

[3]*Amity Institute of Pharmacy, Amity University Uttar Pradesh, Lucknow Campus, Lucknow, Uttar Pradesh, India*

[4]*Department of Pharmacognosy & Phytochemistry, School of Pharmaceutical Sciences, Delhi Pharmaceutical Sciences & Research University, New Delhi, Delhi, India*

*Corresponding author

ABSTRACT

Herbal products have played a vital role in traditional medicine across ancient civilizations such as Mesopotamia, Egypt, China, and India. These natural remedies, derived from various plant parts, are valued for their cultural relevance, perceived safety, and therapeutic efficacy. The chapter comprehensively explores the formulation, production, and management of herbal products, beginning with herb selection and identification through advanced methods like high-performance thin-layer chromatography,

Herbal Drug Industry: From Cultivation to Innovation and Global Impact.
Abhishek Tiwari, Varsha Tiwari, and Ajay Sharma (Eds.)

DOI: 10.1201/9781779640994-4

high-performance liquid chromatography, and DNA barcoding. It details biological analyses to ensure safety and quality, followed by various extraction techniques including maceration, percolation, infusion, distillation, expression, Soxhlet extraction, and supercritical fluid extraction. The chapter further discusses types of herbal formulations such as decoctions, tinctures, glycerites, tablets, capsules, ointments, creams, oils, and powdered preparations, highlighting formulation considerations, stability, and shelf life. Manufacturing processes encompass raw material selection, quality control, extraction, standardization, packaging, and finished product testing to ensure regulatory compliance and product integrity. The chapter also highlights India's contribution to herbal product development, showcasing globally recognized formulations like neem, turmeric, Ashwagandha, Triphala, and BGR-34. These products demonstrate the integration of ancient Ayurvedic knowledge with modern scientific practices, enhancing India's prominence in the global herbal market.

4.1 INTRODUCTION

Herbal or plant-based products have often been used in health and medical treatment since ancient times [1]. Plants have been a basis for the treatment and the development of drugs in traditional medicine methods [2]. The word herbal is used to refer to the use of the plant or its parts from the plant for medicinal purposes [3]. Herbal medicine, which is also known as botanical medicine or phytomedicine, is the name of a very wide spectrum of natural remedies that are prepared from various parts of plants like leaves, roots, flowers, seeds, or stems. Those substances have served as an essential component of the age-old practices of traditional medicine throughout the world for centuries. The popularity of herbal medicines is based on the fact that they are natural, have cultural roots, and are perceived as safe by people in comparison to synthetic drugs. They are used to prevent, reduce, or cure different health problems. These are often implemented as part of general wellness strategies that take into account the close linkage of the body, mind, and spirit [4]. Several commercially available herbal products are dietary supplements, herbal teas, herbal extracts, herbal cosmetics, and other products that are prepared from plant materials [5]. Traditional herbal medicines are usually taken with the purpose of either changing the outcome of a disease or as a complement to conventional medicine and are highly valued because of their natural sources and presumed health benefits [6]. They can be provided in tablets, liquids, creams, or other forms that fit their intended use and dosing frequency [7].

The popularity of herbal products dates back thousands of years, as we can see in the herbal products of ancient times in Mesopotamia, Egypt, China, and India. In the ancient Mesopotamian civilization, the use of herbs in medicine dates back to almost 2600 BC. The clay tablets of that era even talk about the use of thyme and laurel as curing plants [8]. The papyrus of ancient Egypt not only tells us about the process of herbal preparation to treat different diseases, but also about the production of medicine of those times [9]. Traditional Chinese medicine (TCM) is the oldest medical system in the world, which is traced back to more than 2000 years ago when the first pharmacopeia was compiled around 200 BC. This famous TCM text contains over 300 medical plants and their applications, which are the foundation of TCM today. Herbalism was a common thing in the Middle Ages where many monastery gardens were set up to grow medicinal herbs to cure different diseases [10]. India is home to several herbs used in traditional medicine systems such as Ayurveda, Siddha, and Unani. The Indian contribution to herbal medicine can be traced to Ayurveda texts as early as 3000 BC [11]. The Rigveda, which is a very ancient holy book of India, is about various medicinal plants and their healing powers. *Charaka Samhita* and *Sushruta Samhita*, the main treatises of Ayurveda, also deal with significant detail on phytotherapeutics and their preparation [12]. Additionally, India, as the abode of a large number of plants and a well-known herbal medicine practitioner, is a significant player in the global herbal products market. Increasingly, Indian herbal products such as herbal supplements, teas, and skin-care products are coming to the forefront in the world market for their perceived effectiveness and safety. Apart from that, India has also significantly contributed to scientific research of herbal medicine with numerous research institutions and pharmaceutical companies working on research of medicinal plants and the development of herbal products for modern medical practice. Hence, herbal treatment has been popular since the older days, and many regions have been using this as their primary source of medical treatment before the arrival of modern medicine [13]. However, a shift from synthetic drugs to herbal products has been observed lately, mainly because people have become more aware of the negative impact of synthetic drugs and the need for natural remedies [14]. Additionally, plant-based drugs and products are becoming widely used nowadays as substitutes to boost health and serve as a way of therapy alone or in combination with other medications. People believe that herbal medicines are safer and do not cause any side effects; therefore, they choose herbal medicines more often [15]. In Asia and Africa, more than 80% of the people still rely on traditional methods of healing as their primary source of healthcare [16]. Moreover, it is important to mention that nearly 25% of modern medications that are traditionally used were first isolated from plants or plant extracts [17].

Herbal products are a rich and varied group and are commonly classified into three categories according to their use, composition, and methods of preparation [18]. Medicinal herbs comprise a major section as they possess healing properties that can be used for curing common diseases as well as to improve the person's overall health such as gingko, turmeric, ginseng, echinacea, and others [19]. Culinary herbs, on the other hand, are the major ingredients used for flavoring and aroma of foods and beverages and may also contribute to health benefits in the form of taste and smell such as basil, parsley, oregano, and others [20]. Aromatic herbs have a natural place in perfumes and aromatherapy, as their charming scents make them useful for relaxation and mental clarity examples include mint, lemongrass, rosemary, and lavender [21]. Cosmetic herbs are used in making beauty products for the skin and personal care, which serve as natural substitutes for other beauty needs [22]. Compositionally, herbal products can be broadly classified into two main categories: single herbs and complex herbal formulas. As for single herbs, these herbs are derived from just one plant species and are generally used in whole or powdered form. They are identified for their unique medicinal or flavoring qualities. On the other hand, herbal mixtures are a combination of different herbs to get synergistic effects or at the same time to solve different health problems. The blends are specifically created to have a balance of properties and are well-rounded with these herbs. There are diverse production processes for herbal products and they all result in different forms and degrees of the herbs. Dried herbs are used predominantly for brewing teas or encapsulated for easy consumption. Extracts are the concentrated forms of herbal constituents. They are available in liquid or powder form with increased potency as compared to the original plant. Tinctures are another well-liked form, produced by infusing herbs in alcohol or glycerine to take out their active components, offering a concentrated and also easily absorbed form of the herb. Thus, depending upon the usage, composition, and methods used for the preparation they are classified [23].

The recognition and acceptability of herbal products have been increasing fast in recent years, due to several reasons such as the growing trend of natural remedies, worries about the side effects of synthetic drugs, and the need for safe and environmentally friendly healthcare options [24]. There are various herbal products which include dietary supplements, teas, tinctures, and topical preparations that are produced from natural plant sources [25]. The main reason why herbal products are liked by many people is because of their perceived safety and mild character. Many people prefer herbal medicines because they are considered to be safer than synthetic drugs and because they are derived from natural sources [26]. This opinion is echoed by the fact that the use of some herbs in traditional medicine systems has a long history with only a few reported adverse effects. The demand for herbal products is significantly affected by the growing information sharing about their health benefits by the expansion of the internet and social media [27]. As a result, it has become easier for people to obtain herbal knowledge, which has in turn increased the popularity of herbal medicine among the common people. In consequence, the demand for herbal remedies is increasing. Herbal products have a unique quality of versatility because many herbs provide multiple benefits and can treat digestive problems, skin diseases, and stress. This diversity consequently adds to the simplicity and affordable nature of herbal remedies, which are desirable to people who are looking for natural healing methods [28]. Furthermore, herbal products are appreciated for their sustainability and eco-friendly nature. On the contrary, natural medicinal products, which in most cases are obtained from renewable plant-based sources, are able to satisfy the market demand for eco-friendly products. The ever-increasing demand for natural, safe, and efficient healthcare solutions is expected to keep the popularity of herbal products at a high level. The ongoing research dedicated to the health benefits of herbs will probably be able to fuel this trend; thus, herbal products will be more and more present in the healthcare sector in the future [29].

This chapter includes the selection and identification of herbs, various methods of extraction of herbs, types of herbal formulation, and manufacturing considerations regarding product development of herbal products. Additionally, it also includes Indian commercially available herbal products.

4.2 SELECTION OF HERBS

The choice of herbal products is an important factor because it ensures their efficacy, safety, and suitability of the needs [30]. The various criteria for the selection of herbs include the following.

4.2.1 INTENDED USE

While choosing herbs that are going to be used for a certain purpose, it is very important to know their distinctive medicinal properties. Herbs vary in activity as they contain different compounds that contribute to their therapeutic effects. For example, ginger and peppermint are well-known for their ability to enhance digestion activity [31]. Ginger is known as a carminative, as it contains gingerol that helps to stimulate digestion and ease the feeling of nausea, which makes it a good remedy for dyspepsia and motion sickness [32]. Peppermint includes menthol that relaxes the stomach muscles and can bring relief from symptoms of irritable bowel syndrome and flatulence [33]. Similarly, chamomile and valerian are well-known for their calming effect that may help you to relax and have better sleep. Chamomile has apigenin, the compound that binds to some receptors located in the brain and therefore facilitates sleep and reduces anxiety. The valerian plant contains valerenic acid which can help ease the start of sleep and improve sleep quality [34]. Furthermore, herbal remedies such as echinacea and elderberry are known for supporting the immune system and fighting off infections. Echinacea contains important active compounds such as echinacoside and alkamides which are known for being able to boost the immune system, thus reducing the severity and duration of colds and flu. Elderberry is rich in flavonoids, which are antioxidants and anti-inflammatory in nature that can help strengthen the immune system of the body and decrease the chances of infections. Thus, knowledge of herbs and their mechanism of action on the body will be the key factor in selecting the right herbs to resolve your health issues [35].

4.2.2 SAFETY

Evaluating herbs' safety is crucial for people who suffer from other health problems or are under medication that can be combined with herbs and from allergic reactions. The fact that some plants can cause side effects or interactions that may be hazardous, especially in large doses or for a longer duration of time [36]. For example, St. John's Wort which is frequently used for the treatment of depression, can interfere with medications such as antidepressants, birth control pills, and blood thinners [37]. Consequently, it can also enhance the sun sensitivity of some people, thus provoking sunburn or skin irritation. In addition, immune system-enhancing herbs like echinacea which is commonly used to treat colds and other infections, echinacea may cause allergic reactions in some people who are allergic to plants like ragweed or other daisy family plants. People having allergies should avoid echinacea or use it with extreme caution while being under medical supervision. Thus, it is crucial that one does an in-depth study of herbs and then consults with a healthcare professional or an herbalist before using herbs, particularly for individuals with specific health problems or those taking medications. They can offer instructions on the safe and appropriate application of herbs based on particular health conditions [38].

4.2.3 QUALITY

The selection of herbs for medicinal purposes has to pay the highest priority to the quality of the products to guarantee their safe and effective use. Choosing organic herbs can reduce the risk of exposure to pesticides, heavy metals, and other contaminants that may be harmful to health [39]. Fresh herbs should exhibit vibrant colors, which indicate their freshness and potency. Signs of wilting or decay should be avoided, as they can indicate a loss of flavor and medicinal properties [40]. For example, while selecting fresh rosemary or thyme, pick herbs with vibrant colors and strong aromas as these are proof that they are fresh and of good quality. Herbs that look wilted or have dark spots should be avoided, as they may have begun to degrade and lose their essential properties. Through careful selection of the best herbs, it will be able to get the most out of their health benefits while at the same time minimizing the risk of exposure to harmful contaminants [41].

4.2.4 POTENCY

When it comes to herbs or plant-based products, the potency of herbal products is essential, because it can be affected by such factors as growing conditions, harvesting methods, and different processing techniques. Potency represents the concentration of active substances in the herb which implies its efficacy to provide health benefits. The environmental factors that influence the growth of herbs also contribute greatly to the strength of herbs. For example, herbs that are grown in nutrient-rich soil and under proper sunlight exposure tend to be more potent than those grown in poor soil or shaded areas [42]. Organic farming techniques can potentially preserve potency by refraining from the application of harmful synthetic compounds that may diminish the herb's natural compounds [43]. The methods of harvesting can also influence potency. Harvesting herbs at the right time will help to produce the maximum potency [44]. For example, picking chamomile flowers when they are in full bloom, results in the highest number of essential oils which are responsible for their calming nature [21]. The technique of processing, including drying and storage, may affect the potency of herbs. The right drying methods, like air drying or using low temperatures, can be useful for keeping the herb's active compounds intact. Storing in airtight containers out of light and humidity will also help retain potency throughout the period. Selecting herbs that are powerful enough and properly stored will maintain their healing potential. By keeping the above factors in mind, people can choose herbs that provide the greatest health benefits [45].

4.3 METHODS FOR IDENTIFYING AND AUTHENTICATING HERBS

The quality, safety, and effectiveness of herbs can only be guaranteed by the accurate identification and authentication of them. Several ways are used for the identification of herbs which include, the physicochemical method, macroscopic analysis, microscopic analysis, chemical analysis, and biological analysis as shown in Figure 4.1 [46]. Through the use of these different methods, manufacturers and herbalists can certainly prove the authenticity of herbs, which will guarantee the quality and increase consumer trust.

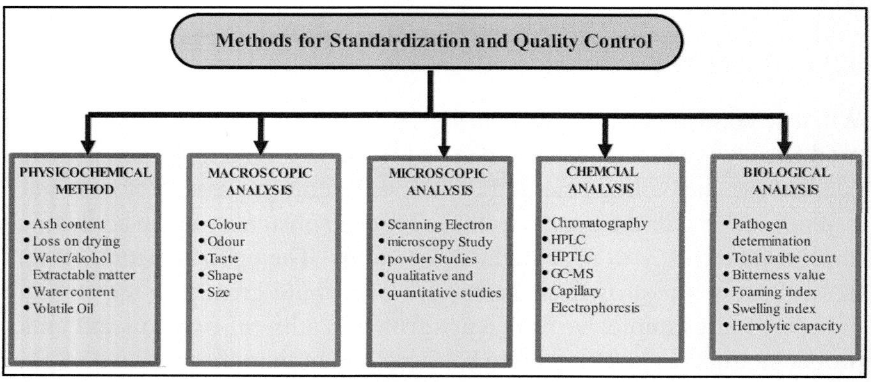

FIGURE 4.1 The methods for standardization and quality control.

4.3.1 MACROSCOPIC ANALYSIS

It is a basic technique that is used to identify herbs by their physical features that are easily seen by the naked eye. This technique consists of the observation of the attributes such as color, size, shape, and texture, which are specific to each herb species. For example, the special serrated edges of mint leaves or the purple spots on sage leaves can be used to tell the difference between these two herbs [47]. Through the careful analysis of these features, herbalists and botanists can precisely identify herbs and differentiate them from similar-looking species. The macroscopic examination is especially useful in the case of dried herbs because their physical characteristics do not change much. Nevertheless, it is necessary to mention that even though the macroscopic examination can be a useful tool, it is usually used together with other methods, such as the microscopic examination and chemical analysis, to make sure that the herbs are correctly identified and authenticated [48].

4.3.2 MICROSCOPIC ANALYSIS

It is an indispensable method applied in the identification and authentication of herbs. This technique is based on the cellular structure of the herb which is studied using a microscope to reveal the unique features that are characteristic of the herb species. Through the study of the size, shape, and arrangement of cells, as well as the presence of specific structures such as trichomes, stomata, and glandular hairs, researchers can precisely determine which herbs are being referred too [49]. For example, microscopic examination is used in herb identification and differentiating between the various kinds of mint. All mint species belong to the genus *Mentha*, but each species has its particular cellular structure that can be seen under a microscope [50]. For example, peppermint and spearmint can be distinguished by the fact that the leaves of the former have more glandular hairs which are more abundant in the former [51]. The microscopic examination is the best way to identify powdered herbs or herbal extracts because it shows the cellular structure of the herb in detail [52]. Besides, this method can also be employed to identify the adulteration or the contamination of herbs, as the foreign materials will have a different cellular structure than the real herb. Hence, the microscopic examination of herbs is a strong tool in the identification and authentication of herbs; thus, it gives information about their cellular composition and it is the way to ensure their quality and safety [48].

4.3.3 CHEMICAL ANALYSIS

These tests are a crucial method in the identification and authentication of herbs, providing valuable information about their composition [53]. Techniques such as chromatography and spectroscopy are commonly used to identify the presence of specific chemical compounds in herbs, which are often unique to certain species and can be used for authentication purposes. One of the chemical analysis techniques applied in herb identification is gas chromatography-mass spectrometry (GC–MS). GC–MS is a powerful analytical tool that enables the separation, identification, and quantification of the chemical elements of an herb. It is very commonly used in the field of herbal identification and authentication because of its high sensitivity and capability of analyzing the mixture of compounds. The GC–MS process mainly involves two main steps that are gas chromatography and mass spectrometry. In gas chromatography, the herb sample is vaporized and then injected into a column that is filled with a stationary phase. These vaporized compounds travel through the column where they interact with the stationary phase, resulting in separation based on factors such as their size, polarity, and others. This process of separation is responsible for the removal of individual compounds from the herb sample. After they are separated, these compounds go to a mass spectrometer where they are ionized and fragmented into smaller ions. A mass spectrometer determines the mass-to-charge ratio (m/z) of the ions and produces a mass spectrum that represents the unique molecular fingerprint of the herb sample. To identify the herb, the mass spectrum of the sample is scanned through the database of the known mass spectra of the authentic herbs. This comparison helps researchers ascertain the identity of the compounds present in the sample and affirm the authenticity of the herb. GC–MS is also good at detecting any adulterants or contaminants present in the sample as they will have different mass spectra from the authentic herb. GC–MS is a useful tool in the identification and authentication of herbs. It provides chemical composition information about a sample and helps to ensure the quality and safety of herbal products [54]. Moreover, thin-layer chromatography (TLC) is one of the most commonly used techniques in herbal analysis, which is utilized for separating and identifying chemical compounds. The TLC plates have a thin layer of stationary phase (silica gel or cellulose) coated on a glass or plastic plate. The herb extract or sample is spotted onto the plate and then placed in the developing chamber. The solvent is introduced into the developing chamber. With the solvent moving up the plate, it brings the molecules in the sample along. Various substances have different rates of travel, thus producing separation of substances based on their chemical characteristics. The identification of the herbs is made possible by comparing the spots on the TLC plate to the known standards. One of the applications of TLC is the identification of artemisinin in sweet wormwood which has antimalarial properties. The unique blue fluorescence of artemisinin under ultraviolet (UV) light can be seen on TLC plates, making it easier to identify [55]. Techniques like high-performance thin-layer chromatography (HPTLC) are an advance version of TLC, which is used for the identification and quantification of chemical components in herbs. HPTLC is a continuation of the traditional TLC with higher resolution and sensitivity, making it very useful for complex herbal extracts. For HPTLC, a small amount of the herbal extract is applied as a spot on a TLC plate, the same as for TLC. The plate is then positioned in a development chamber, which has a solvent system that moves up the plate using capillary action. In its course, the solvent takes the herbal extract constituents along with it, separating them based on their chemical properties. One of the main benefits of using HPTLC is the fact that it can separate and identify multiple compounds in one run, which makes it a useful tool in herbal analysis. HPTLC plates are usually observed with a UV lamp or a densitometer to see the separated compounds as spots on the plate. Such spots are then compared to reference standards that aid in the identification of specific compounds. HPTLC is widely used in the identification of marker compounds or chemical components peculiar to one particular plant. They are used to identify the herb and its quality. For example, in the case of Ginkgo biloba extracts, the presence of ginkgolides and bilobalide can be used as markers for authenticity. Moreover, high-performance liquid chromatography (HPLC) is a highly sophisticated chromatographic method used for the chemical analysis of herbs. HPLC utilizes a high-pressure pump to run a liquid solvent that carries the herb extract through a column filled with a stationary phase [56]. The extract compounds are separated according to their interaction with the stationary phase and then detected by a detector like the UV–Vis spectrophotometer or the mass spectrometer. HPLC is a good tool for the analysis of various compounds in herbs. As such, HPLC can be utilized to determine the quantity of active ingredients, such as ginsenosides in *Panax ginseng* that are responsible for its pharmacological effects [57].

4.3.4 THE DNA BARCODING

It is a molecular technique that is based on the use of selected gene sequences for species identification. It can thus help with herbal identification, especially if morphological features are not enough or it is difficult to shape up differences between closely related species [58]. In this method, a standardized DNA sequence from a specific gene is selected as a molecular barcode. This barcode is unique for each species of herbs and once compared with the reference database, it can identify the herb species. The two DNA barcodes for plants that are being used the most frequently are the barcode region of the rRNA found in the Internal Transcribed Spacer and maturase K regions. This technique is not only suitable for herbal medicine but is also essential to identify species to guarantee the safety and effectiveness of herbal products. It also aids in detecting adulteration or substitution of herbs, as well as confirmation of proper identification of herbs used in traditional medicine practices. Thus, DNA barcoding is a highly strong tool for herbal identification as it offers an exact and reliable method of differentiation among species of herbs through their DNA barcodes [59].

4.3.5 BIOLOGICAL ANALYSIS

The analysis of herbal products on a biological basis consists of a group of different tests that are chosen to evaluate the safety and effectiveness of the products. An essential component of it is the assessment of microbial contamination, which implies testing on the existence of bacteria, fungi, and any other microorganism [60]. This is a particular concern to avoid the production of products contaminated with invisible insects or harmful pathogens like bacteria that can cause infections or other health problems. Another major aspect is pharmacological experiments, which have bitterness value, foaming index, swelling index, and hemolytic activity in the details [61]. The bitterness value refers also to the level of "bitterness" presence of such substance which beyond all doubt is an important parameter in determining the acceptability of herbal products [62]. The foaming index can also be helpful when working with shampoos and soaps, which are foaming substances. On the other hand, the swelling index indicates in what proportion the substance swells in a solvent which may, in turn, help to elucidate its physicochemical features [63]. Hemolytic activity analysis helps determine whether a substance may lead to the break of red blood cells which is considered significant when considering toxicity [64]. Many of these pharmacological tests alongside microbial contamination analysis are made to ascertain product quality and safety meanwhile giving assurance of quality to consumers and regulatory agencies.

4.4 EXTRACTION TECHNIQUES OF HERBALS

Several extraction methods are used in herbal medicine to extract bioactive compounds from herbs depending upon the type of herbals used in the formulation. Some of the most common techniques used in extractions include the following.

4.4.1 MACERATION

It is a simple but efficient extraction technique, that is applied to obtain bioactive compounds from herbs. This involves soaking the herb in a solvent, like alcohol or oil, to extract the desired constituents over an extended period. Maceration is particularly suitable for the extraction of heat-sensitive substances because it does not involve heating the herb [65]. For example, maceration is a commonly used method of preparation of herbal tinctures in herbal medicine. Tincture is an herbal extract made by soaking herbs in alcohol. The alcohol is a solvent that extracts the medicinal compounds from the plant. The mixture is then allowed to macerate for a certain period, during which the alcohol draws out the desired components. The liquid is strained after maceration to remove the solid plant material, and what is left is a potent herbal extract [66]. Another example of maceration is oil extraction from herbs. In this process, the herb is immersed in a carrier oil, such as olive oil or coconut oil, to extract the essential oils. The mixture is then left to macerate for several weeks, during which time the carrier oil can extract the aromatic compounds from the herb. The oil is then strained to separate the solid herb material from the infused oil, which is rich in essential oils. Thus, maceration is a gentle extraction approach that is broadly applied in herbal medicine for the extraction of a wide variety of bioactive compounds from plants [67].

4.4.2 PERCOLATION

In this process, herbs are fluently and thoroughly passed through the solvent. It is the same procedure as maceration but it makes the more complete extraction and is more time-efficient. Through percolation, the herb is tightly contained within a vertical column, and continuously the solvent is added to the top of the column. The solvent used in the extraction goes through all parts of the herb and picks up the compounds that are needed. These components are carried down into the column by the solvent. The essence is accumulated in the column's bottom, while the remainder of the plant is discarded. Additionally, percolation is popular in the pharmaceutical and herbal medicine fields to reveal the useful components of plants [68]. Percolation is performed to isolate active components from herbs to produce herbal extracts and tinctures. This method ensures the best possible extraction of bioactive compounds, which is one of the reasons this method is preferred for creating consistent herbal products with the same high potency [69].

4.4.3 INFUSION

It is one of the most popular methods of extraction that involves cooling down of the herb in hot water to extract of water-soluble compounds. With this softening process, the plant material releases their active components that are then extracted into the water [70]. Eventually, the herbal infusion, which is another name for the herbal tea, is obtained. Chamomile tea, which is the tea that is most common and infusion, is probably one of the most well-known. Chamomile flowers are placed into hot water so that water-soluble compounds including flavonoids and oil are extracted [71]. Another example of infusion is peppermint tea which is brewed by letting dry peppermint leaves infuse in boiled water. Peppermint tea is refreshing and helps in digestion, relieves stomach problems, and alleviates tension headache. It is a widely used method that makes the extraction of water-soluble compounds easier, facilitating the preparation of healthful drinks with varied tastes and therapeutic benefits [72].

4.4.4 DISTILLATION

It is an old method that has been used for a long time for the separation of essential oils and aromatic compounds from herbal materials. This procedure implies the heating of the herb or plant material to evaporate its volatile components, afterward cooling the vapor to condense it back into a liquid form. Steam distillation, which is one of the common types of distillation, is the process where steam passes through the herb material, carrying the volatile compounds along with it. Through the cooling of the steam, it becomes liquid and thus separates from the essential oils [73]. Extraction of lavender essential oil is a great example of distillation. The Lavender flowers are placed in a distillation apparatus and the steam is passed through them. The heat makes the volatile oils in the lavender vaporize and the steam to evaporate with it. Thus, it serves as a way of utilizing the aromatic and therapeutic properties of herbs and plants for medicinal purposes [74].

4.4.5 EXPRESSION

It a process usually preferably applied to fruits in order to extract their herbal oils or juicy pulps, is a simple extraction method. Over a series of steps, the fruit peel is pressed to release the essential oils which then get collected into a container. This is a common technique in the processing of the essences of citrus as in the production of juices. In this method, no solvents or heat is used thus making an efficient way for getting the oils and juices from fruits. Although this process is known for most peeled and high-oil fruits, such as citrus fruits [75].

4.4.6 SUPERCRITICAL FLUID EXTRACTION

It is an advanced method of extraction that uses supercritical CO_2 as a solvent to extract compounds from different substances, including herbs and botanicals. The process involves the pressurization and heating of CO_2 beyond its critical point to become a supercritical fluid, which has properties of both gas and liquid. An instance of supercritical fluid extraction is the extraction of caffeine from coffee beans. In this process, supercritical CO_2 is sent through coffee beans, it selectively extracts caffeine while other compounds remain untouched. This way, the decaffeinated coffee is produced while keeping the flavor and aroma of the beans [75]. The second example is the production of essential oils from plants such as lavender or peppermint. Supercritical CO_2 is the technique of extracting volatile aromatic compounds from the plant material, thus obtaining highly concentrated essential oils with minimal solvent residues. This method of extraction has several advantages compared to the traditional methods of extraction, such as high efficiency, selectivity, and the fact that it can be carried out at low temperatures, thus preserving the integrity of heat-sensitive compounds. Besides, CO_2 is nontoxic, nonflammable, and easily available, which is why it is the favored solvent for extraction in the food, pharmaceutical, and herbal industries [76].

4.4.7 SOXHLET EXTRACTION

It is a procedure that is used for the extraction of compounds from solid herb materials by continuous extraction with a solvent using a specialized apparatus, which is the Soxhlet extractor. This technique is especially applicable for the extraction of compounds that are not easily soluble in the solvent and need to be repeated a lot of times to get the best extraction efficiency [77]. For instance, Soxhlet extraction is the usual method in herbal medicine to extract lipophilic compounds, such as essential oils, from botanical materials like seeds, bark, or roots. The compounds are placed in a porous thimble, which is inserted into the Soxhlet extractor. The solvent, which is usually a nonpolar solvent such as hexane or ethanol, is heated and let to evaporate, thus the extracted compounds are taken along with the solvent. The vapor condenses and falls back into the herb, thus creating a chain of extraction [78]. Another example of Soxhlet extraction is the extraction of fat from food samples for the purpose of analysis. Soxhlet extraction is utilized to extract lipids from food matrices such as nuts or seeds, with a nonpolar solvent like petroleum ether or hexane. The extracted lipids are then examined for their structure and content. Soxhlet extraction is a flexible and effective method of obtaining a variety of compounds from solid materials, and it is widely used in different industries, such as herbal medicine, food, and environmental analysis [79]. Table 4.1 shows various extraction methods, their advantages, disadvantages, and examples of herbal compounds that can be extracted using each method.

TABLE 4.1 The Advantages and Disadvantages of Various Types of Extraction Techniques

Extraction Method	Advantages	Disadvantages	Examples of Herbal Compounds Extracted
Maceration	Simple and inexpensive method; suitable for delicate plant materials	Longer extraction time; lower efficiency compared to other methods	Capsaicin from chili peppers; allicin from garlic
Percolation	Faster extraction process; allows for continuous extraction	Requires specialized equipment; higher initial investment	Caffeine from coffee beans; Echinacea extract from Echinacea roots
Infusion	Easy and commonly used method; suitable for water-soluble compounds	Limited extraction of nonwater-soluble compounds; lower extraction efficiency compared to other methods	Chamomile tea; peppermint tea
Distillation	Produces highly concentrated extracts; can separate volatile compounds	High energy consumption; loss of heat-sensitive compounds	Lavender essential oil; eucalyptus essential oil
Expression	Simple and efficient method for extracting oils from citrus fruits	Limited to extracting oils from plant parts with high oil content; not suitable for extracting water-soluble compounds	Lemon oil from lemon peels; orange oil from orange peels
Supercritical fluid extraction	High extraction efficiency; selective extraction of compounds; environmentally friendly	Requires specialized equipment and expertise; higher initial investment; limited scalability	Curcumin from turmeric; cannabidiol from hemp
Soxhlet extraction	Suitable for extracting compounds with low solubility; continuous extraction process	Long extraction time; potential loss of heat-sensitive compounds; requires large amounts of solvent	Capsaicin from chili peppers; artemisinin from *Artemisia annua*

4.5 TYPES OF FORMULATION AND ITS CONSIDERATIONS

Herbal products come in various forms to cater to different preferences and needs. These include decoctions, herbal teas, tinctures, glycerites tablets, and capsules for oral consumption. Additionally, there are herbal soaps, creams, and ointments for external use. The choice of formulation type often depends on the desired outcome and the properties of the herb.

4.5.1 DECOCTIONS

These are herbal preparations created by boiling herbs in water to extract their soluble constituents, commonly used in traditional herbal medicine for hard plant materials like barks and roots, or herbs with sparingly soluble constituents. Typically, a mixture of 2–12 herbal materials is boiled to create a decoction, intended for immediate use within 24 h. For longer storage, preservatives may be added to prevent spoilage, and stability testing is advised to determine the product's shelf-life under specific storage conditions. To improve taste, decoctions can be sweetened with syrup or honey [80]. For instance, Sijunzi decoction, a Chinese herbal remedy, includes *P. ginseng*, *Poria cocos*, *Atractylodes macrocephala*, and *Glycyrrhiza uralensis* when analysis through LC/MS revealed that the concentration ratios of active compounds in the decoction differed from those in individual herb extracts, indicating the decoction process influences the extracted active components amount. Stability studies have demonstrated that decoctions can remain chemically stable for extended periods under specific storage conditions [81].

4.5.2 TINCTURES

It is a herbal extract manufactured by plant materials in a mixture of alcohol and water. This method is particularly effective in extracting a wide range of compounds from the plants. Quality control for tinctures involves using analytical techniques like nuclear magnetic resonance and MS to ensure consistency and purity. Alcohol acts as a preservative in tinctures, allowing them to have a long shelf life. The alcohol content in tinctures typically ranges from 25% to 90% v/v, depending on the solubility of the active compounds [82]. For example, water-soluble compounds like tannins and mucilage require lower alcohol concentrations, while compounds like alkaloids and essential oils require higher concentrations. Proper storage is essential for maintaining the quality of tinctures. Most tinctures can last up to five years when stored correctly [83]. However, some tinctures, such as Passionflower and milk-thistle, have shorter shelf lives due to the low thermal stability of their constituents. It is important to store tinctures properly to avoid degradation and ensure their efficacy. Improperly stored tinctures can lead to changes in their chemical composition, reducing their effectiveness [84].

4.5.3 GLYCERITES

These are herbal extracts made with glycerine instead of alcohol and water, catering to those preferring alcohol-free remedies. However, they have a shorter shelf life, typically lasting six months to two years compared to tinctures [85]; thus, it is recommended to store glycerites in the refrigerator for best results. To maintain glycerite potency, the glycerine concentration should be at least 50–60% in the final product. Moreover, glycerine also serves as an effective preservative for fresh plant juices when mixed in equal parts, creating a succus that keeps the juice green and suspended better than alcohol. This preparation is useful for children's medicines and soothing throat, digestive, or cough remedies. Despite being less potent and having a shorter shelf life than alcohol-based extracts, glycerites offer an alcohol-free alternative for those seeking herbal remedies. They are particularly beneficial for individuals looking for gentle, soothing herbal preparations [86].

4.5.4 TABLETS

These are solid medications, typically shaped round, oval, or square, and are formed through compression. They consist of active pharmaceutical ingredients along with excipients or formulation additives like binders, glidants, and lubricants, which aid in the efficient process of tableting [87]. Disintegrants ensure the tablet disperses in the gastrointestinal tract, while sweeteners or flavors mask any unpleasant tastes, and pigments enhance their visual appeal. Additionally, tablets may be coated to improve taste, ease of swallowing, protect against stomach acid, and enhance stability for a longer shelf life [88]. Herbal tablets, designed for oral consumption, incorporate various herbal materials to achieve specific therapeutic effects. These materials can be in the form of finely powdered plant material or extracts obtained using suitable solvents. The stability of herbal tablets is of utmost importance, as it directly impacts their shelf life [89]. For instance, tablets containing *Rhodiola rosea* L. extract were found to remain stable for six months under conditions of 25°C/60% relative humidity (RH). However, these tablets failed the stability test when subjected to 40°C/75% RH due to a decrease in hardness [90].

4.5.5 CAPSULES

These are solid dosage forms containing a drug and filler enclosed in a gelatin container. They can be hard gelatin capsules for dry powdered herbal ingredients or granules, or soft gelatin shells for herbal oils or ingredients dissolved or suspended in oil. Upon oral administration, the gelatin shell dissolves, releasing the contents. Capsules are often preferred over tablets as they can mask the taste of their contents and achieve uniform dosage more easily [91]. Herbal capsules typically use hard-shelled gelatin capsules filled with finely milled and sifted plant material or extracts mixed with appropriate excipients like fillers. They offer better stability compared to aqueous preparations like decoctions or infusions. Determining the stability and shelf life of herbal capsules is crucial for providing proper storage instructions. For instance, an accelerated stability study of herbal capsules for immunomodulation and stress showed that the quantifiable active components remained within 90% of the initial amount, indicating stability at room temperature for two years [92].

4.5.6 OINTMENTS AND CREAMS

Semisolid and greasy formulations can be applied to the skin, rectum, or nasal mucosa. Typically, they have a hydrophobic base that does not mix with skin secretions. Ointments are used as emollients or carriers for applying medications to the skin, either suspended or dissolved. Incorporating finely sifted or extracted plant materials into the base, herbal ointments should not be used for deep wounds. While ointments are relatively stable compared to other liquid forms, the presence of herbal materials can lead to quicker deterioration. Hence, it is crucial to determine the stability of herbal ointments to provide appropriate storage and shelf-life instructions [93]. For instance, a study evaluated an ointment with herbal tinctures of calendula and arnica for hemorrhoid treatment using a stability-indicating TLC technique. The ointment was found to have a shelf life of one month at 25°C/60% RH and two months at 5°C when protected from light. This highlights the importance of assessing the stability of herbal ointments to ensure their efficacy and safety [94].

Similarly, herbal creams are semisolid emulsions consisting of a mixture of oil and water, making them hydrophilic. They typically incorporate herbal materials either in finely sifted form or as extracts. Due to the presence of water in the base, herbal creams usually contain antimicrobial preservatives and may have a relatively shorter shelf life compared to ointments. It is important to distinguish between creams and ointments in herbal formulations. Herbal creams specifically refer to those with a hydrophilic base. If the base is purely hydrophobic, then the preparation is classified as an ointment. This differentiation ensures clarity in product categorization and helps users understand the composition and properties of the herbal preparation they are using [95].

4.5.7 HERBAL OILS

It consists of herbal materials suspended or dissolved in an oily base, often referred to as infused or macerated oils. They are distinct from essential oils, which are aromatic oils obtained through distillation. Primarily intended for external use, herbal oils are commonly used as liniments, although some formulations may be suitable for oral use, albeit less frequently. These oils often include herbal materials like leaves containing essential oils. The stability and shelf life of a herbal oil primarily depend on the type of oil used in the extraction process. Different oils possess varying degrees of stability, which directly impacts the overall stability of the herbal oil product. Hence, selecting oils with appropriate stability characteristics is crucial to ensure the quality and efficacy of the herbal oil preparation [96].

4.5.8 POWDERED HERBAL PREPARATION

These preparations are intended for direct use or incorporation into foods, beverages, insufflations, or wound care. They may consist of finely sifted herbal materials from various plant parts, aimed at achieving specific therapeutic effects. Similar to herbal teas, the stability of these powders depends on the type and nature of the herbal material, as well as the moisture content within the packaging. For example, the dried herb and extract of the root of *Nauclea latifolia* S.M., a plant with antimalarial properties found in Africa, remained stable under tropical room temperature conditions for over one year when stored in sealed glass containers. This underscores the importance of proper storage and packaging to maintain the stability of herbal powder preparations [97].

4.6 MANUFACTURING PROCESSES FOR HERBAL PRODUCTS

In the manufacturing of herbal products, the initial step involves meticulous sourcing and quality-control measures to ensure the final product's quality, efficacy, and safety. The formulation of herbal products involves a variety of steps which are depicted in Figure 4.2.

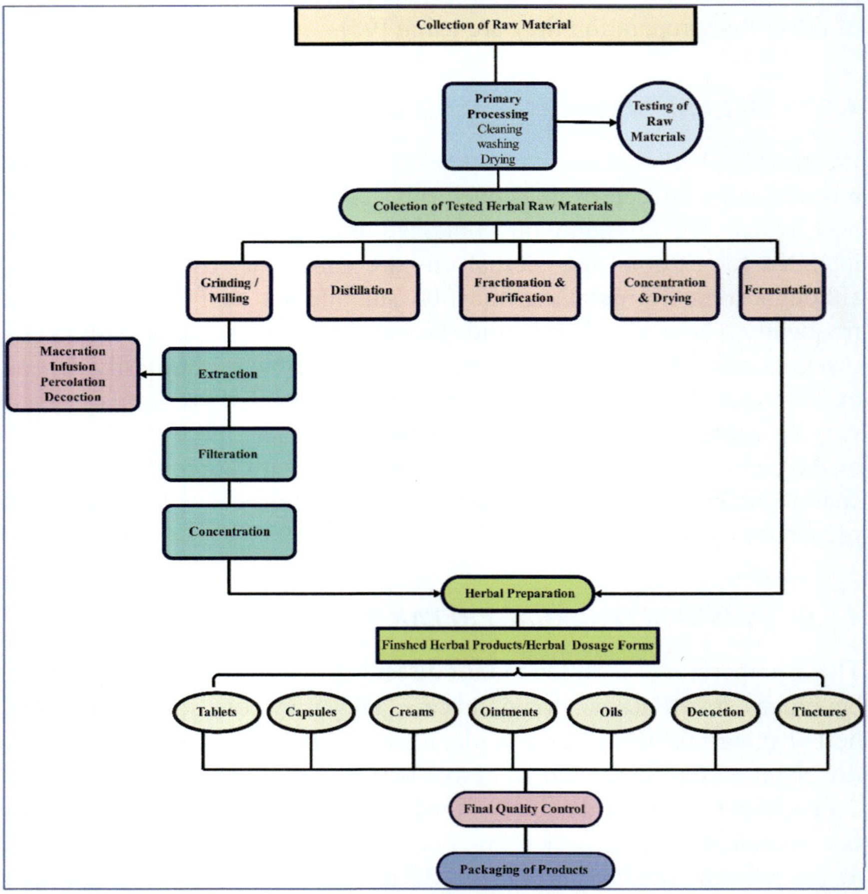

FIGURE 4.2 The whole process of manufacturing herbal products.

Raw material selection is a critical process where manufacturers carefully choose herbs from reputable sources. These sources are selected based on their adherence to stringent quality standards and regulatory requirements.

This ensures that the herbs used are of high quality and free from contaminants. Following raw material selection, quality-control testing is performed to verify the identity, purity, and potency of the herbs. This testing process involves various methods such as visual inspection, microscopic analysis, and chemical analysis. By adhering to these rigorous sourcing and quality-control practices, manufacturers can maintain the integrity and quality of their herbal products [98]. In the preparation phase of herbal product manufacturing, careful steps are taken to ensure the raw herbs are properly cleaned, dried, and processed for extraction or formulation. The herbs are inspected and cleaned to remove any foreign materials, dirt, or contaminants. This is typically done by hand or using mechanical methods to ensure the herbs are pure and free from impurities. After cleaning, the herbs are dried to reduce their moisture content and preserve their quality. Various drying methods can be used, including air drying, sun drying, or mechanical drying. Each method is chosen based on the specific requirements of the herbs and the desired end product. Once dried, the herbs are ground or milled into a suitable form for extraction or formulation. This step helps to break down the herbs into smaller particles, making it easier to extract their beneficial compounds. The grinding or milling process is carefully controlled to ensure the herbs are not damaged and that their properties are preserved [99].

After the grinding and milling process comes that is extraction. It is a pivotal process in herbal product manufacturing, where bioactive compounds are extracted from the herbs using various methods such as maceration, percolation, distillation, infusion, supercritical fluid extraction, Soxhlet extraction, and expression. Each of these extraction methods has its advantages and is chosen based on the specific properties of the herbs and the desired end product. By carefully selecting and implementing the appropriate extraction method, manufacturers can ensure that they extract the maximum number of bioactive compounds from the herbs, resulting in high-quality herbal products [54].

In the formulation stage of herbal product manufacturing, the extracted herbal components are combined with other ingredients to create the final product. This involves careful mixing and standardization to ensure consistency and efficacy. Herbal extracts or powders are blended with excipients such as fillers, binders, and disintegrants, among others. These ingredients are mixed in specific proportions to achieve the desired consistency and form of the product. The choice of excipients and their proportions are critical in ensuring the product's stability, bioavailability, and effectiveness [100].

Standardization is the process of ensuring that the final product contains consistent levels of active ingredients across different batches. This is crucial for maintaining the product's efficacy and safety. Standardization involves testing the product to determine the concentration of the active ingredients and adjusting the formulation as needed to meet the specified standards. Standardization and stability of herbal products depends upon various factors which are mentioned in Figure 4.3.

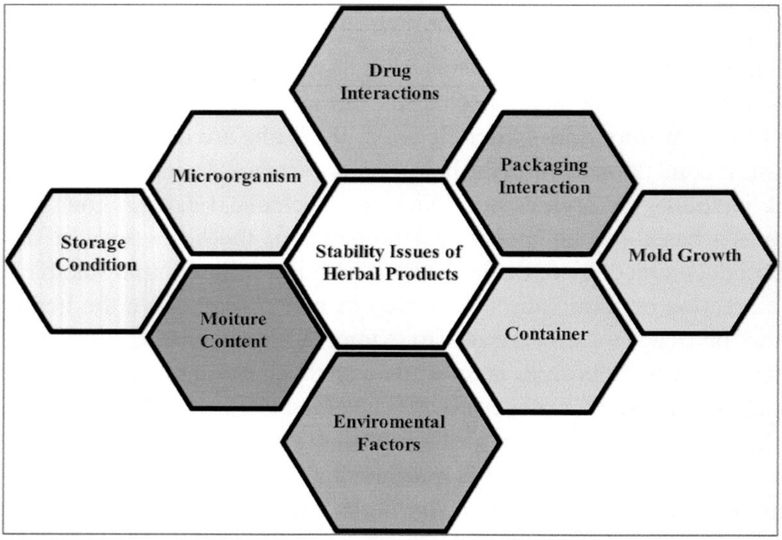

FIGURE 4.3 The stability issues of herbal products.

By standardizing the product, manufacturers can ensure that consumers receive a reliable and consistent product with each use. Then comes the packaging stage which is a critical aspect of herbal product manufacturing, ensuring that the final product remains safe, effective, and compliant with regulatory standards. This stage involves careful selection of containers and meticulous labeling, backed by comprehensive quality-assurance measures. Container selection is an essential process as containers provide optimal protection for the herbal products. Factors such as protection from light, moisture, and contamination are carefully considered. Dark, airtight containers may be chosen to shield the product from light and moisture, preserving its potency and quality. Additionally, containers with tamper-evident seals further ensure product integrity and consumer safety. Moreover, clear and comprehensive labeling is essential for informing consumers about the herbal product. Labels should include essential information such as the list of ingredients, recommended dosage, expiry date, and storage instructions. Lastly, when the final products are produced tests should be performed to evaluate the product's compliance with specifications for identity, purity, potency, and safety. These tests typically encompass a range of analyses, including chemical, physical, and microbiological testing. By conducting thorough finished product testing, manufacturers can confirm that the product meets regulatory standards and is safe for consumer use [101].

4.7 INDIAN DEVELOPED AND COMMERCIALIZED HERBAL PRODUCTS

India has a long history of herbal medicine and the country has, over time, developed and commercialized a variety of herbal products that are now recognized both nationally and internationally. These products are usually made from plants and herbs that have been used for a long time in Ayurveda, the ancient Indian medicine system [102]. An example of this is the products containing neem. Neem, also scientifically called *Azadirachta indica*, is a plant that has been traditionally used in India for its medicinal properties. Today, neem-based products like neem oil, neem soap, and neem toothpaste are very popular due to their antiseptic, antifungal, and antibacterial properties [103]. Another case is products that are made of turmeric. Turmeric, or *Curcuma longa*, is a main ingredient in Indian cuisine and medicine. Turmeric-containing products, including turmeric supplements, turmeric tea, and turmeric skin-care products, are famous for their anti-inflammatory and antioxidant characteristics. Indian herbal items have also found a place in the global market [104]. Products like Brahmi (*Bacopa monnieri*) supplements for memory enhancement [105], Ashwagandha (*Withania somnifera*) supplements for stress relief [106], and Triphala formulations for digestive health have become famous in the world [107]. Furthermore, BGR-34 is an Ayurvedic herbal supplement approved by CSIR for managing diabetes [108]. It consists of a blend of natural ingredients, including Daruharidra (*Berberis aristata*), Manjistha, Vijaysar (*Pterocarpus marsupium*), Methi (fenugreek), Guduchi, Gudmar, and other herbal components [109].

The commercialization of these herbal products has not only aided the development of the Indian herbal industry but has also promoted the traditional knowledge of herbal medicine. Besides, the consumption of these products has resulted in the progress in research and development of Indian herbal products that are now available on the international market and meet quality standards. On the whole, Indian-developed and commercialized herbal products prove that the country is willing to keep its traditional medicinal heritage and at the same time, it also adopts modern scientific advancements. Table 4.2 includes various marketed available herbal products with active constituents and their uses or claims.

TABLE 4.2 Commercially Available Herbal Products in India

S. No.	Herbal Product	Active Constitutes	Use/Claims
01	Pudin hara pearls	*Mentha piperita* and *Mentha spicata*	For indigestion, gas, and stomach ache
02	Spirulina plus capsule	Phycocyanin	Antioxidant and anti-inflammatory properties
03	Galakol tablet	*Smilax chinensis*, *Caesalpinia bonduc*, *Acacia melanoxylon*, *Mucuna puriens*	Immune system and fungal infections
04	Bresol syrup	Holy basil, Malabar nut, and turmeric	Treatment and prevention of respiratory troubles
05	Himcolin gel	*Jyotishmati*, *Lathakasthuri*, *Nirgundi*, *Vathada*, *Karpasa*	Erectile dysfunction
06	Koflet lozenge	Honey, Trikatu, *Terminalia chebula*	Relieves cough, alleviates mucosal irritation, soothes throat
07	Anantavati tablet	*Withania somnifera*, *Centella asiatica*, *Convolvulus pluricaulis*, *Nardostachys jatamansi*	Reduce stress and to help maintain a balanced mood
08	Livomyn tablet	*Andrographis paniculata*, *Picrorhiza kurroa*	Stimulating liver functions as well as to correct any liver pathology
09	Sumenta tablet	*Bacopa monnieri*, gooseberry, Shankha vati, sweet flag, staff tree	Help in reduction of stress
10	Manjishtha tablets	Purpurin, munjistin, xanthopurpurin, pseudopurpurin	Used in treatment of arthritis

4.8 FUTURE PERSPECTIVES AND CHALLENGES

Current trends in herbal product development show the increasing popularity of natural and eco-friendly alternatives to conventional medicine. A major trend is the combination of ancient herbal knowledge with modern scientific research which in turn leads to the creation of standardized herbal extracts with proven efficacy and safety profiles. Another trend is the implementation of newer technology like nanotechnology and biotechnology in order to increase the bioavailability and therapeutic effectiveness of herbal products. This contains the production of nanoformulations and phytophospholipid complexes that enhance the delivery of herbal components to the target tissues. Besides, there is now an increasing interest in herbal products that have multiple health benefits, such as adaptogenic herbs that assist the body in coping with stress and enhance the overall health. These products usually blend various herbs that work together to increase their beneficial effects. In addition to this, the use of herbal products in personalized medicine, where treatments are made according to individual genetic, physiological, and lifestyle factors, is also a new trend. The goal of this way of thinking is to make herbal therapies more effective and at the same time to reduce the possibility of side effects. Moreover, there is an increasing demand for herbal products for the purpose of preventive medicine, and a lot of attention is being given to the maintenance of health and the prevention of chronic diseases. As a result, the creation of herbal supplements and functional foods that boost the immune system, cognitive function, and cardiovascular health has been done. Hence, the herbal product development trends show a move toward evidence-based herbal medicine, innovative formulation technologies, and holistic approach to health and wellness.

Regardless of these advancements, the herbal products industry has to cope with numerous problems that affect its growth and development. The most significant problem is the absence of the uniform laws and the control of the quality. Different from drugs, herbal products are usually not under any regulations, and thus, quality, effect, and safety standards of them will be different in different products and markets. Another major issue is regarding adulteration and contamination. The increase in demand for herbal products poses a risk of adulteration with lower quality herbs, synthetic substances, or contaminants. This can affect the efficacy and effectiveness of herbal products, which may cause the consumers to be exposed to possible health hazards. Moreover, scientific investigation and clinical trials on herbal products are the other difficulties. Though the traditional herbal knowledge is deep, there is a necessity for more scientific research to prove the effectiveness, safety, and the way the herbal products work of the herbal products. The absence of scientific data can make it difficult for herbal medicine to be recognized in mainstream healthcare. In addition to that, the marketing and education are also very important in the herbal products sector. Manipulating advertising, making false statements, and the absence of consumer's knowledge about the risks and benefits of herbal products can destroy consumer trust and confidence in these products. The changes to be done to solve these challenges need the cooperation of the governments, the industry stakeholders, and the scientific communities to create clear rules, to improve the quality-control measures, to support sustainable practices, and to enhance the consumer education and awareness about herbal products.

KEYWORDS

- **herbal medicine**
- **Indian herbal products**
- **Ayurvedic formulations**
- **herbal manufacturing**

REFERENCES

1. Pandey, M., et al., Phytomedicine: An ancient approach turning into future potential source of therapeutics. *J Pharmacogn Phytother* 2011, 3(3), 27–37.
2. Yuan, H., et al., The traditional medicine and modern medicine from natural products. *Molecules* 2016, 21(5), 559.
3. Wachtel-Galor, S., & Benzie, I. F. Herbal medicine: An introduction to its history, usage, regulation, current trends, and research needs. In Iris F.F. Benzie and Sissi Wachlet-Galor (Eds.). *Herbal Medicine: Biomolecular and Clinical Aspects*. 2nd edition. CRC Press/Taylor & Francis: Boca Raton, FL, USA, 2012.
4. Qadir, S. U., & Raja, V. Herbal medicine: Old practice and modern perspectives. In: *Phytomedicine*, Elsevier, 2021, pp. 149–180.
5. Mosihuzzaman, M. Herbal medicine in healthcare—An overview. *Nat Prod Commun* 2012, 7(6), 807–812, 1934578X1200700628.

6. Organization, WHO. *WHO Global Report on Traditional and Complementary Medicine* 2019, World Health Organization, 2019.
7. Kumadoh, D., & Ofori-Kwakye, K. Dosage forms of herbal medicinal products and their stability considerations—An overview. *J Crit Rev* 2017, 4(4), 1–8.
8. Pan, S.- Y., et al., Historical perspective of traditional indigenous medical practices: The current renaissance and conservation of herbal resources. *Evid Based Complement Altern Med* 2014, 2014, 525340.
9. Leake, C. D. *The Old Egyptian Medical Papyri*, University of Kansas Press: Lawrence, Kan, 1952.
10. Chan, K. The evolutional development of Traditional Chinese Medicine (TCM) outside the Chinese Mainland: Challenges, training, practice, research, and future development. *World J Tradit Chin Med* 2016, 2(4), 6–28.
11. Sen, S., & Chakraborty, R. Toward the integration and advancement of herbal medicine: A focus on traditional Indian medicine. *Botanics: Targets Ther* 2015, 5, 33–44.
12. Krishnaswamy, N. *AYURVEDA*.
13. Ravishankar, B., & Shukla, V. J. Indian systems of medicine: A brief profile. *Afr J Tradit Complement Altern Med* 2007, 4(3), 319–337.
14. Cohen, K., & Weinstein, A. M. Synthetic and non-synthetic cannabinoid drugs and their adverse effects—A review from public health prospective. *Front Public Health* 2018, 6, 349132.
15. Najmi, A., et al., Modern approaches in the discovery and development of plant-based natural products and their analogues as potential therapeutic agents. *Molecules* 2022, 27(2), 349.
16. Karunamoorthi, K., et al., Traditional medicinal plants: A source of phytotherapeutic modality in resource-constrained health care settings. *J Evid-Based Complement Alternat Med* 2013, 18(1), 67–74.
17. Gurib-Fakim, A. Medicinal plants: Traditions of yesterday and drugs of tomorrow. *Mol Aspects Med* 2006, 27(1), 1–93.
18. Choudhary, N., & Sekhon, B. S., An overview of advances in the standardization of herbal drugs. *J Pharm Educ Res* 2011, 2(2), 55.
19. Sofowora, A., Ogunbodede, E., & Onayade, A. The role and place of medicinal plants in the strategies for disease prevention. *Afr J Tradit Complement Alternat Med* 2013, 10(5), 210–229.
20. Pal, R. S., et al., A review on the recent flavoring herbal medicines of today. *Open Med J* 2020, 7(1).
21. Worwood, V. A. *The Complete Book of Essential Oils and Aromatherapy, Revised and Expanded: Over 800 Natural, Nontoxic, and Fragrant Recipes to Create Health, Beauty, and Safe Home and Work Environments*, New World Library, 2016.
22. Sumit, K., et al., Herbal cosmetics: Used for skin and hair. *Inven J* 2012, 2012, 1–7.
23. Li, F.- S., & Weng, J.- K. Demystifying traditional herbal medicine with modern approach. *Nat Plants* 2017, 3(8), 1–7.
24. David, B., Wolfender, J. - L., & Dias, D. A. The pharmaceutical industry and natural products: Historical status and new trends. *Phytochem Rev* 2015, 14, 299–315.
25. Alamgir, A., & Alamgir, A. Herbal drugs: Their collection, preservation, and preparation; evaluation, quality control, and standardization of herbal drugs. In:

Therapeutic Use of Medicinal Plants and Their Extracts: Volume 1: Pharmacognosy, 2017, pp. 453–495.
26. Hart, B. L. The evolution of herbal medicine: Behavioural perspectives. *Anim Behav* 2005, 70(5), 975–989.
27. RH, R. U. Traditional herbal medicine, pharmacognosy, and pharmacopoeial standards: A discussion at the crossroads. In: *Evidence-based Validation of Herbal Medicine*, Elsevier, 2015, pp. 45–85.
28. Khan, M. S. A., & Ahmad, I. Herbal medicine: Current trends and future prospects. In: *New Look to Phytomedicine*, Elsevier, 2019, pp. 3–13.
29. Shahid, M., & Mohammad, F. Perspectives for natural product based agents derived from industrial plants in textile applications—A review. *J Cleaner Prod* 2013, 57, 2–18.
30. Yalavarthi, C., & Thiruvengadarajan, V. A review on identification strategy of phyto constituents present in herbal plants. *Int J Res Pharm Sci* 2013, 4(2), 123–140.
31. Rubió, L., Motilva, M.- J., & Romero, M.- P. Recent advances in biologically active compounds in herbs and spices: A review of the most effective antioxidant and anti-inflammatory active principles. *Crit Rev Food Sci Nutr* 2013, 53(9), 943–953.
32. Remadevi, R., Surendran, E., & Ravindran, P. Properties and medicinal uses of ginger. In: *Ginger*, CRC Press, 2016, pp. 509–528.
33. Balakrishnan, A. Therapeutic uses of peppermint—A review. *J Pharm Sci Res* 2015, 7(7), 474.
34. Herbert, C. *Sleep, the Elixir of Life: How to Restore Sleep with Herbs and Natural Healing*. Aeon Books, 2021.
35. CINGI, C., et al., Efficacy of traditional herbal formulas on human immunity. *Eur Rev Med Pharmacol Sci* 2023, 27, 27–40.
36. Haq, I. Safety of medicinal plants. *Pak J Med Res* 2004, 43(4), 203–210.
37. Schulz, V. Safety of St. John's Wort extract compared to synthetic antidepressants. *Phytomedicine* 2006, 13(3), 199–204.
38. Giles, J. T., et al., Evaluation of echinacea for treatment of the common cold. *Pharmacother: J Hum Pharmacol Drug Ther* 2000, 20(6), 690–697.
39. Reinholds, I., et al., Mycotoxins, pesticides and toxic metals in commercial spices and herbs. *Food Addit Contam: Part B* 2017, 10(1), 5–14.
40. Antunes, M. D. C., & Cavaco, A. M. The use of essential oils for postharvest decay control. A review. *Flavour Fragr J* 2010, 25(5), 351–366.
41. Green, A. *Field Guide to Herbs & Spices: How to Identify, Select, and Use Virtually Every Seasoning on the Market*, Quirk books, 2006.
42. Youn, W. B., Hernandez, J. O., & Park, B. B. Effects of shade and planting methods on the growth of Heracleum moellendorffii and Adenophora divaricata in different soil moisture and nutrient conditions. *Plants* 2021, 10(10), 2203.
43. Magkos, F., Arvaniti, F., & Zampelas, A. Organic food: Buying more safety or just peace of mind? A critical review of the literature. *Crit Rev Food Sci Nutr* 2006, 46(1), 23–56.
44. Canter, P. H., Thomas, H., & Ernst, E. Bringing medicinal plants into cultivation: Opportunities and challenges for biotechnology. *Trends Biotechnol* 2005, 23(4), 180–185.

45. Orphanides, A., Goulas, V., & Gekas, V. Drying technologies: Vehicle to high-quality herbs. *Food Eng Rev* 2016, 8, 164–180.
46. Upton, R., et al., Botanical ingredient identification and quality assessment: Strengths and limitations of analytical techniques. *Phytochem Rev* 2020, 19(5), 1157–1177.
47. Rungsung, W., Dutta, S., & Hazra, J. Pharmacognostical approach towards authentication and quality evaluation of medicinal plants-A compendious description. *Res J Pharmacogn Phytochem* 2013, 5(2), 77–83.
48. Govindaraghavan, S., & Sucher, N. J. Quality assessment of medicinal herbs and their extracts: Criteria and prerequisites for consistent safety and efficacy of herbal medicines. *Epilepsy Behav* 2015, 52, 363–371.
49. Khadhraoui, B., et al., Histo-cytochemistry and scanning electron microscopy for studying spatial and temporal extraction of metabolites induced by ultrasound. Towards chain detexturation mechanism. *Ultrason Sonochem* 2018, 42, 482–492.
50. Ayaz, A., et al., Systematics study through scanning electron microscopy; a tool for the authentication of herbal drug Mentha suaveolens Ehrh. *Microsc Res Tech* 2020, 83(1), 81–87.
51. Maffei, M., Bertea, C., & Mucciarelli, M. Anatomy, physiology, biosynthesis, molecular biology, tissue culture, and biotechnology of mint essential oil production. In: *Mint: The Genus Mentha*. CRC Press: Boca Raton, 2007, pp. 41–85.
52. Liu, W. J. *Traditional Herbal Medicine Research Methods: Identification, Analysis, Bioassay, and Pharmaceutical and Clinical Studies*, John Wiley & Sons, 2011.
53. Gad, H. A., et al., Application of chemometrics in authentication of herbal medicines: A review. *Phytochem Anal* 2013, 24(1), 1–24.
54. Balekundri, A., & Mannur, V. Quality control of the traditional herbs and herbal products: A review. *Fut J Pharma Sci* 2020, 6, 1–9.
55. Jain, A., et al., High performance thin layer chromatography (HPTLC): A modern analytical tool for chemical analysis. *Curr Res Pharm Sci* 2014, 8–14.
56. Cañigueral i Folcarà, S., et al., High performance thin-layer chromatography (HPTLC) in the quality control of herbal products. In: Muñoz-Torrero, D., Cajal, Y., & Llobet, J. M., (Eds.), *Recent Advances in Pharmaceutical Sciences VIII, 2018*, Research Signpost, 2018, pp. 119–136. ISBN: 978-81-308-0579-5. Chapter 7.
57. de Rijke, E., et al., Analytical separation and detection methods for flavonoids. *J Chromatogr A* 2006, 1112(1–2), 31–63.
58. Ferri, G., et al., Species identification through DNA "barcodes". *Genet Test Mol Biomark* 2009, 13(3), 421–426.
59. Purty, R., & Chatterjee, S. DNA barcoding: an effective technique in molecular taxonomy. *Austin J Biotechnol Bioeng* 2016, 3(1), 1059.
60. de Sousa Lima, C. M., et al., Microbial contamination in herbal medicines: A serious health hazard to elderly consumers. *BMC Complement Med Ther* 2020, 20, 1–9.
61. Gaitén, Y. I. G., Lizama, R. S., & Payrol, J. A. Importance of pharmacognosy studies in the quality control of herbal drugs. In: *Medicinal Plants of Ecuador*, CRC Press, 2022, pp. 3–17.
62. Bone, K., & Mills, S. *Principles and Practice of Phytotherapy: Modern Herbal Medicine*, Elsevier Health Sciences, 2012.
63. Ritota, M., & Manzi, P. Natural preservatives from plant in cheese making. *Animals* 2020, 10(4), 749.

64. Wadhwa, R., et al., Red blood cells as an efficient in vitro model for evaluating the efficacy of metallic nanoparticles. *3 Biotech* 2019, 9, 1–15.
65. Stéphane, F. F. Y., et al., Extraction of bioactive compounds from medicinal plants and herbs. *Nat Med Plants* 2021.
66. Vinatoru, M., An overview of the ultrasonically assisted extraction of bioactive principles from herbs. *Ultrason Sonochem* 2001, 8(3), 303–313.
67. Shankar, S., et al., Essential oils, components and their applications: A review. *Plant Arch* 2021, 21(1), 2027–2033.
68. Srivastava, R., & Parambil, J. V. Evolution of extraction technique for the separation of bioactive compounds from Aegle marmelos. *Sep Sci Technol* 2023, 58(4), 667–681.
69. Meuninck, J. *Medicinal Plants of North America: A Field Guide*, Rowman & Littlefield, 2016.
70. Fonmboh, D. J., et al., An overview of methods of extraction, isolation and characterization of natural medicinal plant products in improved traditional medicine research. *Asian J Res Med Pharm Sci* 2020, 9(2), 31–57.
71. Etheridge, C. J., & Derbyshire, E. Herbal infusions and health: A review of findings from human studies, mechanisms and future research directions. *Nutrit Food Sci* 2020, 50(5), 969–985.
72. Thiagarajah, K., et al., Plants infused water as preferred healthy drinks. In: *Bottled and Packaged Water*, Elsevier, 2019, pp. 367–402.
73. Mohammad Azmin, S. N. H., et al., Herbal processing and extraction technologies. *Sep Purif Rev* 2016, 45(4), 305–320.
74. Morro Pérez, N. Distillation and extraction of herbs from Lamiaceae family. 2021.
75. Mamma, D., & Christakopoulos, P. Biotransformation of citrus by-products into value added products. *Waste Biomass Valorization* 2014, 5, 529–549.
76. Jyotirmayee, B., & Mahalik, G. *Essential Oils Extracted from CO_2 and Its Benefits*, 2021, Renu Publishers, New Delhi, p. 85.
77. Palma, M., et al., Extraction of natural products: Principles and fundamental aspects. In *Natural Product Extraction*, 2013.
78. Hudaib, M., et al., Recovery evaluation of lipophilic markers from Echinacea purpurea roots applying microwave-assisted solvent extraction versus conventional methods. *J Sep Sci* 2003, 26(1–2), 97–104.
79. López-Bascón, M., & De Castro, M. L. Soxhlet extraction. In: *Liquid-phase Extraction*, Elsevier, 2020, pp. 327–354.
80. Ody, P. *The Complete Medicinal Herbal: A Practical Guide to the Healing Properties of Herbs*, Simon and Schuster, 2017.
81. Pu, Z., et al., Multiple approaches to characterize and visualize the chemical composition of Sijunzi Decoction comprehensively. *J Sep Sci* 2023, 46(8), 2200737.
82. Turzhigitova, S., et al., Technology for obtaining dosage forms (tinctures, extracts) from local plant raw materials and studying their toxicity. *Res J Pharm Technol* 2022, 15(8), 3540–3548.
83. Rodino, S., & Butu, M. Herbal extracts—new trends in functional and medicinal beverages. In: *Functional and Medicinal Beverages*, Elsevier, 2019, pp. 73–108.
84. Bone, K. *A Clinical Guide to Blending Liquid Herbs: Herbal Formulations for the Individual Patient*, Elsevier Health Sciences, 2003.

85. Dog, T. L. *Healthy at Home: Get Well and Stay Well Without Prescriptions*, National Geographic Books, 2014.
86. Bruton-Seal, J., & Seal, M. *Backyard Medicine for All: A Guide to Home-Grown Herbal Remedies*, Skyhorse, 2018.
87. Awad, A., Trenfield, S. J., & Basit, A. W. Solid oral dosage forms. In: *Remington*, Elsevier, 2021, pp. 333–358.
88. Pavani, M. *Formulation and Evaluation of Orodispersible Tablets of Taste Masked Nizatidine*, Nandha College of Pharmacy: Erode, 2012.
89. Devi, V. K., Jain, N., & Valli, K. S. Importance of novel drug delivery systems in herbal medicines. *Pharmacogn Rev* 2010, 4(7), 27.
90. Gels, A. L. T. I. S. P1-Dermal and transdermal delivery. In: Pharmaceutics for Pharmacy Students, 2024.
91. Benza, H. I., & Munyendo, W. L., A review of progress and challenges in soft gelatin capsules formulations for oral administration. *Int J Pharm Sci Rev Res* 2011, 10(1), 20–24.
92. Swathy, B., Menaka, M., & Veerareddy, P. R. An overview of plant medicines in novel form. 2019.
93. Bharat, P., et al., A review: Novel advances in semisolid dosage forms & patented technology in semisolid dosage forms. *Int. J. PharmTech Res* 2011, 3, 420–430.
94. Zdoryk, O. A., et al., Investigation of physical and chemical stability of ointment with herbals. *Int J Pharm Compd* 2014, 18(3), 248–252.
95. Valarmathi, S., et al., Formulation and Evaluation of Herbal Face Cream. *Res J Pharm Technol* 2020, 13(1), 216–218.
96. Das, K. *Essential Oils and Their Application*, New India Publishing Agency, 2013.
97. Visht, S., & Chaturvedi, S. Isolation of natural products. *J Curr Pharm Res* 2012, 2(3), 584.
98. Pan, S., et al., A proposal for a quality system for herbal products. *J Pharm Sci* 2013, 102(12), 4230–4241.
99. Pan, J., et al., The development of an herbal material quality control strategy considering the effects of manufacturing processes. *Chin Med* 2019, 14, 1–12.
100. Kunle, O. F., Egharevba, H. O., & Ahmadu, P. O. Standardization of herbal medicines-A review. *Int J Biodivers Conserv* 2012, 4(3), 101–112.
101. Kumari, R., & Kotecha, M. A review on the Standardization of herbal medicines. *Int J Pharma Sci Res* 2016, 7(2), 97–106.
102. Sharma, A., et al., Herbal medicine for market potential in India: An overview. *Acad J Plant Sci* 2008, 1(2), 26–36.
103. Eid, A., Jaradat, N., & Elmarzugi, N., A Review of chemical constituents and traditional usage of Neem plant (Azadirachta Indica). *Palest Med Pharm J*, 2017, 2(2), 3.
104. Vaughn, A. R., Branum, A., & Sivamani, R. K. Effects of turmeric (Curcuma longa) on skin health: A systematic review of the clinical evidence. *Phytother Res* 2016, 30(8), 1243–1264.
105. Shankar, P. S., et al., Brahmi (Bacopa monnieri) as functional food ingredient in food processing industry. *J Pharmacog Phytochem* 2018, 7(3), 189–194.
106. Smith, S. J., Lopresti, A. L., & Fairchild, T. J. Exploring the efficacy and safety of a novel standardized ashwagandha (*Withania somnifera*) root extract (Witholytin®) in

adults experiencing high stress and fatigue in a randomized, double-blind, placebo-controlled trial. *J Psychopharmacol* 2023, 37(11), 1091–1104.
107. Ahmed, S., Ding, X., & Sharma, A. Exploring scientific validation of Triphala Rasayana in ayurveda as a source of rejuvenation for contemporary healthcare: An update. *J Ethnopharmacol* 2021, 273, 113829.
108. Gupta, B., et al., Preliminary clinical assessment and non-toxicity evaluation of an ayurvedic formulation BGR-34 in NIDDM. *J Tradit Complement Med* 2018, 8(4), 506–514.
109. Prasad, P. Diagnosis and Management of Diabetes Through Ayurveda (the Ancient Indian System of Medicine). *Socio-Scientific Interaction in Diabetes and Cancer and Its Management* 2023, 213.

CHAPTER 5

Regulatory Requirements for Herbal Drug Industries

GEETANJALI SAINI,[1] BHUPENDRA SINGH,[1*] MANISH VYAS,[2] NARESH RANGRA,[3] PRASHANT KUMAR,[4] and SUMIT DURGAPAL[5]

[1]NGI College of Pharmacy, Neelkanth Group of Institutions, Modipuram, Uttar Pradesh, India

[2]Research and Development Cell, Parul University, Vadodara, Gujarat, India

[3]School of Pharmacy, Chitkara University, Baddi, Himachal Pradesh, India

[4]SRM Modinagar College of Pharmacy, SRM Institute of Science and Technology Delhi-NCR Campus, Delhi-Meerut Road, Modinagar, Ghaziabad, Uttar Pradesh, India

[5]Department of Pharmaceutics, Uttaranchal University, Dehradun, Uttarakhand, India

*Corresponding author

ABSTRACT

The global interest in herbal medicines has surged over the past two decades, with the phytopharmaceutical market projected to reach approximately $10 billion annually. Phytotherapeutic agents standardized herbal preparations composed of raw or processed plant materials are gaining attention for their potential therapeutic value. Despite this growth, significant challenges remain in ensuring the safety, efficacy, and quality of herbal products. Contrary to the common perception that herbal medicines are inherently safe, many plants contain potent compounds,

Herbal Drug Industry: From Cultivation to Innovation and Global Impact.
Abhishek Tiwari, Varsha Tiwari, and Ajay Sharma (Eds.)

DOI: 10.1201/9781779640994-5

such as digitalis and pyrrolizidine alkaloids, which can pose serious health risks. The lack of comprehensive scientific data for many medicinal plants limits their clinical reliability. Current regulatory frameworks vary widely, encompassing categories such as prescription drugs, over-the-counter products, traditional medicines, and dietary supplements. However, the herbal industry continues to face obstacles including inadequate good manufacturing practices (GMP), poor agricultural and collection practices, and insufficient regulatory oversight. To enhance the credibility and global acceptance of herbal products, it is essential to harmonize and strengthen regulatory standards. Improving quality assurance systems and investing in research and development will not only ensure product safety and consistency but may also lead to the discovery of novel therapeutic applications. A well-regulated and research-driven herbal industry holds great promise for future healthcare systems.

5.1 INTRODUCTION

Herbal products are becoming increasingly popular due to their numerous benefits [1]. They are used to cure and prevent various illnesses, including antimicrobial, antifertility, antiaging, antispasmodic, antianxiety, anti-inflammatory, analgesic, vasodilatory, anti-HIV, and hepatoprotective therapies [2]. They are also used to treat chronic tiredness caused by Alzheimer's disease, cirrhosis, acne, asthma, menopause, impotence, gallstones, migraine, and to boost memory. Herbal remedies have been used since ancient times, and their pros and cons are considered to create new medicines with minimal negative impact on health [3]. Natural products have given rise to various medical systems such as traditional Chinese, Indian, European, Japanese Kampo, traditional Arabic and Islamic medicine, and folk medicines. These systems make use of not only herbal remedies but also pharmaceuticals made from minerals, metals, and animals, or from physical processes such as Panchkarma [4].

Plants, plant parts, and phytochemicals derived from them have been used for centuries in traditional medicine to treat various illnesses. These natural substances have played a vital role in modern medicine as well, with more than 100 active plant-derived chemicals accounting for 25% of all prescription medications worldwide. Out of the 252 drugs included in the WHO's essential medicine list, 11% are solely derived from plants [5]. Traditional medicines are relied upon as primary healthcare by over 80% of the population in Africa and Asia, while in India, nearly 80% of rural residents use traditional medicine or medicinal plants. India's herbal sector utilizes over 960 plant species, with 178 of them having large volume production levels exceeding 100 metric tons per year [6].

Herbal drugs are classified into three groups based on the type of active metabolites. The first group includes drugs used in their crude form, while the second group consists of active ingredients separated from plant extracts, which are generally pure compounds with higher pharmacological activity. For the third group, data on the acute and chronic toxicity of herbal drugs in animals are available to ensure their safety [7]. In 2003, the WHO regional office for South East Asia held a workshop on herbal medicine regulation. During the workshop, a system for categorizing herbal pharmaceuticals was proposed, which divided them into four categories: imported herbal medicines, modified herbal medicines, indigenous herbal medicines, and herbal medicines within established systems. Indigenous herbal remedies are well known for their composition, methods of application, and dosage due to their long history of use in the local population. Therefore, efficacy evaluations for local use are not necessary due to time constraints. Meanwhile, modified herbal medicines refer to herbal medicines that have been altered from their original form, either in dose or form, administration method, herbal medicinal components, production techniques, or medical purposes [2]. These modified herbal medicines must meet national regulatory safety and effectiveness standards, and preclinical and clinical data may or may not be necessary depending on the changes made. Imported herbal medicines, including raw components and finished goods, must be registered and sold in their country of origin and must provide data on efficacy and safety to the national authorities of the country importing them. The final two types of herbal medications must comply with good manufacturing procedures (GMP). The safety and effectiveness of herbal products depend on their quality, which is affected by problems such as adverse reactions, adulterations, substitutions, misidentification, mislabeling of herbal ingredients, and contamination by heavy metals, pesticides, and microbes. To minimize these quality risks, it is important to implement appropriate quality control measures during the manufacturing process. GMP is an essential tool to ensure that the manufacturing process adheres to guidelines, uses sufficient quality control measures, and produces goods of satisfactory quality before they can be sold. However, regulatory agencies face technical challenges when developing GMPs for herbal products, leading to different regulatory requirements across different countries. For instance, the GMP established by the European Union (EU) is exclusive to European areas, while the US federal government regulates the production of herbal products intended for use as nutritional supplements. In China, where herbal products are utilized according to the principles of Traditional Chinese Medicine (TCM), they are referred to as TCMs and are subject to the same laws as conventional pharmaceuticals [9]. India is recognized for exporting standardized herbal extracts and raw materials, as well as herbal medications in the form of Ayurvedic pharmaceuticals, to various regions of the globe [10]. Although the use of herbal medications has grown globally, concerns about their widespread use and the impact on their commercialization have been raised by reports of negative effects and adulteration. This chapter aims to identify the regulatory framework for the commercialization of herbal drugs as well as the development of technical standards in the manufacturing of herbal drugs [11].

5.2 THE GLOBAL MARKET OF HERBAL DRUGS

Over the past few decades, the general public's interest in natural remedies, especially herbal therapy, has grown significantly. This trend is particularly evident in affluent nations but is also observed in developing countries. Consequently, the trade in herbal medicine has gained a lot of traction globally, attracting the attention of numerous pharmaceutical corporations, including multinationals. Until a few years ago, only a few small businesses were interested in marketing herbal medications. However, the situation has changed, and now most significant international corporations are intrigued by the prospects of herbal medicine [12]. In March 2020, the WHO declared COVID-19 a worldwide pandemic. The pharmaceutical and health industries have been severely affected by the epidemic, with both short- and long-term consequences. Additionally, there have been delays in noncritical projects and programs, which have impacted R&D and manufacturing activities. The drug shortage has led to varying impacts on hospital and retail medicine sales worldwide. The *DARU Journal of Pharmaceutical Sciences* reports that starting in January 2020, the amount of medications used in hospitals to treat COVID-19 patients increased by around 100–700%. These medications included sedatives, respiratory treatments, and pain relievers. Pharmaceutical corporations are responding to the global epidemic and attempting to recover lost revenue, even though the full impact is still uncertain. Since there is no specific medication available to treat COVID-19, consumers are focusing more on boosting their immunity. Boosting immunity has become a priority for many people, especially in Asian countries where herbs are easily available. Raw herbs and locally made treatments have gained attention for their ability to suppress the COVID-19 attack on the body. Herbal tea, turmeric, coriander, cumin, and garlic are key constituents in many medicines and nutritional supplements that are widely marketed [13]. Despite supply chain disruptions, the global herbal medicines industry achieved average growth during the first quarter of 2020.

The demand for natural ingredients in the cosmetics industry is constantly increasing, driven by the growing awareness of consumers regarding natural cosmetics and the preference of cosmetics manufacturers for natural herbal substitutes over synthetic ingredients. This trend is expected to continue in the foreseeable future as consumers' demand for natural ingredients in cosmetics and toiletries keeps increasing [14]. Cosmetic product manufacturers are replacing synthetic chemicals with natural ingredients, mostly in response to customer demand and a shift toward more sustainable raw materials. As a result of the consumer desire for chemical-free personal care products and toiletries, the market for herbal remedies is expected to grow. The market for herbal beauty products is expected to grow at a compound annual growth rate (CAGR) of about 6.3% from 2023 to 2033. By 2023, it is estimated to be worth approximately US$73.0 billion, representing over 5% of the entire beauty goods market. With the increasing popularity of natural remedies and the focus on healthy skin and hair, the market for herbal beauty products is projected to reach US$134.0 billion by 2033. As the industry continues to expand, competition is expected to intensify. According to future market insights's estimate, leading herbal beauty product companies are expected to account for only 2–5% of total sales [15, 16] (Figure 5.1).

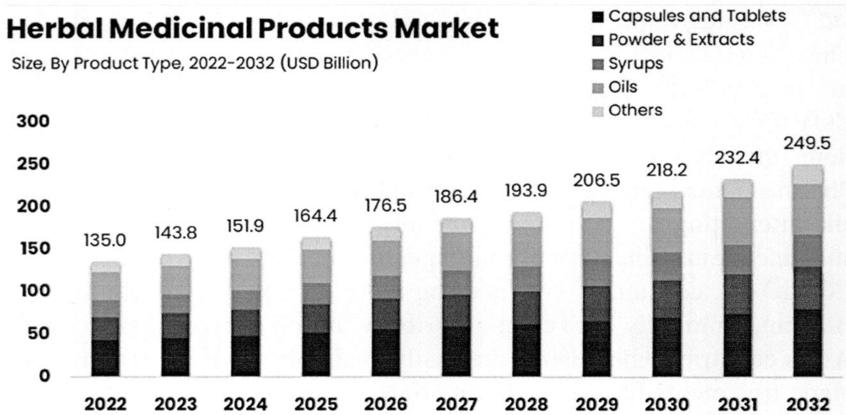

FIGURE 5.1 Herbal medicinal products market report.

Source: Retrieved August 7, 2025, from https://marketresearch.biz/report/herbal-medicinal-products-market/accessed-on-07-08-2025

The global market for herbal medicine was valued at US$185.86 billion in 2020 and is projected to grow at a CAGR of 11.32% from US$230.03 billion in 2021 to reach US$430.05 billion by 2030. Between 2023 and 2028, the European herbal medicine market is expected to grow at a CAGR of 6.02%. The German market is expected to dominate the European herbal medicine market during the projection period. This sector is expected to contribute significantly to the overall European market in the coming years. By 2028, the e-commerce delivery channel is projected to generate more revenue due to its wider exposure, growing usage of mobile phones and the internet, wider coverage regions, and ability to sell products at reduced rates. Additionally, in 2022, the herbal medications category held a significant portion of the total market. From 2023 to 2028, the herbal medicine market in the United Kingdom is expected to grow at the fastest pace. The country's market growth is influenced by a developed healthcare infrastructure, increasing healthcare spending, and an ageing population. The Indian Herbal Drugs Market is expected to grow significantly, reaching a size of $2.6 billion by 2027. The industry is projected to expand at a CAGR of 11.7% from 2022 to 2027. The growth of the Indian herbal drugs industry can be attributed to several factors, including the increasing demand for ready-to-eat food and ready-to-drink beverages, changing consumer preferences, the potential health benefits of herbal extracts, and the rise in disposable income.

5.2.1 IMPORTANCE OF REGULATORY REQUIREMENTS IN ENSURING SAFETY AND EFFICACY

Herbal products can have several adverse effects. Well-controlled randomized clinical trials (RCTs) have shown that the use of herbal medications can lead to unfavorable side effects. Ephedra usage can cause cardiovascular difficulties; kava-kava use can result in hepatotoxicity; Datura metal-containing asthma treatments can lead to anticholinergic effects, resulting in lower visceral activity; and liquorice can cause water retention [17]. In response to an increase in complaints of negative effects, regulatory and monitoring bodies in several countries have issued warnings on the use of herbal medications. In 1993, the American Herbal Products Association imposed restrictions on the use of comfrey, a herbal remedy containing pyrrolizidine alkaloids (PAs), for external applications. Later in 2001, the United States Food and Drug Administration (USFDA) removed comfrey from all dietary supplements due to reports of hepatotoxicity. Similarly, in 2004, the USFDA banned Chinese herbs containing ephedra because of reports of cardiovascular events associated with its usage in the United States for weight loss [18]. The United Kingdom's Medicines and Healthcare Products Regulatory Agency issued a warning to all herbal interest groups in 2007 to discontinue any unlicensed proprietary products that may include hepatotoxic PAs derived from *Senecio* species. In China, the use of three herbal remedies containing aristolochic acids (AAs), including Radix Aristolochiae Fangchi (Guangfangji), Caulis Aristolochiae Manshuriensis (Guanmutong), and Radix Aristolochiae (Qingmuxiang), has been prohibited since 2004 due to the possible danger of nephrotoxicity [19].

The use of herbal medicines has become a prevalent practice worldwide, but it has also brought about several issues that need attention [20]. One of these issues is the presence of hazardous heavy metals exceeding the allowable limit set by national regulatory agencies. Reports of toxic pollutants have been documented at every stage of production, from raw material procurement to manufacture. Heavy metal toxicity linked to Ayurvedic treatment was first documented in the United Kingdom in 1978, and since then, more than 50 published reports on heavy metal poisoning have emerged from various parts of the world, such as the Middle East, Western Europe, Australia, North America, and the Indian subcontinent [14]. The main pollutants include arsenic, copper, lead, and mercury. The mercury concentration of 31 Ayurvedic medicines was examined, and it was discovered that all but one surpassed the permissible threshold of 1 ppm mercury, with 16 preparations exceeding the limit by more than two times. Furthermore, significant variations in the amount of mercury present in a single, identical medication produced by many firms were noted, indicating a lack of consistency in the product and potential hazards. In Indian herbal medicines made from nine plants, a buildup of heavy metals (Pb, Cd, Cu, and Zn) over WHO-acceptable levels was detected. This issue further highlights the need for better regulation and monitoring of herbal medicine production to ensure consumer safety [21].

The growth and globalization of traditional herbal medicine have been negatively affected by the discovery of pesticide residues in natural products. There are increasing reports of contaminated crude medical herbs, as well as their preparations and products such as tinctures, infusions, decoctions, and essential oils. Many countries have regulations in place regarding the use of pesticides on medicinal plants. The WHO has set maximum residue limits for these pesticides in wild or farmed medicinal plants. Different countries' pharmacopoeias provide residual limits and assay procedures for organochlorine pesticides. To ensure the safety of herbal medicines, highly sensitive analytical techniques must be used for both qualitative and quantitative assessments of pesticide residues. Various analytical techniques, such as GC, HPLC, GC/MS, HPLC/MS, SFC, capillary electrophoresis, and enzyme-linked immunosorbent assay, can be used to determine pesticide residues. The complex compositions of natural medicines and the variety of pesticide residue forms make it difficult to develop a pesticide residue removal technique for herbal medicines that do not compromise the active components or result in secondary contamination from the organic solvent [22].

In light of reports on adulteration and contamination with heavy metals, pesticides, and microorganisms in herbal treatments, the development of efficient identification methods for herbal materials and their constituent parts has become necessary. This is essential to ensure the purity and quality of herbal medications. Therefore, procedures that guarantee their safety and quality must be devised [23].

Herbal pharmaceuticals are often classified as dietary supplements or traditional medicines and are subject to national legislation. They must be proven to be of good quality, safe, and have traditional usage. Synthetic medications, on the other hand, are subjected to stringent regulations that ensure their quality, safety, and efficacy through preclinical research and clinical trials. Plant materials' identification, purity, and potency are checked using tests like spectroscopy and chromatography to meet the quality control demands for herbal medications. Standardization is difficult due to natural ingredient diversity. Safety is usually established based on conventional usage, but more modern research is required. Human clinical trials are not typically required for efficacy investigations, especially in the case of traditional herbal treatments [24]. However, *in vitro* and animal studies may be included. Long-duration studies track safety and efficacy after commercialization. Component lists, dosage recommendations, and any adverse effects must be accurately listed on the labels. Regulations for herbal medications may be less strict than those for synthetic medications, but health claims are often restricted and must be supported. Manufacturers must record adverse occurrences, and postmarketing monitoring must track side effects, effectiveness, and long-term safety [22]. Regulatory bodies may require more research or label revisions in response to fresh information.

5.3 REGULATORY AGENCIES FOR HERBAL DRUGS

5.3.1 INDIA

In India, herbal pharmaceuticals are governed by the Drug and Cosmetic Act (D and C) of 1940 and the Rules of 1945. These regulations explicitly cover Ayurvedic, Unani, and Siddha treatments. The Department of Ayurveda, Yoga and Naturopathy, Unani, Siddha and Homoeopathy (AYUSH) handles the regulations and requires that the manufacturing or sale of herbal medications only take place after obtaining a manufacturing license, if necessary. The D and C Act covers licensing, formulation composition, production, labeling, packing, quality, and export control [25]. The GMP guidelines for producing herbal medications are outlined in Schedule "T" of the Act. The official formularies and pharmacopoeias for drug quality standards are available (Table 5.1). The D and C Act's first schedule includes mandatory requirements for licensing any herbal product that falls under either of the two categories:

1. Ayurvedic, Siddha, and Unani Medicine
2. Patent and Proprietary Medicine

TABLE 5.1 Herbal Drug Regulation in Different Countries

Sr. No.	Country	Regulatory Authority	Specific Regulations	Specific Regulations	References
	United States	Food and Drug Administration	Herbal drugs are regulated as dietary supplements	The DSHEA sets regulations for labeling, manufacturing practices, and safety standard cGMP regulations apply to herbal product manufacturers	[25]
	United Kingdom	MHRA	Herbal drugs are regulated as THMPs or as OTC medicines	The THMPD set standards for the safety and efficacy of herbal medicines OTC herbal products are regulated under the human medicines regulations	[26]
	Canada	Health Canada	Herbal products are regulated as NHPs	NHPs regulations govern the safety, efficacy, and quality of herbal products NHPs must have a product license and include an NPN on the label	[27]
	Australia	TGA	Herbal medicines are regulated as complementary medicines	Complementary Medicines (CMI) regulations ensure the safety, efficacy, and quality of herbal products Products must be listed on the ARTG before they can be sold	[28]
	India	Ministry of Ayush	Herbal medicines are regulated as Ayurvedic, Siddha, and Unani medicines	Drugs and Cosmetics Act 1940 and Rules 1945 provide the regulatory framework for herbal drugs Products must comply with the standards set by the Pharmacopoeia of India	[24]
	China	CFDA	Herbal medicines are regulated as TCM	Regulations include the GMP standards for herbal products TCM products must be registered and approved before they can be sold	[21]
	Japan	MHLW	Herbal medicines are regulated as Kampo medicine	Kampo medicines must meet the standards set by the Japanese Pharmacopoeia Regulations also cover manufacturing and quality control standards	[9]

Notes: DSHEA: Dietary Supplement and Education Act; cGMP: Current good manufacturing practice; MHRA: Medicines and Healthcare products Regulatory Agency; THMPs: traditional herbal medicinal products; OTC: over-the-counter; THMPD: traditional herbal medicinal products directives; NHPs: natural health products; NPN: natural product number; TGA: Therapeutic Goods Administration; ARTG: Australian Register of Therapeutic Goods; CFDA: China Food and Drug Administration; TCM: traditional Chinese medicine; GMP: good manufacturing practice; MHLW: Ministry of Health, Labour and Welfare.

5.3.2 UNITED STATES OF AMERICA

The US Food and Drug Administration (FDA) categorizes botanical products into three groups: foods, medications, and dietary supplements. The classification of a product is based on the claims made about it or its intended use. A product is categorized as medication if it aims to reduce, identify, cure, or prevent a medical condition. Medicinal supplements and pharmaceuticals are two categories of botanical products that aim to change the composition or operation of the human body. Before they can be commercialized, medications require an FDA-approved new drug application. On the other hand, dietary supplements fall under the Dietary Supplement Act of 1994, which does not require premarket clearance from the FDA. Marketers are responsible for ensuring that their products are safe and that their labels comply with legal requirements [26]. Claims made about dietary supplements must follow the FDA's regulatory criteria, and the current GMP guidelines should be followed while producing them.

5.3.3 EUROPEAN UNION

The European Medicine Agency has established two methods for registering herbal medicines. The first method is to obtain full marketing authorization according to Directive 2001/83/EC. This involves submitting a dossier containing data from clinical trials, pharmacological, toxicological, and physicochemical testing, as well as information on the quality, safety, and efficacy of the medicinal products. The second method is to follow a simpler protocol in accordance with Directive 2004/24/EC [27]. This method applies to traditional herbal medicinal preparations that do not require medical supervision. In cases where there is sufficient scientific material to support a well-established medicinal use but no evidence of a lengthy traditional medicinal use, evidence of the product's historic use is recognized as proof of its effectiveness. However, authorities may request proof of safety. Product specifications must contain physicochemical and microbiological testing as part of quality control requirements. The item must adhere to the quality requirements in the applicable European Pharmacopoeia or member state pharmacopoeias. The substance should have been used medicinally for at least 30 years, including at least 15 years in the EU, according to the bibliographic evidence society [28].

If the product has been available for less than 15 years but otherwise meets the requirements for the streamlined registration process, the application for traditional use registration will be sent to the Committee for Herbal Medicinal Products as per the instructions.

5.3.4 CANADA

Since January 1, 2004, Health Canada has regulated herbal remedies and traditional medicines, including Ayurvedic medicine, under the natural health products (NHPs) laws. Any producer, packer, labeler, or importer must first register with Health Canada before commencing any such project. This requires registering the product(s) and the manufacturing site(s), as well as providing information on the microbiological, chemical, standardization, stability, and composition of the product. The Natural Health Product Directorate (NHPD) is responsible for receiving reports on contaminant testing procedures, tolerance limits, safety, and efficacy, as well as ingredient characterization and quantity by assay or input. The NHPD enforces that NHPs must comply with contaminant limits and be produced in accordance with GMP guidelines [29].

5.3.5 AUSTRALIA

In Australia, the Therapeutic Goods Administration regulates herbal products that fall under the umbrella of alternative medicine. This category includes TCM, Ayurvedic medicine, and indigenous Australian remedies. Complementary medications that do not require monitoring by a doctor must be registered on the Australian Register for Therapeutic Goods (ARTG) before being marketed. While medications intended for therapeutic conditions with higher risk must be registered on the ARTG, medications for low-risk diseases must also be included. Only claims supported by evidence that are registered on the ARTG are accepted [30].

5.3.6 MALAYSIA

In Malaysia, herbal products are considered as controlled goods. Before introducing herbal products into the market, marketers are required to register the product. The applicant must be listed in one of two categories with Suruhanjaya Syarikat Malaysia, which is the Registrar of Businesses in Malaysia.

1. Traditional products
2. Health supplements

Functional claims made in supplements must be approved by the authority, and only those claims can be made. However, for traditional products, the authorities only need the label "traditionally used for" to appear before any claim is made on the product [31].

5.3.7 SAUDI ARABIA

Herbal items in Saudi Arabia are classified as traditional goods. To be considered acceptable, they must have been used traditionally for at least 50 consecutive years and prepared using the same technique and dosage that have been customarily employed. Depending on the evidence presented, they may be classified as nonpharmacological evidence for traditional goods or pharmacopoeial evidence for traditional products. For the former classification, the dosage form, duration of use, recommended dose, mode of administration, quantity, and risk information should all match those found in the Pharmacopoeia, and the production technique must be conventional. For the latter classification, two separate references that support the safety and effectiveness of the product must be supplied. These references can come from peer-reviewed published articles, clinical studies, pharmacopoeias, textbook references, data from nonclinical studies on pharmacokinetics and pharmacodynamics, toxicity information, reproductive effects, and the possible genotoxicity or carcinogenicity of an ingredient, as well as information based on prior finished product marketing experience [8].

5.3.8 PHILIPPINES

Herbal medicines in the Philippines are subject to the same regulations as other conventional herbal products. The regulatory body, Bureau of Food and Drugs (BFAD), mandates that products made from plant materials should be marketed under this category, even if their use is based only on the traditional experience of at least five decades, as documented in medical, historical, and ethnological literature. BFAD requires traditional herbal items to be registered before manufacturing, importing, or marketing. Companies' brand names fall under BFAD's management and are considered conventional herbal products as well. Prior approval from BFAD is required for product registration [32].

5.3.9 NIGERIA

In Nigeria, the National Agency for Food and Drug Administration and Control (NAFDAC) is in charge of regulating the trade of herbal products and has categorized them as "Herbal Remedies and Associated Items." The premarketing registration of herbal medicines and allied items is mandatory in Nigeria. Additionally, all advertising for these products must be approved by NAFDAC. According to the Food and Drug Act of 1990, the promotion of any illness condition listed in "Schedule 1" as a cure is prohibited [33].

5.4 INTERNATIONAL HARMONIZATION

Efforts have been made to ensure that herbal pharmaceuticals meet consistent pharmacopoeial standards, standardization, and categorization across nations. Although similar herbal remedies are included in the pharmacopoeias of China, Japan, and Korea, their details vary somewhat. Therefore, harmonization activities have been started to guarantee that the same herbal medicines are of the same quality, safety, and efficacy worldwide [34]. The same raw plant material may still be described even if the original plant's family or species has changed. However, the component employed for the herbal medication, or the term conveyed by the Latin binomial pharmacopoeia name, or the Chinese character, may change, even when the same basic plant material is given [35]. To support the international commercialization of safe and efficacious herbal medications, the Western Pacific Regional Forum for the Harmonization of Herbal Medicine attempted to harmonize the crude drug monographs in the pharmacopoeias of six Asian nations (Japan, China, Korea, Singapore, Vietnam, and Hong Kong). Similarly, the American nations started to harmonize their procedure criteria for herbal product registration in 2000.

The Pan American Network of Drug Regulatory Harmonization working group on medicinal plants aims to advance awareness of the many categories of herbal products, definitions of terminology, and identification of procedures and minimal specifications for herbal product registration [36].

A standardized nomenclature has been developed for the "WHO International Standard Terminologies on Traditional Medicine in the Western Pacific Region." This will aid in establishing a shared scientific foundation across various traditional medicine systems. The compilation includes around 4000 traditional medicine phrases, and it is believed that this would help in creating clinical practice guidelines based on evidence. It has been suggested to classify herbal treatments using an anatomical therapeutic chemical (ATC) approach that is compatible with prescription medications. This approach has been accepted and published in the Herbal ATC Index and Guidelines for Herbal ATC Classification, with a few changes. In India, there are over 8000 herbal medication firms, out of which 5000 are GMP-compliant manufacturing facilities [37]. Thirty percent of the herbal sector exports consist of finished goods, including herbal extracts, while the remaining 70% comprises raw materials. Fifty-five major enterprises in India export herbal drugs. We conducted an initial investigation using a 25-item questionnaire to determine the difficulties faced by these businesses when producing and shipping herbal medications. One of the main obstacles to commercialization is compliance with various national regulatory norms. A third of the industries polled said that it is very difficult and time-consuming to achieve regulatory compliance with diverse country requirements [38].

5.4.1 LABELING OF HERBAL DRUGS

The quality of customer education regarding herbal products is just as important as the final product itself. Warnings on the label or packet can help reduce the risk of improper usage and negative side effects. The product label is the primary source of information about herbal products. However, currently, no government agency or organization confirms whether a supplement or plant has been accurately labeled. Studies have shown that labeling for herbal remedies often does not accurately reflect the contents of the bottle. Consumers have less than a 50% chance of receiving what is advertised on the label of a herbal product.

Additionally, published examinations of herbal supplements have revealed significant discrepancies between what is advertised and what is actually in the bottle. The term "standardized" does not have a legal definition, so seeing it on a product label does not necessarily mean that the quality of the product will be higher. It is often up to the consumer to determine what is safe and effective for them, and inconsistent labeling on herbal products can be frustrating for customers [39].

All herbal products and their packaging must display specific information on the label. The information should include a statement that the product has been manufactured according to Pharmacopoeia standards, a description of the active ingredients and their levels, and instructions on how frequently and how much to take the medicine. The label should also indicate the extraction technique used, the ratio of menstruum and macerate utilized, and any potential negative effects. Moreover, the label should specify the amount of a particular biochemical component added to the product's composition through standardization [40]. Customers can use the potency metric provided by standardization to compare dosages with those recommended by clinical research and assess the product's quality. The label should also ensure that the correct herb was used and list the product's name, origin, intended use, net quantity of contents, additional ingredients (such as herbs and amino acids) and additives (for which no daily values have been established), storage guidelines, shelf life or expiration date, warnings, disclaimer, and the name and address of the manufacturer, packer, or distributor.

Herbs that are classified as nutritional supplements cannot list any health benefits or "disease claims" on their labels, which often leaves customers uninformed. Herbal product usage is heavily influenced by marketing, and media plays an important role in educating people about NHPs. However, there is an issue with "propaganda" in the media, leading to scientific incoherence. Herbal products are not reviewed by any government agency unless there is a medical claim on the package. The FDAs, responsible for prescription medications, only examine herbal products if they believe they may be hazardous or if the label makes medical claims. Botanical dietary supplements are evaluated by researchers for possible health benefits and safety hazards using a variety of methods, including historical usage and in-lab research with animal or cell models. Studies involving human subjects can also provide relevant data about the application of botanical dietary supplements.

5.4.2 GOOD MANUFACTURING PRACTICE FOR HERBAL DRUGS

India boasts approximately 10,000 licensed pharmacies that produce ISM and herbal medications. Unfortunately, the increased commercialization of this industry has led to dishonest manufacturing methods becoming prevalent (Table 5.2). This includes subpar manufacturing practices such as inadequate and incorrect labeling, shortcuts being taken instead of necessary but time-consuming operations, and others. As a result, the ISM drug-manufacturing sectors have been required to implement GMPs. The Drugs and Cosmetics Amendment Rules, 2000, outlines the specifics of the GMP provision for Ayurvedic, Siddha, and Unani medications. In June 2002, the Government of India developed recommendations for the implementation of GMP standards. These standards ensure that the drugs are manufactured using genuine, prescribed-quality raw materials that are free from contamination; manufacturing processes adhere to prescribed standards; appropriate quality control measures are implemented; and manufactured drugs that are released for sale are of acceptable quality.

TABLE 5.2 Key Differences in the Regulatory Requirements for Herbal and Synthetic Drugs

S. N.	Aspects	Herbal Drugs	Synthetic Drugs	Reference
1.	Source	Plants or plant extracts	Chemical synthesis	[19]
2.	Composition	A complex mixture of compounds	Well-defined, consistent chemical composition	
3.	Regulation of ingredients	Difficult due to multiple active compounds	Well-defined chemical structure, stringent standards for purity and quality	
4.	Safety and efficacy	Safety and efficacy studies required; reliance on traditional use in some cases	Rigorous preclinical and clinical trials required	
5.	Regulatory pathways	Varied, sometimes simplified for traditional medicines	Established, involving rigorous testing phase	
6.	Labeling requirements	Accurate ingredient lists, dosage instructions, and potential side effects	Detailed information on active ingredients, dosage administration, contraindications, warnings	
7.	Health claims	Limited and may require scientific evidence	Closely regulated, requiring strong clinical evidence	
8.	Postmarketing surveillance	Continuous monitoring for safety and efficacy	Monitoring adverse events, updating information based on new data	

It is important to allocate enough space at the factory where medicines are manufactured to perform the following activities: (1) receive and store raw materials, (2) carry out processing and manufacturing activities, (3) have a quality control section, (4) store finished products, and (5) maintain records in a suitable office, including rejected drugs and goods.

5.4.3 SAFETY OF HERBAL DRUGS

Before using any medical intervention, it is important to evaluate its benefits and risks for a specific patient. However, analyzing the benefits and risks of supplementary medications can be challenging due to the lack of data in certain safety-related areas.

Overall, there is a lack of adequate information available on the effectiveness of herbal drugs on:

1. Active metabolites
2. Pharmacokinetics
3. Pharmacology
4. Toxicology
5. Adverse effects and their frequencies
6. Effect of long-term use
7. Drug–herb interactions: interactions with food, alcohol
8. Use in specific patient groups: children, elderly, patients with renal or hepatic conditions, gender effects
9. Use in pregnancy
10. Contraindications and warnings

It can be difficult to compare the benefit-risk ratio of herbal treatments to conventional medications, even when studies have shown similar effectiveness. This is because there is insufficient information. Clinical trials have shown that some herbal remedies have a better safety profile than conventional medications with similar efficacy. For example, St. John's wort extracts have been found to have fewer side effects than other antidepressants in randomized controlled studies involving individuals with depression. Similarly, randomized controlled trials comparing saw palmetto extracts to finasteride in males with BPH have been published. However, benefit-risk analyses must be conducted on a case-by-case basis, and it cannot be assumed that herbal remedies will always have a better benefit-risk ratio than prescription medications. Additionally, it should not be assumed that a benefit-risk analysis applies to every method of preparing a particular plant. Evidence of safety should be considered specific to an extract or, at most, to similar herb preparations with substantially similar chemical profiles.

Herbal treatments are often misunderstood in terms of their frequency and harmful effects. It is a common misconception that herbs are always safe because of their natural origin. However, this is not entirely true as many plants are naturally toxic, and using therapeutic herbs can sometimes have negative effects. These side effects may not be mild and can be different from type A adverse drug reactions, which are predictable, dose-related, and frequent. Herbal medicines can cause type B reactions (rare, erratic, dose-independent, and typically severe reactions), as well as long-term use and delayed effects that may appear years after drug use (e.g., carcinogenic and teratogenic reactions).

5.4.4 EVALUATION OF EFFICACY AND SAFETY OF HERBAL DRUGS

Herbal products used for diagnosing, treating, mitigating, preventing, or curing illnesses are sometimes classified as medicines based on the laws of the specific country. However, in several countries, including the United States, botanical products are marketed as "dietary supplements." In other countries, herbal medicines are treated as pharmaceuticals and must pass safety and clinical effectiveness tests before they can be registered [41]. The WHO Guidelines for the Assessment of Herbal Medicines recommend that more programs be established to investigate the effectiveness and safety of herbal medicines, but currently, only a few exist. Although it is possible to conduct clinical studies using herbal pharmaceuticals, few well-controlled double-blind (placebo-controlled) trials have been conducted using herbal medicines, according to a review of the literature. A recent meta-analysis of reviews published in prestigious medical publications, including the *British Medical Journal*, the *Lancet*, the *Annals of Internal Medicine*, the *Journal of the American Medical Association* (JAMA), and the *British Journal of Clinical Pharmacology*, supports this assumption. Such disparities might be explained by a number of variables, including:

1. The quality control and standardization of herbal medications used in clinical studies are often inadequate.
2. Herbal medications are used in various doses, but most studies lack sufficient randomization and proper patient selection.
3. Additionally, the number of patients in most studies is inadequate to achieve statistical significance.
4. Creating suitable placebos can be challenging due to differences in flavors, scents, and other factors.
5. Significant differences in the duration of herbal medicine treatments.

Research on herbal medications is limited due to various challenges, resulting in a lack of well-controlled double-blind clinical trials to demonstrate their effectiveness and safety. Nevertheless, numerous clinical studies have been conducted on various herbal medications, such as *Ginkgo biloba* extract, used to treat cardiovascular and central nervous system (CNS) diseases, and *Hypericum perforatum*, commonly known as St. John's wort, used as an antidepressant [42]. However, most of these clinical trials have faced criticism similar to those previously highlighted. Therefore, well-controlled randomized double-blind studies are still required to determine the therapeutic effectiveness of these herbal medications, even though clinical trials have demonstrated that they are quite safe and do not have any significant adverse effects.

Additional botanical medications include *Panax ginseng*, used as a tonic herb; *Tanacetun parthenium*, also known as feverfew and used as a migraine headache remedy; *Allium sativum*, commonly known as garlic and used to treat cardiovascular disorders such as low-density protein cholesterol; *Valeriana officinalis*, used as a sedative and sleep aid; *Matricaria chamomilla*, suggested as a carminative, anti-inflammatory, and antispasmodic; and *Silybium marianun*, commonly known as milk thistle and useful for mending liver function including cirrhosis. The herbal medicines with the largest global market include *Piper methysticum*, commonly known as *Kava kava*; *Aesculus hippocastanum*, also known as horse chestnut; *Cassia acutifolia*, commonly known as Senna; and *Rhamnus purshiana*, commonly known as cascara sagrada, all used as laxatives. Other herbal medicines include *Echinacea purpurea*, commonly known as Echinacea and used as an anti-inflammatory and immunostimulant; *Arnica montana*, commonly known as arnica and used to treat post-traumatic and postoperative conditions; and *Serenoa repens*, commonly known as saw palmetto and used to treat benign prostatic hyperplasia. All these herbal medicines have been evaluated in various clinical trials, but more appropriate and well-controlled RCTs are still required to confirm their effectiveness.

5.5 LACK OF REGULATORY GUIDELINES

The lack of regulatory requirements is one of the primary reasons for the low quality of herbal medical products. As per the study conducted among the stakeholders revealed that over 60% of them advised developing criteria for quality control of herbal medicines. The report also recommends creating guidelines for standardizing the preparation of herbal drugs and identifying active components through marker-based identification, despite the release of guidelines for preclinical safety evaluation of Ayurveda, Siddha, and Unani (ASU) and other traditional medicines. Good storage and agricultural practices are as critical as quality control in the production of herbal drugs. The National Medicinal Plants Board created standards for excellent field collecting and agriculture methods in India in 2009 in line with the WHO's Good Agricultural and Collection Practices (GACP). However, most manufacturers and those dealing with raw materials remain unaware of these rules. The farmers' lack of awareness of these requirements and the related operating costs make it impractical for many groups or firms to comply with them. The report recommends establishing government-certified raw material supply centers in each state to assist firms in obtaining genuine raw materials. The respondents have proposed more detailed regulatory rules for the standardization of raw materials and quality control throughout the manufacturing process to produce high-quality medications.

The sale of traditional medicines in India is mostly done through over-the-counter (OTC) medications. The market for herbal OTC drugs is driven by advertising and consumer demand, while the market for prescription medications is mainly governed by physician preference. Interestingly, 12% of surveyed firms conduct formal clinical trials at different medical institutions, while almost half of the companies undertake general safety research for the drugs. However, there are currently no guidelines in India for the assessment or conduct of clinical studies on herbal medication. To address this, the Medicines and Cosmetics 4th Amendment Rule 2008

(Rule 170) provides rules for assessing ASU medicines. The new regulation divides ASU medications into four major groups based on clinical research requirements. No clinical evidence is needed for ASU products prepared in accordance with the formula, as defined in Section 3(a) of the Drugs and Cosmetics Act (DCA), and medications based on aqueous extracts of medicinal plants for certain purposes. However, safety and effectiveness investigations are required for unique ASU medicines, medications based on Indian ethnomedicine, and drugs based on hydroalcoholic extract. Ayurveda recognizes a diverse category of extracts through crude powders, decoctions, or aqueous extracts of medicinal plants; this is not the case with hydroalcoholic extracts. It is thought that the production procedure for hydroalcoholic extracts deviates from the core ideas of traditional preparation. For this reason, formulations claiming to be Ayurvedic should not contain any sort of hydroalcoholic extract. Clinical research is also required for medications based on aqueous extracts, even for novel indications.

The introduction of the DCA regulations has dealt another significant blow to the Indian herbal business. Despite the fact that GMP compliance has been mandatory since 2006, only 107 out of the enterprises evaluated in the field research were found to meet the requirements for it. Moreover, survey results showed that the States Food and Drug Administration interprets the DCA differently, which has led to a scenario where a medication or formulation that is prohibited in one state is allowed in another. The poll also revealed that one of the significant problems is the variation in medication registration deadlines between different states. To address these issues, the development of uniform processes, clear timetables, and specific standards defining the meetings with regulators could facilitate the elimination of irregularities with regard to state licensing agencies and the establishment of a national system.

Many companies have faced difficulties in commercializing their products due to the need to comply with various regulatory norms of different countries. To simplify and speed up the clearance process, more than half of the respondents suggested the creation of a standard technical dossier format [43]. It is also recommended to establish uniform requirements for dossier submission and drug registration processes for herbal drugs. Harmonizing pharmacopoeia and recognizing Indian monographs in other countries would be beneficial for international drug registration. For example, in the United States, promoting herbal products has been a challenge for producers because the Indian Pharmacopoeia (IP) does not have a specific section on dietary supplements, unlike the US Pharmacopoeia (USP). According to IP 2007 general notifications, the inclusion of a monograph in the IP does not mean that the formulation has received FDA approval for use as a medication. Even if a chemical is not intended for the drug market, a drug license is required if a manufacturer wants to declare any product to be IP grade. Additionally, drug regulations state that a location cannot produce an IP-grade material or use machinery used in the production of a non-IP chemical. Small and medium-sized producers cannot afford to set up medium-sized production facilities dedicated to IP/USP-grade herbal extracts and preparations. To ensure the safety, effectiveness, and quality of herbal medicines across national borders, pharmacopoeia must be harmonized. Harmonization of the filing of dossiers and registration procedures for herbal drugs is necessary to advance international trade. Most of the respondents emphasized the necessity of receiving scientific counsel before developing new drugs and formulations, starting clinical trials, and submitting a dossier [44].

5.6 CHALLENGES AND ISSUES

5.6.1 IMPACT OF REGULATORY GUIDELINES ON THE STATUS AND SAFETY OF HERBAL DRUGS

The issues related to the use of herbal medicines are mostly caused by their classification as food or dietary supplements by some governments. This classification allows herbal remedies to be marketed immediately without any requirement for proof of their efficacy, safety, or quality. As a result, the criteria for quality testing and manufacturing of herbal medicines are generally less stringent or structured. In some cases, even practitioners of traditional medicines lack proper licensing or registration. Due to these reasons, both the public and medical professionals are increasingly concerned about the safety of traditional and herbal therapies. In many countries, herbal treatments and related products are introduced into the market without undergoing adequate safety or toxicological evaluation [45]. As a result, there is a lack of instruments to oversee quality control and production processes. These preparations are often easily accessible to customers without a prescription, and they may not be aware of the potential risks associated with using a herbal remedy.

Different countries have different definitions and laws regarding food and herbal preparations. As a result, medicinal plants can be categorized as a meal, a therapeutic food, a nutraceutical, or a herbal remedy. This confuses consumers and patients when herbal medications are added to the list of controlled substances. For instance, in the United States, natural remedies are governed by the Dietary Supplement Health and Education Act of 1994. A dietary supplement is defined as a substance that includes a "dietary element" for consumption, such as vitamins, minerals, herbal products, and more phytochemicals from additional toxicity studies if the herb was available for purchase before 1994. Regulatory specialists in different countries and pharmacovigilance centers frequently do not share regulatory expertise regarding herbal products [46].

5.6.2 CHALLENGES ASSOCIATED WITH HERBAL–ALLOPATHIC DRUG INTERACTION

Different plants contain varying amounts of active phytoconstituents, each with its unique pharmacology, metabolism, and binding properties [47]. These constituents can interact with allopathic medications, leading to pharmacokinetic or pharmacodynamic interactions. Allopathic medications with a limited therapeutic window are more likely to have interactions with herbal drugs. For instance, patients on warfarin may experience increased bleeding due to the inhibitory effects of garlic and ginger on platelets. There are other instances of interactions between herbal drugs and allopathic medications that should be taken into consideration.

1. Ephedrine prolongs the sympathomimetic impact (hypertensive crises) by interacting with MAO inhibitors and beta-blockers.
2. Increased CNS depression with a combination of valerian and sedatives.
3. Ginseng has been found to increase the metabolism of GABA and dopamine levels in the brain by interacting with MAO inhibitors.
4. The combination of acetaminophen and kava may have adverse effects, and the use of azole antifungals can increase liver toxicity.

5.6.3 CHALLENGES RELATED TO HERBAL DRUG SAFETY

The safety of herbal medicines is a concern for consumers, regulators, and medical professionals. An adverse action analysis is more complicated for these medicines than for traditional pharmaceuticals. Various factors, such as the geographical origin, handling techniques, administration route, difficulties, and interactions with other prescription medications, make it difficult to evaluate their safety. In addition, the lack of knowledge or attention to taxonomy and classification creates a unique problem during the authentication and collection of herbal material for medicinal treatment. Producers of herbal remedies need to provide proper paperwork to ensure the safety of their products. Using commonly accepted scientific nomenclature, including synonyms, is crucial to avoid confusion caused by different names of herbal plants [48]. For example, *Artemisia absinthium* L. has 11 different common names, seven of which are completely unrelated to their biological names. The similarity in names of plants such as *V. officinalis* and *Heliotropium europaeum* (garden heliotrope) can be confusing. Hence, it is essential to use the plant's true biological name, the ingredient used, the brand name, and any adverse drug effect reactions when dealing with herbal treatments. Effective surveillance of medicinal plant safety requires collaboration among botanists, phytochemists, pharmacologists, and other key stakeholders.

5.6.4 CHALLENGES ASSOCIATED WITH CLINICAL RESEARCH

Studying herbal pharmaceuticals presents a number of challenges that must be addressed before developing a unique drug and conducting major phase III trials. These challenges include economic, moral, quality control, study plan, and regulatory concerns. In 2005, the WHO published an operational strategy outlining the regulatory requirements necessary for scientific studies on herbal products. In RCTs, blinding is the most effective way to minimize bias and remove the influence of a placebo. Typically, this procedure is carried out in a double-blind fashion, meaning that neither the analyst nor the patient is informed about the allocation of treatment. Double-blind studies are challenging to maintain with herbal preparations, however, because the therapeutic process involves a variety of therapeutic modalities, such as lifestyle counseling, listening, explaining, and lifestyle and dietary advice in addition to herbal remedy suggestions. Therefore, single blinding can be applied in which only the analyst, but not the patient, is aware of the therapeutic allocation. Other variables may impact the results of clinical studies and should be taken into consideration [49].

- When conducting a clinical trial, it is important to choose controls that are as similar as possible to the intervention group to ensure that the study can provide evidence of the specific effects of the herbal drug being tested. However, for some natural chemicals, such as ginger, finding a suitable control group may be difficult due to its distinctive odor.
- Determining the appropriate sample size is also a crucial step in the clinical trial process.
- It has been recognized that occupational harmonization is essential, particularly in research involving herbal products, where the role of the therapist is critical.

5.7 FUTURE DIRECTIONS AND CONCLUSION

While the contemporary healthcare market is worth billions of dollars, herbal medicine still has a relatively small role to play. This study examines the breadth and potential of herbal medicines, along with the issues and challenges that firms producing herbal pharmaceuticals face today. However, as things change, the popularity of herbal remedies is growing due to their high level of safety, efficacy, and synergistic impact. The stability of the formulation of herbal medications is important as it affects the drug's quality and effectiveness. Innovative approaches, such as suspension, biodegradable cellulose, therapeutic proteins, nanoparticles, and emulsifiers, can help reduce medication instability. Preventing drug degradation due to environmental variables is a major issue when it comes to medicine stability. To guarantee medication stability, all specifications, including those related to packing and containers, must be met [50]. It is crucial to conduct research on pharmacokinetics, ADME, and neonatal mortality to ensure the safety, toxicity, and effectiveness of herbal medicines, given their potential toxicity and adverse effects, including kidney damage, the development of stones, and acute neuropathy. The most critical phase in the creation of herbal medications is clinical studies and ethical considerations, which confirm safety, toxicity levels, and efficacy. Such proof is necessary to compete with existing allopathic medicines and to thrive in the global pharma market. Competent authority rules for safety and quality standards are essential for herbal producers to maintain the quality of their products. However, many herbal producers, industries, and farmers are not aware of acceptable agricultural and collection techniques (GACP) or proper storage processes due to the lack of rules and regulations. The only herbal medications that have a chance for success and global recognition are those that adhere to international regulations and GACP standards.

The commercialization and marketing of herbal treatments are challenging in today's drug era due to defects and weaknesses in quality manufacturing, standardization, business legislation, and regulatory requirements. Indian herbal medicine is hindered by low-quality raw materials, microbial contamination, and heavy metal deposition throughout the production process, from manufacturing to horticulture. These concerns hinder the expansion of the herbal sector, and the FDA prohibits low-quality and contaminated medications from reaching the international market. The production of herbal drugs is an ongoing process that adheres to the WHO's advice to use GACP and GMP to ensure the quality and standard of herbal medications. The correct implementation of drug-controlled authority regulations through establishment harmonization is necessary to prevent any delays in the registration of new drugs. Herbal firms, manufacturers, and entrepreneurs should understand the government's business and market growth plan and promote safe, high-quality pharmaceuticals that undergo frequent updates. The lack of research motivation, technological and regulatory hurdles, and the industry's low level of market participation are the causes of the small role herbal medicine plays in the contemporary healthcare market.

KEYWORDS

- **efficacy**
- **herbal drugs**
- **pharmaceutical industries**
- **regulatory requirements**
- **safety**

REFERENCES

1. World Health Organization. *WHO Guidelines for Assessing Quality of Herbal Medicines with Reference to Contaminants and Residues*. World Health Organization, 2007.
2. World Health Organization. *Research Guidelines for Evaluating the Safety and Efficacy of Herbal Medicines*. WHO Regional Office for the Western Pacific, 1993.
3. Payyappallimana, U. Role of traditional medicine in primary health care: An overview of perspectives and challenging. *Yokohama Int Soc Sci Res* 2010, 14(6), 723–743.
4. Sharma, A. K., & Pundarikakshudu, K. Regulatory aspects of Traditional Indian Medicines (TIM) in India and in international purview. *J AOAC Int* 2019, 102(4), 993–1002.
5. Gao, P., & Watanabe, K. Introduction of the world health organization project of the international classification of traditional medicine. *J Chin Integr Med* 2011, 9(11), 1161–1164.
6. Thomford, N. E., Senthebane, D. A., Rowe, A., et al., Natural products for drug discovery in the 21st century: Innovations for novel drug discovery. *Int J Mol Sci* 2018, 19(6), 1578. http://dx.doi.org/10.3390/ijms19061578
7. Sahoo, N. C., Manchikanti, P., & Dey, S. Herbal drugs: Standards and regulation. *Fitoterapia* 2010, 81(6), 462–471.
8. Bent, S. Herbal medicine in the United States: Review of efficacy, safety, and regulation. *J Gen Intern Med* 2008, 23(6), 854–859.
9. Brantley, S. J., Argikar, A. A., Lin, Y. S., Nagar, S., & Paine, M. F. Herb--Drug interactions: Challenges and opportunities for improved predictions. *Drug Metab Dispos* 2013, 42(3), 301–317.
10. Chawla, R., Thakur, P., Chowdhry, A., et al., Evidence based herbal drug standardization approach in coping with challenges of holistic management of diabetes: A dreadful lifestyle disorder of 21st century. *J Diabetes Metab Disord* 2013, 12(1), 12–35
11. Zhou, X., Li, C. G., Chang, D. H. T., & Bensoussan, A. Current status and major challenges to the safety and efficacy presented by Chinese herbal medicine. *Medicines* 2019, 6(1), 14.
12. Tilburt, J. C., & Kaptchuk, T. J. Herbal medicine research and global health: An ethical analysis. *Bull World Health Organ* 2008, 86(8), 594–599.
13. Calixto, J. B. Efficacy, safety, quality control, marketing and regulatory guidelines for herbal medicines (phytotherapeutic agents). *Braz J Med Biol Res* 2000, 33(2), 179–189.
14. Luqman, S., Rizvi, S. I., Beer, A. M., Khare, S. K., & Atukeren, P. Efficacy of herbal drugs in human diseases and disorders. *Evid-Based Complement Altern Med* 2014, 2014, 1–2.
15. Mathur, M. Phyto-complex and their role in enhancing efficacy of herbal drugs. *Med Plants* 2013, 5(3), 118.
16. Herbal Medicinal Products Market. (2025, August 7). Herbal medicinal products market report. MarketResearch.biz. Retrieved August 7, 2025, from https://marketresearch.biz/report/herbal-medicinal-products-market/accessed-on-07-08-2025

17. Choi, D., Kim, J. H., Cho, S. Y., Kim, D. H., & Chang, S. Y. Regulation and quality control of herbal drugs in Korea. *Toxicology* 2002, 181–182, 581–586.
18. Muyumba, N. W., Mutombo, S. C., Sheridan, H., Nachtergael, A., & Duez, P. Quality control of herbal drugs and preparations: The methods of analysis, their relevance and applications. *Talanta Open* 2021, 4, 100070.
19. Shinde, V., Dhalwal, K., Potdar, M., & Mahadik, K. R. Application of quality control principles to herbal drugs. *Int J Phytomed* 2009, 1(1), 4–8.
20. Evans, W. C. Trease and Evans' Pharmacognosy. 1978. http://182.160.97.198:8080/xmlui/handle/123456789/547.
21. Kuchta, K., Schmidt, M., & Nahrstedt, A.. German kava ban lifted by court: The alleged hepatotoxicity of kava (*Piper methysticum*) as a case of ill-defined herbal drug identity, lacking quality control, and misguided regulatory politics. *Planta Med* 2015, 81(18), 1647–1653.
22. Yan, B., Li, Y., Guo, Z. T., & Qu, H. Quality by design for herbal drugs: A Feedforward control strategy and an approach to define the acceptable ranges of critical quality attributes. *Phytochem Anal* 2013, 25(1), 59–65.
23. Kunle. Standardization of herbal medicines—A review. *Int J Biodivers Conserv* 2012, 4(3).
24. Rashid, S., Zafar, M., Ahmad, M., et al., Microscopic investigations and pharmacognostic techniques used for the standardization of herbal drug Nigella sativa L. *Microsc Res Tech* 2018, 81(12), 1443–1450.
25. Gautam, A., Kashyap, S. J., Sharma, P. K., Garg, V., Visht, S., & Kumar, N. Identification, evaluation and standardization of herbal drugs: A review. *Der Pharm Lett* 2010, 2(6), 302–315. https://www.cabdirect.org/abstracts/20113033868.html.
26. Bansal, A., Chhabra, V., Rawal, R. K., & Sharma, S. Chemometrics: A new scenario in herbal drug standardization. *J Pharm Anal* 2014, 4(4), 223–233.
27. Mandal, M., Misra, D. S., Ghosh, N. N., & Mandal, V. Physicochemical and elemental studies of Hydrocotyle javanica Thunb. for standardization as herbal drug. *Asian Pac J Trop Biomed* 2017, 7(11), 979–986.
28. Chawla, R., Thakur, P., Chowdhry, A., et al. Evidence based herbal drug standardization approach in coping with challenges of holistic management of diabetes: a dreadful lifestyle disorder of 21st century. *Journal of Diabetes & Metabolic Disorders*. 2013, 12(1).
29. Lazarowych, N. J., & Pekos, P. Use of fingerprinting and marker compounds for identification and standardization of botanical drugs: Strategies for applying Pharmaceutical HPLC analysis to herbal products. *Drug Inf J* 1998, 32(2), 497–512.
30. Dhiman, A., Sharma, K., Sharma, A., & Sindhu, P. A review on the status of quality control and standardization of herbal drugs in India. *Drug Development and Therapeutics* 2016, 7(2), 107.
31. Ajay, K. S., Jyoti, N., Rajak, H., Rajesh, K., & Kapoor, V. Standardization of herbal drugs: Need of the day for global competition. *J Pharm Res* 2013, 12(3), 103.
32. Brantley, S. J., Argikar, A. A., Lin, Y. S., Nagar, S., Paine, M. F. Herb–drug interactions: Challenges and opportunities for improved predictions. *Drug Metabolism and Disposition*. 2013, 42(3), 301–317.
33. Liu, S. H., Chuang, W., Lam, W., Jiang, Z., & Cheng, Y. Safety surveillance of traditional Chinese medicine: Current and future. *Drug Saf* 2015, 38(2), 117–128.

34. Morris, C. A., & Avorn, J. Internet marketing of herbal products. *JAMA* 2003, 290(11), 1505. http://dx.doi.org/10.1001/jama.290.11.1505
35. Zhou, S., Gao, Y., Jiang, W., Huang, M., Xu, A., & Paxton, J. W. Interactions of herbs with cytochrome P450. *Drug Metab Rev* 2003, 35(1), 35–98.
36. Santini, A., Cammarata, S. M., Capone, G., et al., Nutraceuticals: Opening the debate for a regulatory framework. *Br J Clin Pharmacol* 2018, 84(4), 659–672.
37. De Lima Moreira, D., Teixeira, S. S., Monteiro, M., De-Oliveira, A. C. A. X., & Paumgartten, F. J. R. Traditional use and safety of herbal medicines1. *Revista Brasileira De Farmacognosia* 2014, 24(2), 248–257.
38. Chegu, S., & Nagabhushanam, M. V. A comprehensive study on regulation of herbal drugs in India, US and European Union. *Int J Drug Regul Aff* 2021, 9(1), 78–86.
39. Parveen, A., Parveen, B., Parveen, R., & Ahmad, S. Challenges and guidelines for clinical trial of herbal drugs. *J Pharm Bioallied Sci* 2015, 7(4), 329.
40. Sen, S., Chakraborty, R., & De, B. Challenges and opportunities in the advancement of herbal medicine: India's position and role in a global context. *J Herb Med* 2011, 1(3–4), 67–75.
41. Vikaas, B., Yadav, S., Choudhary, M., & Author_Id, N. A comprehension study on regulation of herbal drugs in USA, European Union and India. *Int J Drug Regul Aff* 2017, 5(4), 8–17.
42. Rousseaux, C. G., & Schachter, H. Regulatory issues concerning the safety, efficacy and quality of herbal remedies. *Birth Defects Res* 2003, 68(6), 505–510.
43. Benzi, G., & Ceci, A. herbal medicines in European regulation. *Pharmacol Res* 1997, 35(5), 355–362.
44. Verma, N. Current regulatory challenges and approaches in the registration of herbal drugs in Europe. *Clin Res Regul Aff* 2016, 33(1), 9–24.
45. Ekor, M. The growing use of herbal medicines: Issues relating to adverse reactions and challenges in monitoring safety. *Front Pharmacol* 2014, 4, 177.
46. Alostad, A., Steinke, D., & Schafheutle, E. International comparison of five herbal medicine registration Systems to inform regulation development: United Kingdom, Germany, United States of America, United Arab Emirates and Kingdom of Bahrain. *Pharm Med* 2018, 32(1), 39–49.
47. Wang, M., & Franz, G. The role of the European pharmacopoeia (Ph Eur) in quality control of traditional Chinese herbal medicine in European member states. *World J Tradit Chin Med* 2015, 1(1), 5–15.
48. Tachjian, A., Maria, V., & Jahangir, A. Use of herbal products and potential interactions in patients with cardiovascular diseases. *J Am Coll Cardiol* 2010, 55(6), 515–525.
49. Fabricant, D. S., & Farnsworth, N. R. The value of plants used in traditional medicine for drug discovery. *Environ Health Perspect* 2001, 109(suppl 1), 69–75.
50. Mukherjee, P. K., Harwansh, R. K., Bahadur, S., & Banerjee, S., Kar, A. Evidence based validation of Indian traditional medicine—Way forward. *World J Tradit Chin Med* 2016, 2(1), 48.

CHAPTER 6

Quality Standards and Monographs for Herbal Drugs

ARYA LAKSHMI MARISETTI[1*], GANA MANJUSHA K.[2], SAURABH DAHIYA[3], M. V. N. L. CHAITANYA[4], D. S. N. B. K. PRASANT[5], VENKATESWARA RAO AMARA[6], and RITU KARWASRA[7]

[1]*Department of Pharmacognosy & Phytochemistry, School of Pharmaceutical Sciences, Delhi Pharmaceutical Sciences & Research University, New Delhi, Delhi, India*

[2]*Vignan Institute of Pharmaceutical Technology, Visakhapatnam, Andhra Pradesh, India*

[3]*Delhi Institute of Pharmaceutical Sciences and Research, Delhi Pharmaceutical Sciences and Research University, New Delhi, Delhi, India*

[4]*School of Pharmaceutical Sciences, Lovely Professional University, Punjab, India*

[5]*School of Pharmacy and Technology Management, SVKM's Narsee Monjee Institute of Management Studies (NMIMS), Polepally SEZ, TSIIC, Hyderabad, Telangana, India*

[6]*Department of Regulatory Toxicology, National Institute of Pharmaceutical Education and Research (NIPER), Hajipur, Bihar, India*

[7]*Central Council for Research in Unani Medicine (CCRUM), Ministry of AYUSH, Government of India, New Delhi, Delhi, India*

*Corresponding author

Herbal Drug Industry: From Cultivation to Innovation and Global Impact.
Abhishek Tiwari, Varsha Tiwari, and Ajay Sharma (Eds.)

DOI: 10.1201/9781779640994-6

ABSTRACT

Many developed and developing countries have policies that support the widespread use of medicinal plants, frequently as nonprescription medicines. These herbal remedies, which are significant in both history and culture, are essential for maintaining health. Herbal remedies are becoming more and more common in alternative healthcare practices around the world, even in spite of the availability of contemporary pharmaceuticals. Protection of these treatments' efficacy, safety, and quality has grown to be a major global concern. When creating comprehensive herbal monographs, pharmacognostical research plays a crucial role in guaranteeing the efficacy and safety of these medications. The scientific names, parts used, geographic distribution, and tests for authenticity and purity are only a few of the detailed details about the plants that are included in these monographs. They also comply with WHO criteria by providing information on active ingredients, dosage forms, therapeutic applications, pharmacology, and any interactions. Herbal monographs are incorporated into a number of international pharmacopeias, such as the United States Pharmacopeia, the European Pharmacopoeia, and the International Pharmacopoeia. Additionally, these monographs can be found in publications like books, journals, and databases. Additional resources on certain medicinal plants can be found from groups like the German Commission and the European Scientific Cooperative on Phytotherapy. Additional information on herbal products can be sourced from databases such as the Natural Medicines Comprehensive Database, NAPRALERT, and publications by Bhat, among others.

6.1 GENERAL PARAMETERS OF MONOGRAPHS FOR HERBAL DRUGS

An herbal monograph serves as a scientific document providing a comprehensive description of a medicinal herb, detailing its nomenclature, parts used, constituents, therapeutic applications, contraindications, side effects, potential unsuitability with other medications, dosage recommendations, and the herb's mode of action. This document plays a crucial role in establishing quality control measures for the herb in question.

Within the realm of herbal pharmacopeia, qualitative and therapeutic monographs on botanicals are outlined. These monographs establish specific standards governing the quality of distinct herbal products [1]. Herbal monographs are an essential component of quality control procedures since they are the most thorough and meticulously reviewed source of information about herbal medicine.

Over the years, the WHO has played a pivotal role in introducing monographs for medicinal plants globally. The WHO Guidelines for the Assessment of Herbal Medicines has driven the development of these monographs, aiming to standardize the quality control of herbal medicines. Between 1999 and 2009, WHO published approximately 116 monographs on both organized (e.g., whole plants or their parts) and unorganized drugs (e.g., oil, latex, juice, and secretions), categorizing them by terms like Herba, Folium, Bulbus, Radix, Flos, Fructus, Cortex, Rhizoma, or Olium.

Noteworthy publications, such as the *Complete German Commission E Monographs*, *Herbal Medicine: Expanded Commission E Monographs*, the *ABC Clinical Guide to Herbs*, and the *Identification of Medicinal Plants* by the American Botanical Council, have further contributed to the field of herbal monographs. In the European Union (EU), the Community herbal monograph provides a scientific opinion on the safety and efficacy of herbal substances intended for medicinal use. These monographs, evaluated by the Committee on Herbal Medicinal Products (HMPC), distinguish between well-established use (requiring marketing authorization [MA]) and traditional use (simplified registration).

Herbal monographs are often compiled by regulatory authorities and include scientific conclusions regarding the safety and efficacy of herbal medicine. They aim to standardize technologies and evaluation standards, promoting consistency in the review process. The herbal monograph offers scientific information on safety, efficacy, and quality control, serving as a valuable resource for appropriate herbal use across countries, research laboratories, and industries. Moreover, it provides models for countries to develop their own monographs or formularies and facilitates information exchange globally [2].

6.2 COMPONENTS OF MONOGRAPHS

Pharmacopeial monographs for herbal medicines encompass crucial information, including identity, purity, and content specifications. Each monograph typically consists of the following:

1. Monograph title
   - May include Latin names or common local and English names.
   - Specifies relevant plant part(s), state, type of preparation, and dosage form.
2. Definition
   - Offers detailed information, including Latin binomial name, taxonomic authority, plant family name, and common names.
   - Describes plant part(s), material state, type of preparation, dosage form, and harvesting season as per Good Agricultural and Collection Practices (GACP).
   - Includes names and molecular formulae of relevant constituents.
3. Identification
   - Ensures the examined herbal medicine matches the label.
   - Utilizes macroscopic and microscopic characteristics.
   - Employs chemical tests, fingerprinting, DNA-based tests, and tests for contaminants/impurities.
   - Macroscopic characteristics.
   - Specifies important botanical features for clear identification.
   - Highlights differences between species when applicable.
4. Microscopic characteristics
   - Utilizes microscopic examination for identification.
   - Crucial for herbal materials where macroscopic identification is challenging.
5. Chemical tests
   - Ensures presence and quality, avoiding nonspecific tests.
   - May include fingerprinting using chromatography or spectroscopy.
6. DNA-based tests
   - Uses polymerase chain reaction and DNA sequencing for identification.
7. Tests for contaminants/impurities
   - Covers foreign matter, elemental contaminants, microbiological quality, mycotoxins, toxic substances, and residual solvents.

8. Specifications
   - Tailored to individual herbal medicines.
   - Sets limits for undesirable constituents and includes additional tests to detect potential adulterants.
   - Addresses safety-related compounds when necessary.
9. Assay
   - Quantitatively determines constituents responsible for therapeutic activity.
   - Establishes assay limits for each constituent.
10. Physicochemical tests
    - Provides characterization standards.
    - Evaluates water and/or alcohol extractable matter, ash content, loss on drying, water content, and volatile oils, among others.
11. Other tests:
    - May include swelling index, bitterness values, particle size, or specific tests relevant to the herbal medicine.
12. Additional information
    - Covers packaging, labeling, and storage requirements consistent with regulations.
    - Offers guidance on packaging in specific cases (e.g., oils or oleoresins).
13. Reference standards
    - Describes the use of reference standards (RS) in the analysis.
    - RS may be pure substances or extracts for comparison.
14. Utilization
    - Pharmacopeial monographs establish specifications crucial for ensuring proper quality in herbal products.
    - They play a pivotal role in safeguarding patient safety.
    - Contribute to securing the global drug supply chain.
    - Accelerate product development, foster competition, and enhance patient access to quality herbal medicines.

6.3 REGULATORY CONTEXT

6.3.1 BRITISH PHARMACOPOEIA

- Role: The British Pharmacopoeia (BP), published by the British Pharmacopoeia Commission Secretariat of the Medicines and Healthcare Products Regulatory Agency, is a leading collection of standards for herbal medicinal products and pharmaceutical substances in the United Kingdom (UK).
- Function: It sets publicly available standards for the quality of medicines, contributing significantly to public health. The BP is utilized globally and is a key reference in pharmaceutical research, development, manufacturing, and testing.

6.3.2 WHO

- Role: WHO is a global health agency that has undertaken the publication of monographs on medicinal plants.
- Function: WHO's monographs provide information on the safety, efficacy, and quality of selected medicinal plants. The organization follows guidelines for the assessment of herbal medicines adopted by the International Conference of Drug Regulatory Authorities (ICDRA).

6.3.3 EUROPEAN MEDICINES AGENCY AND COMMITTEE ON HERBAL MEDICINAL PRODUCTS

- Role: The European Medicines Agency (EMA) is responsible for the scientific evaluation of medicines in the EU. HMPC is a committee within EMA focusing on herbal medicinal products.
- Function: The EU herbal monograph, created by HMPC, contains scientific opinions on safety and efficacy data about herbal substances and their preparations. EU monographs form the basis for regulatory decisions on medicinal products containing specific herbal substances or preparations in the EU.

6.3.4 INTERNATIONAL CONFERENCE OF DRUG REGULATORY AUTHORITIES

- Role: ICDRA is a forum for drug regulatory authorities worldwide.
- Function: WHO developed monographs on selected medicinal plants following the guidelines adopted by ICDRA. These guidelines guide the assessment of herbal medicines and aim for international harmonization in regulatory approaches.

6.3.5 NATIONAL PHARMACOPEIAS (E.G., US PHARMACOPEIA, INDIAN PHARMACOPOEIA)

- Role: National pharmacopeias, such as the US Pharmacopeia and Indian Pharmacopoeia (IP), provide standards for herbal medicinal products within their respective countries.
- Function: They play a crucial role in ensuring the quality and safety of drugs and herbal products. Compliance with these standards is often a requirement for regulatory approval and market access.

6.4 CHALLENGES AND THE NEED FOR HARMONIZATION

1. Divergent standards: The text highlights that monographs developed in different countries do not always conform to international standards, particularly those of ESCOP or WHO.
2. Importance of harmonization: Harmonization of standards is essential for ensuring consistency in quality, safety, and efficacy assessments globally.

Regulatory bodies like WHO, EMA, ICDRA, and national pharmacopeias play pivotal roles in establishing and enforcing standards for herbal medicines. The collaboration and harmonization efforts among these bodies are crucial for promoting global public health and facilitating international trade in herbal products.

6.5 COMPARATIVE STUDY OF MONOGRAPHS (IP, USP, AYURVEDIC PHARMACOPEIA, SIDDHA, UNANI, ETC.)

6.5.1 OVERVIEW OF DIFFERENT PHARMACOPEIAS

Herbal pharmacopeias play a vital role in fostering the responsible use of herbal medicines, aiming for the utmost efficacy and safety. This involves the establishment of rigorous standards, encompassing identity, purity, and analytical criteria for botanicals. Both traditional wisdom and scientific insights contribute to shaping these standards [3]. In the past, pharmacopeias dedicated to herbal medicines centered on plant sources and specific plant parts. This approach heavily relied on detailed macroscopic and microscopic descriptions [4]. Over time, the evolution of analytical techniques, such as chromatographic fingerprints and impurity tests, has significantly enhanced the quality of pharmacopeial monographs. This shift reflects a commitment to more precise and advanced methodologies [4]. The growing recognition of herbal drugs with robust pharmacological activities has underscored the importance of including an assay in pharmacopeial monographs. This ensures a thorough understanding and quantification of the active components, contributing to a comprehensive assessment of herbal medicines [5]. The latest guidelines, encapsulated in the "Good Pharmacopoeial Practices: Draft Chapter on Monographs on Herbal Medicines" by the WHO, stress the need for harmonizing the information in monographs. This involves aligning the definition with the monograph title and specifying crucial quality parameters, including identity, purity, and content [5].

6.5.1.1 INDIAN PHARMACOPOEIA

IP serves as a cornerstone in regulating pharmaceutical standards within India. Published by the Indian Pharmacopoeia Commission (IPC) under the Ministry of Health & Family Welfare, Government of India, IP plays a crucial role in upholding the quality of drugs as mandated by the Drugs and Cosmetics Act, 1940, and Rules 1945 [6].

6.5.1.1.1 Legal Authority and Recognition

IP stands as the official compendium of standards for drugs manufactured and marketed in India. The standards set forth in IP, which include procedures of analysis and drug specifications covering identity, purity, and strength, are of authoritative nature. These standards are not only integral during routine quality assurance processes but also hold legal acceptability in dispute resolution within the court of law [6].

6.5.1.1.2 Historical Roots (1833–1927)

The genesis of IP dates back to 1833 when a committee from the East Indian Company's Dispensary advocated for the publication of a pharmacopeia. The journey continued with the Bengal Pharmacopoeia and General Conspectus of Medicinal Plants in 1844. IP 1868 integrated drugs from both BP 1867 and indigenous sources, laying the foundation for subsequent editions. In 1927, a government-appointed Drug Enquiry Committee recommended the establishment of a National Pharmacopoeia [6].

6.5.1.1.3 Postindependence Developments (1948 Onward)

Postindependence, the IP Committee was established in 1948, with the primary objective of publishing IP. The subsequent editions, starting from the inaugural edition in 1955 to the latest in 2022, showcase a commitment to evolving pharmaceutical standards in India. Noteworthy editions include IP 1996, which introduced a supplement for Veterinary Products, and IP 2010, the sixth edition accompanied by a DVD. The most recent IP 2022, the ninth edition, continues this legacy [6].

6.5.1.1.4 Standards and Monographs

IP expresses its standards through detailed specifications and test methods. These standards, encapsulated in monographs, are applicable to various pharmaceutical articles. These monographs compile specifications relevant to ensuring compliance with IP standards [6].

6.5.1.2 BRITISH PHARMACOPOEIA

The BP stands as the authoritative compendium, setting standards for medicinal and pharmaceutical substances within the UK. Enforced by law, these standards hold sway not only in the UK but also across a significant part of the Commonwealth [7].

6.5.1.2.1 Historical Pillars (Since 1864)

Since its inception in 1864, the BP has been a stalwart provider of official standards for medicines. Over time, it has evolved into an encompassing repository, offering a comprehensive collection of standards for UK pharmaceutical substances and medicinal products. Notably, it incorporates all monographs and texts of the European Pharmacopoeia (EP) (Ph. Eur.) [7].

6.5.1.2.2 Legal Status and Effectivity

Pharmacopoeias holding legal status in the UK include the BP, which extends to the BP (Veterinary), and the Ph. Eur. Published annually in August, the BP becomes legally effective on January 1st of the ensuing year, contributing significantly to the regulatory framework [7].

6.5.1.2.3 Role in Public Health (Medicines and Healthcare products Regulatory Agency)

The BP plays a pivotal role in safeguarding public health by contributing to the functions of the Medicines and Healthcare products Regulatory Agency. Serving as a vital reference tool, it guides individuals and organizations engaged in pharmaceutical realms, spanning research, development, manufacture, and quality control and analysis [7].

6.5.1.2.4 Global Influence and Collaboration

The impact of the BP reverberates globally, reaching over 100 countries. Its influence is embedded in the medicines legislation of Commonwealth countries. Beyond national boundaries, the BP actively engages with the EP, offering expert advice and contributing significantly to the standard-setting processes in Europe. Additionally, it extends its expertise to the WHO, fostering international discussions on maintaining the quality of medicines [7].

6.5.1.3 EUROPEAN PHARMACOPOEIA

The EP stands as the pinnacle of official standards for medicines in Europe. Covering a spectrum from bulk drug substances to analytical methods, it is meticulously maintained and distributed by the European Directorate for the Quality of Medicines [8].

6.5.1.3.1 Comprehensive Quality Control

Serving as a single reference work, the EP is the linchpin for ensuring the quality control of medicines within the signatory states of the Convention on its elaboration. The standards enshrined within provide both a legal and scientific foundation, guiding the entire trajectory from development to production and marketing processes [8].

6.5.1.3.2 Scope of Standards

The EP standards encapsulate the qualitative and quantitative composition of medicines. They delineate the requisite tests for medicines, the raw materials integral to production, and the intermediates involved in synthesis. It mandates that all producers of medicines and substances for pharmaceutical use adhere to these stringent quality standards to bring their products to market within the signatory states [8].

6.5.1.3.3 Legal Mandate

The mandatory nature of the EP is fortified by a robust legal framework. Several key documents underpin this compulsion, including the Convention developed by the Council of Europe on the Elaboration of a EP. The protocol adopted in 1994 amended the Convention in preparation for the accession of the EU, outlining the powers of the EU and its member states within the EP Commission. Additionally, EU Directive 2001/83/EC and Regulation (EU) 2019/6 on veterinary medicinal products substantiate the mandatory character of EP monographs, especially in the context of seeking MA [8].

6.5.1.3.4 Undertakings of the Convention

The contracting parties of the Convention commit to a progressive elaboration of a pharmacopeia common to the concerned countries, aptly titled the "EP." Simultaneously, they pledge to take requisite measures, either through direct implementation in national legislation or indirect implementation via national translation, to ensure that EP monographs become the official standards within their respective countries [8].

6.5.1.4 UNITED STATES PHARMACOPEIA

6.5.1.4.1 Introduction

The United States Pharmacopeia (USP) stands as the official compendia of the United States, dedicated to establishing standards for excipients, drug substances, and drug products. Published annually by the United States Pharmacopeial Convention, it plays a pivotal role in ensuring the quality, safety, and efficacy of medicines [9].

6.5.1.4.2 USP–National Formulary: A Comprehensive Resource

The USP–National Formulary (NF), a cornerstone of the USP, encompasses over 5000 quality standards for medicines, covering chemical and biologic entities, active pharmaceutical ingredients, and excipients. Regarded as the most comprehensive source for medicine quality standards globally, it serves as a linchpin for safeguarding the well-being of patients [9].

6.5.1.4.3 Global Impact and Utilization

The influence of USP extends far beyond US borders. It is not only an official quality standard for medicines marketed in the United States but is also extensively utilized in over 140 countries worldwide. Integrated into the laws of more than 40 countries, USP has become a universal benchmark for medicine quality standards [9].

6.5.1.4.4 Three-Tiered Quality Standards in USP-NF

The USP-NF employs a three-tiered approach to quality standards for prescription medicines:

1. Monographs: These specify the identification, potency, purity, and efficacy requirements that should be met by a medication. Furthermore, monographs describe the crucial examinations necessary to guarantee that a medication and its constituent parts fulfill these exacting standards.
2. General chapters: These chapters provide industry-wide information that is crucial for promoting the development and manufacturing of novel, generic, and biosimilar medications. They do this by outlining accepted procedures, tests, and methodologies.
3. Material reference standards: These requirements verify the capacity of a medication and its constituent parts to pass testing, guaranteeing tight adherence to quality standards when combined with monographs and general chapters.

6.5.2 BRIEF INTRODUCTION TO OTHER PHARMACOPEIAS

1. IP: Enforced by regulatory authorities in India, IP has a rich history dating back to 1833, providing authoritative standards for drugs manufactured and marketed in India [6].
2. EP: Serving as the gold standard for medicines in Europe, EP outlines legal and scientific bases for quality control, with mandatory status in signatory states [8].
3. Government initiatives in India: The Government of India, through the Pharmacopoeia Commission for Indian Medicine & Homoeopathy (PCIM&H), consolidates efforts in developing Pharmacopoeial Standards for Ayurvedic, Unani, Siddha, and Homoeopathic drugs. Acting as a Central Drug Testing cum Appellate Laboratory, PCIM&H ensures the quality and safety of Indian systems of Medicine & Homoeopathy [9].

6.5.2.1 AYURVEDIC PHARMACOPEIA

The API holds the status of a legalized document sanctioned by the Government of India. It serves as a comprehensive guide delineating the quality, purity, and strength standards for specific drugs. These drugs are manufactured, distributed, and sold by licensed manufacturers across India.

6.5.2.1.1 Regulatory Mandate and Compliance

The API, once approved by the authoritative body—the Ayurvedic pharmacopeia Committee—becomes legally binding under the Drugs and Cosmetics Act of 1940. Compliance with the prescribed quality standards outlined in the API is mandatory for all stakeholders involved in the production and distribution of Ayurvedic medicines.

6.5.2.1.2 Two-Part Presentation

The API adopts a two-part structure to encapsulate its standards:

1. Part I: The monographs in this section provide more detail on particular compound formulations that are made from natural sources and are all included in the Ayurvedic Formulary of India.
2. Part II: Including monographs on specific medications obtained from schedule 1 books in accordance with the 1940 Drugs and Cosmetics Act, this section includes insights from popular Ayurvedic classics spanning different periods.

6.5.2.2 SIDDHA AND UNANI PHARMACOPEIA

The Siddha Pharmacopoeia of India holds the status of a legal document, establishing stringent standards for the quality of Siddha drugs and substances. This compilation of standards operates within the regulatory framework defined by the Drugs and Cosmetics Act of 1940.

6.5.2.2.1 Historical Inception

Published for the first time in 2008, the Siddha Pharmacopoeia of India reflects a dedicated effort to codify and regulate the quality parameters of Siddha medicines. This pharmacopeia stands as a vital reference for manufacturers, practitioners, and regulatory bodies.

6.5.2.2.2 Coordination and Publication

The Siddha section of the PCIM&H takes charge of coordinating with the Siddha Pharmacopoeia Committee. This collaboration leads to the publication of official pharmacopeias and formularies, ensuring adherence to established standards.

The Unani Pharmacopoeia serves as a crucial reference book, delineating standards and specifications for the preparation, quality, and identification of medicines within the Unani system of medicine. Unani medicine, rooted in Greco-Arabic traditions, draws from the teachings of Hippocrates and the medical practices of ancient Persia and India.

6.5.2.2.3 Historical and Philosophical Roots

This ancient traditional system finds its origins in the wisdom of Greek physician Hippocrates, seamlessly blending with the medical traditions of ancient Persia and India. The Unani Pharmacopoeia encapsulates these diverse influences, providing a comprehensive guide for practitioners, pharmacists, and manufacturers involved in Unani medicine production (Table 6.1).

6.5.2.3 UNITED STATES PHARMACOPEIA

1. Identity test
   - Microscopic examination of characteristic features.
   - Thin-layer chromatography (TLC) fingerprinting for identity confirmation.
2. Purity tests
   - Heavy metals test for limits on toxic elements.
   - Microbial limits test for microbial contamination.
   - Residue on ignition to assess the inorganic residue after ignition.

TABLE 6.1 Comparative Analysis of Monographs in Various Pharmacopeias

American Herbal Pharmacopoeia	Indian Pharmacopoeia
Monograph contents in format	Definition
Plant name	Statement of purity
Nomenclature	Category
Botanical nomenclature	Usual strength
Botanical family	Description
Pharmaceutical nomenclature	Identification
Definition	Tests
Common names	Foreign organic matter
History	Ethanol soluble/water soluble extractive
Identification	Total ash/acid-insoluble ash/water-soluble ash
Botanical identification	Heavy metals
Macroscopic identification	Loss on drying
Microscopic identification	Microbial contamination
Commercial sources and handling	Weight per ml
Sourcing	Refractive index
Collection	Relative density
Cultivation	Optical rotation
Postharvest handling	Acid value, acetyl value, hydroxyl value, iodine value, saponification value
Drying	Assay
Storage	Storage
Adulterants	Labeling
Qualitative differentiation	
Preparations	

TABLE 6.1 *(Continued)*

American Herbal Pharmacopoeia	Indian Pharmacopoeia
Constituents	HPLC/GC chromatogram
Analytical	TLC chromatogram
High-performance thin layer chromatography (HPTLC)	British Herbal Pharmacopoeia
High performance liquid chromatography (HPLC)	Format
Quantitative standards	Characteristics
Therapeutics	Quantitative standards
Pharmacokinetics	Material of commerce
Pharmacodynamics and clinical efficacy	Powdered material
Animal and *in vitro* studies	
Pharmacological effects—research studies	
Medical indications supported by clinical Trials	
Medical indications supported by traditional and modern experience	
Actions	
Substantiation for structure and functional Claims	
Dosages	
Safety profile	
Adverse reactions	
Interactions	
Reproductive and developmental effects	
Carcinogenicity	
Toxicology	
Contraindications	
Precautions	

TABLE 6.1 *(Continued)*

American Herbal Pharmacopoeia	Indian Pharmacopoeia
Lactation	
Influence on driving	
Overdose	
Treatment of overdose	
Classification of the American Herbal Products Association	
Conclusion	
International status	
References	
Ayurvedic Pharmacopoeia	**International Pharmacopoeia**
Drug names: The Sanskrit name for each drug is listed first in each monograph, and it represents that particular drug	Chemical name
Introduction: The first part of every monograph begins with a synopsis in Sanskrit and the Latin scientific name of the medicine. It also provides a succinct description of the drug's properties, habitat, distribution, and, if relevant, methods of collection. Synonyms	Description
Description	Solubility
Macroscopic	Category
Microscopic	Storage
Identity, purity, and strength	Additional information
Constituents	Requirements
Properties and action	Definition
Important formulations	Macroscopical examination
Therapeutic uses	Microscopical examination
Dose	Identity tests
	Solubility in water and acidity
	Insoluble matter
	Sulfated ash
	Loss on drying

TABLE 6.1 *(Continued)*

Siddha Pharmacopoeia	WHO Monographs
Name of the drugs—The name given on the top of each monograph of the drug is in Tamil	Definition
Introductory para—Each monograph begins with an introductory paragraph indicating the part, scientific name of the drug in Latin with short description about its habit, distribution and method of collection, if any	Synonyms
Synonyms	Selected vernacular names
Description	Description
Macroscopic	Plant material of interest:
Microscopic	General appearance
Identity, purity, and strength	Organoleptic properties
Constituents	Microscopic characteristics
Properties and action	Microscopic characteristics
Important formulations	Geographical distribution
Therapeutic uses	Genera identity tests
Dose	Purity tests
	Microbiology
	Total ash
	Acid-insoluble ash not
	Water-soluble extractive
	Alcohol-soluble extractive
	Pesticide residues
	Heavy metals
	Radioactive residues
	Other purity tests
	Chemical assays
	Major chemical constituents

TABLE 6.1 *(Continued)*

Siddha Pharmacopoeia	WHO Monographs
	Dosage forms
	Medicinal uses
	Uses supported by clinical data
	Uses described in pharmacopeias and in traditional systems of medicine
	Uses described in folk medicine, not supported by experimental or clinical data
	Pharmacology
	Experimental pharmacology
	Clinical pharmacology
	Contraindications
	Warnings
	Precautions
	Carcinogenesis, mutagenesis, impairment of fertility
	Other precautions
	Adverse reactions
	Posology
	References

3. Assay (quantitative analysis)
    - High-performance liquid chromatography (HPLC) for quantification of active constituents.
    - Gas chromatography (GC) for volatile components.
4. Specific tests
    - Specific tests for known adulterants or substitutes.
    - pH determination for acidity or alkalinity.

6.5.2.4 EUROPEAN PHARMACOPOEIA (PH. EUR.)

1. Identity and quality control
    - Macroscopic and microscopic examinations for identification.
    - Limits for microbial contamination, including total aerobic microbial count.
    - Limits for aflatoxins, pesticides, and heavy metals.
2. Chromatographic methods
    - TLC for identification and qualitative analysis.
    - HPLC for quantitative determination of active constituents.
    - GC for volatile components.
3. Therapeutic claims
    - Traditional uses and therapeutic claims may be mentioned.

6.5.2.5 INDIAN PHARMACOPOEIA

1. Botanical description
    - Detailed botanical description, including the macroscopic and microscopic characteristics of the plant source.
2. Chemical constituents
    - Quantitative determination of major chemical constituents, possibly using methods like HPLC or GC.
    - Limits for impurities and contaminants.

3. Pharmacological actions
   - Information on the pharmacological actions and potential therapeutic uses.
4. Safety aspects
   - Contraindications and side effects.
   - Specific safety tests, such as acute toxicity studies.
5. Dosage and use
   - Recommended dosage forms and preparation methods.
   - Dosage recommendations for therapeutic use.

6.5.3 KEY PARAMETERS IN HERBAL DRUG EVALUATION

1. Analytical techniques
   - HPLC and GC are commonly used in all three pharmacopeias for quantitative analysis.
   - TLC is commonly employed for qualitative analysis and fingerprinting.
2. Quality control measures
   - All three pharmacopeias include tests for microbial contamination, heavy metals, and other impurities.
   - Limits for specific contaminants may vary based on regional regulations and practices.
3. Therapeutic claims
   - USP and Ph. Eur. may provide limited information on traditional uses, while IP may include more extensive details.
4. Safety aspects
   - IP places significant emphasis on safety aspects, including contraindications and toxicity studies.
   - USP and Ph. Eur. may focus more on general safety considerations.
5. Dosage and preparation
   - Differences may exist in dosage recommendations and preparation methods, reflecting regional preferences.

6.5.4 COMPARISON OF HERBAL DRUG STANDARDS ACROSS MAJOR PHARMACOPOEIAS

1. Harmonization
   - USP and Ph. Eur.: Similarities may be observed in terms of analytical methods, identity criteria, and dosage form recommendations, reflecting harmonization efforts between these pharmacopeias.
   - IP: While IP may share commonalities, it may also include information specific to the Indian healthcare context.
2. Analytical techniques
   - USP and Ph. Eur.: Both may recommend advanced analytical techniques, such as HPLC or GC, ensuring precision in quantitative analysis.
   - IP: May have variations in recommended analytical methods based on regional preferences or resources.
3. Therapeutic claims and safety
   - IP and Ph. Eur.: Both may provide information on therapeutic claims and safety aspects, reflecting an acknowledgment of traditional uses and safety considerations.
   - USP: May focus more on purity and quality control but may include relevant safety information.
4. Dosage and preparation
   - Consistency: The pharmacopeias may differ in dosage recommendations and preparation methods based on regional practices and historical usage.

6.6 HARMONIZATION EFFORTS IN INDIA

The Ministry of Ayush has embarked on a significant initiative to harmonize the monographs across various pharmacopeias, including API, Siddha Pharmacopoeia of India (SPI), Unani Pharmacopoeia of India (UPI), Homoeopathic Pharmacopoeia of India (HPI), and IP. This undertaking aims at the promotion and facilitation of "One Herb, One Standard."

6.6.1 GOVERNMENT COLLABORATION

In a notable development, the PCIM&H under the Ministry of Ayush and the IPC under the Ministry of Health & Family Welfare formalized this commitment through a Memorandum of Understanding (MoU) signed on August 30, 2022.

6.6.2 REGULATORY SIGNIFICANCE

The standards and analytical methods prescribed in API, SPI, UPI, and HPI are not only regulatory standards but also integral components aligning with global recommendations. These standards aim to synchronize with the guidelines of the WHO and other major national and international pharmacopeias, including the IP.

6.6.3 INCORPORATING ADVANCED TECHNIQUES

The IP introduces modern analytical techniques, such as DNA and high-performance thin-layer chromatography fingerprinting profiles for identification, as well as HPLC for assay techniques. These advancements are reflected in the latest volumes of API, emphasizing the commitment to promoting phytopharmaceuticals with enhanced standards.

6.7 INTERNATIONAL HERBAL PHARMACOPEIAS (AMERICAN, BRITISH, WHO GUIDELINES)

6.7.1 AMERICAN HERBAL PHARMACOPEIA: SHAPING STANDARDS FOR HERBAL MEDICINES

The American Herbal Pharmacopeia (AHP) stands as a significant authority in the realm of herbal medicine, dedicated to setting standards and providing comprehensive monographs for botanicals. Established to ensure the responsible use of herbal medicines, AHP plays a vital role in promoting quality, safety, and efficacy in the herbal industry.

6.7.1.1 MISSION AND OBJECTIVES

1. Promoting responsible use
   - AHP is committed to promoting the responsible use of herbal medicines, emphasizing evidence-based practices and scientific rigor.
2. Scientifically sound monographs
   - AHP develops scientifically sound monographs that serve as detailed reference documents for herbal products, offering guidance on quality, identity, and safety.

6.7.1.2 KEY FEATURES OF AHP

1. Monographs for botanicals
   - AHP provides detailed monographs for a wide range of botanicals used in traditional and modern herbal medicine. These monographs encompass information on botanical identification, parts used, constituents, preparation methods, and quality standards.
2. Quality standards
   - AHP sets stringent quality standards for herbal medicines, ensuring that products meet specified criteria for identity, purity, strength, and composition.
3. Industry guidance
   - AHP's monographs and standards serve as valuable resources for herbal product manufacturers, offering guidance on the development, production, and quality control of herbal formulations.
4. Peer-reviewed publications
   - AHP contributes to the scientific literature through peer-reviewed publications, furthering the understanding of herbal medicines and their applications.

5. Collaborative initiatives

    - AHP engages in collaborative initiatives with industry stakeholders, healthcare professionals, and regulatory bodies to foster a collective commitment to quality in the herbal industry.

6.7.1.3 AHP'S IMPACT ON THE HERBAL INDUSTRY

1. Global recognition

    - AHP's standards are recognized globally, influencing industry practices and contributing to the international harmonization of herbal medicine standards.

2. Trust and credibility

    - Products adhering to AHP standards gain trust and credibility among consumers, healthcare practitioners, and regulatory authorities.

3. Facilitating market access

    - AHP's standards assist herbal product manufacturers in meeting regulatory requirements, thereby facilitating market access and international trade.

6.7.1.4 AHP'S CONTRIBUTION TO HERBAL RESEARCH AND EDUCATION

1. Supporting research

    - AHP's monographs provide a foundation for herbal research, enabling scientists and researchers to build on established standards and explore new avenues in herbal medicine.

2. Educational resources

    - AHP serves as an educational resource for students, healthcare professionals, and herbalists, offering insights into the quality and safety considerations of herbal medicines.

6.7.1.5 CHALLENGES AND FUTURE DIRECTIONS

1. Dynamic nature of herbal medicine
   - AHP faces the challenge of keeping pace with the dynamic nature of herbal medicine, requiring continuous updates and revisions to reflect emerging scientific knowledge.
2. Global collaboration
   - AHP continues to explore opportunities for global collaboration, working with other pharmacopeias and regulatory bodies to further harmonize international standards for herbal medicines.

6.7.2 BRITISH HERBAL PHARMACOPOEIA: SETTING STANDARDS FOR HERBAL MEDICINE

The British Herbal Pharmacopoeia (BHP) stands as a cornerstone in the regulation and standardization of herbal medicines in the UK. It provides a comprehensive set of guidelines and monographs that define the quality, identity, and safety of herbal substances used in medicinal products.

6.7.2.1 MISSION AND OBJECTIVES

1. Quality assurance
   - BHP is committed to ensuring the quality and safety of herbal medicines through the establishment of rigorous standards and guidelines.
2. Pharmacopeial monographs
   - BHP develops detailed pharmacopeial monographs for a wide range of herbal substances, providing a comprehensive reference for herbalists, practitioners, and the herbal product industry.

6.7.2.2 KEY FEATURES OF BHP

1. Comprehensive monographs
   - BHP provides detailed monographs that encompass botanical identification, chemical constituents, therapeutic uses, and quality standards for herbal substances.

2. Quality standards
    - BHP sets stringent quality standards for herbal medicines, covering aspects such as purity, strength, and composition.
3. Traditional and modern medicine integration
    - BHP integrates traditional herbal knowledge with modern scientific principles, ensuring a balanced and evidence-based approach to herbal medicine standards.
4. Legal and regulatory compliance
    - BHP assists in establishing legal and regulatory compliance for herbal products, supporting adherence to standards recognized by regulatory authorities.

6.7.2.3 BHP'S IMPACT ON THE HERBAL INDUSTRY

1. Global recognition
    - BHP's standards are widely recognized internationally, influencing herbal product manufacturers and contributing to global harmonization efforts.
2. Quality benchmark
    - Products meeting BHP standards are considered benchmarks of quality, enhancing the credibility and trustworthiness of herbal medicines in the global market.
3. Facilitating international trade
    - BHP's standards facilitate international trade by providing a common reference for the quality and safety of herbal substances.

6.7.2.4 BHP'S CONTRIBUTION TO HERBAL RESEARCH AND EDUCATION

1. Research support
    - BHP's monographs serve as a foundation for herbal research, supporting scientific investigations into the efficacy and safety of herbal substances.

2. Education resource

    - BHP contributes to herbal education by providing a reliable resource for students, practitioners, and researchers interested in the pharmacopeial standards of herbal medicines.

6.7.2.5 CHALLENGES AND FUTURE DIRECTIONS

1. Dynamic nature of herbal medicine

    - BHP addresses the dynamic nature of herbal medicine by regularly updating and revising monographs to align with emerging scientific knowledge and industry developments.

2. Global collaboration

    - BHP continues to explore opportunities for collaboration with other pharmacopeias and regulatory bodies, fostering global harmonization of herbal medicine standards.

The WHO plays a pivotal role in establishing global guidelines and standards for the development and inclusion of herbal drugs in international pharmacopeias. These guidelines serve as a framework to ensure the quality, safety, and efficacy of herbal medicines on a global scale.

6.7.3 WHO GUIDELINES FOR DEVELOPING MONOGRAPHS OF HERBAL DRUGS

1. Scientific rigor

    - WHO emphasizes the importance of scientific rigor in developing monographs, encouraging the integration of traditional knowledge with evidence-based approaches.

2. Botanical identification

    - Clear guidelines are provided for the accurate botanical identification of herbal drugs, ensuring consistency in the naming and classification of plant materials.

3. Quality standards

    - WHO establishes standards for the quality of herbal drugs, encompassing parameters such as identity, purity, strength, and composition.

4. Safety considerations
   - Guidelines address safety considerations, including potential toxicities, contraindications, and interactions, to ensure the safe use of herbal medicines.
5. Pharmacological actions
   - WHO encourages the inclusion of information on the pharmacological actions and potential therapeutic uses of herbal drugs in monographs.
6. Dosage and administration
   - Clear recommendations for dosage forms, routes of administration, and dosage regimens are outlined to guide healthcare practitioners and consumers.

6.7.4.1 WHO-PUBLISHED MONOGRAPHS

1. Purpose of WHO monographs
   - WHO publishes monographs on selected medicinal plants to provide authoritative information on their safety, efficacy, and quality.
2. Global collaborations
   - WHO collaborates with experts from around the world to ensure that monographs reflect diverse traditional practices and scientific advancements.
3. Inclusion in international pharmacopeias
   - Monographs published by WHO serve as a valuable resource for inclusion in international pharmacopeias, contributing to global harmonization of herbal medicine standards.
4. Comprehensive information
   - WHO monographs offer comprehensive information on medicinal plants, covering botanical characteristics, therapeutic uses, dosage recommendations, and safety profiles.

6.7.4.2 IMPACT ON GLOBAL HERBAL MEDICINE STANDARDS

1. Regulatory alignment
   - WHO guidelines contribute to the alignment of regulatory frameworks globally, fostering consistency in the evaluation and regulation of herbal medicines.
2. Global recognition
   - Herbal products adhering to WHO guidelines and monographs gain international recognition, facilitating acceptance in diverse markets.
3. Capacity building
   - WHO supports capacity-building initiatives, assisting countries in developing the expertise and infrastructure needed to implement herbal medicine regulations.

6.7.4.3 CHALLENGES AND FUTURE DIRECTIONS

1. Diversity of herbal traditions
   - Addressing the diversity of herbal traditions remains a challenge, requiring ongoing efforts to incorporate varied knowledge systems into global standards.
2. Emerging scientific knowledge
   - WHO continuously updates guidelines to reflect emerging scientific knowledge, ensuring that herbal medicine standards remain current and relevant.

6.8 COMPARISON WITH NATIONAL PHARMACOPEIAS

Pharmacopeias, both international and national, play a critical role in establishing standards for the quality, safety, and efficacy of medicinal products, including herbal drugs. A comparative analysis of international pharmacopeias, such as the USP, EP (Ph. Eur.), and national pharmacopeias like the IP and Japanese Pharmacopoeia (JP), sheds light on both differences and similarities in the regulation of herbal drugs.

6.8.1 INTERNATIONAL PHARMACOPEIAS

1. United States pharmacopeia

    - Focus: Emphasizes standards for drugs and healthcare products, including herbal drugs.
    - Influence: Globally recognized and widely used, influencing pharmaceutical practices worldwide.
    - Comprehensive: Addresses identity, purity, strength, and quality control of herbal drugs.
    - Analytical techniques: Utilizes advanced analytical techniques such as HPLC, GC, and TLC.

2. European Pharmacopoeia (Ph. Eur.)

    - Harmonization: Aims at harmonizing pharmaceutical standards across Europe.
    - Multinational recognition: Recognized by numerous countries beyond Europe, contributing to international standards.
    - Herbal emphasis: Provides detailed monographs on herbal drugs, covering botanical identification, purity, and quality control.

3. Japanese Pharmacopoeia

    - Cultural integration: Reflects Japan's unique cultural and traditional approach to medicine.
    - Monographs: Includes monographs for herbal drugs, detailing specifications for quality and safety.
    - Compatibility: Integrates with international standards to facilitate global trade and exchange.

6.8.2 NATIONAL PHARMACOPEIAS

1. Indian Pharmacopoeia

    - Cultural diversity: Reflects the rich tradition of herbal medicine in India, encompassing diverse plant species.
    - Ayurvedic integration: Recognizes and includes Ayurvedic principles in the monographs for herbal drugs.

- Quality standards: Sets stringent quality standards for raw materials and finished herbal products.
- Safety emphasis: Focuses on safety considerations, particularly in the context of traditional herbal formulations.

2. Japanese Pharmacopoeia

   - Herbal tradition: Integrates traditional Japanese herbal practices into the pharmacopeial standards.
   - Kampo medicine: Incorporates standards for Kampo medicines, traditional Japanese herbal formulations.
   - Quality assurance: Emphasizes quality control for herbal drugs used in traditional medicine.

6.8.3 DIFFERENCES AND SIMILARITIES

1. Cultural emphasis

   Difference: National pharmacopeias like IP and JP often reflect the cultural and traditional practices of their respective regions.

   Similarity: Both international and national pharmacopeias prioritize the safety and efficacy of herbal drugs.

2. Analytical techniques

   Difference: Specific analytical techniques may vary between pharmacopeias.

   Similarity: All pharmacopeias utilize advanced analytical methods to ensure accurate quality assessment.

3. Regulatory framework

   Difference: National pharmacopeias are integral to the regulatory frameworks of individual countries.

   Similarity: International pharmacopeias contribute to global regulatory harmonization and facilitate international trade.

4. Integration of traditional medicine

   Difference: National pharmacopeias, especially in countries with rich traditional medicine practices, may integrate traditional knowledge more explicitly.

Similarity: Both international and national pharmacopeias recognize the significance of traditional medicine in healthcare systems.

The differences and similarities among international pharmacopeias (USP, EP) and national pharmacopeias (IP, JP) have profound implications for global trade and standardization in the herbal drug industry.

1. Harmonization challenges
   - Implication: Variability in standards across different pharmacopeias poses challenges for global harmonization.
   - Impact: Inconsistencies may hinder seamless acceptance of herbal products in diverse markets, impacting international trade.
2. Cultural diversity and acceptance
   - Implication: National pharmacopeias, influenced by cultural traditions, may have unique standards not fully aligned with international counterparts.
   - Impact: Products meeting national standards may face acceptance challenges in regions where cultural differences are not adequately recognized.
3. Analytical techniques and compatibility
   - Implication: Differences in recommended analytical techniques may affect the compatibility of herbal drug quality assessment.
   - Impact: Manufacturers may need to adapt their testing methods to meet diverse pharmacopeial requirements, increasing the complexity of international trade.
4. Regulatory compliance
   - Implication: Divergent regulatory frameworks based on different pharmacopeial standards may pose hurdles for businesses.
   - Impact: Manufacturers must navigate varying regulatory requirements, potentially leading to delays and increased costs in product registration and market access.

5. Quality assurance and consumer confidence
    - Implication: Harmonized standards enhance quality assurance and consumer confidence in herbal products.
    - Impact: Products adhering to consistent standards are more likely to gain acceptance in global markets, fostering trust among consumers and regulatory bodies.
6. Integration of traditional knowledge
    - Implication: The integration of traditional knowledge in national pharmacopeias may offer unique perspectives on herbal medicine.
    - Impact: Recognition of traditional practices can enhance the diversity of available herbal products but may require careful consideration to align with international standards.
7. Global regulatory alignment
    - Implication: Collaborative efforts toward global regulatory alignment are crucial for facilitating international trade.
    - Impact: Streamlining regulatory processes based on common standards reduces barriers to market entry and promotes a level playing field for businesses.
8. Capacity building and information sharing
    - Implication: Capacity-building initiatives should address the need for information sharing and training in diverse pharmacopeial standards.
    - Impact: Enhanced expertise and knowledge sharing contribute to a more informed and adaptable herbal industry, supporting global trade.
9. Research and development considerations
    - Implication: Variability in pharmacopeial standards may influence priorities for research and development.
    - Impact: Industry focus on specific markets or regions may influence innovation and investment patterns in herbal drug development.

10. Need for a common framework
    - Implication: The existence of different pharmacopeias underscores the need for a common international framework.
    - Impact: Establishing a universally accepted set of standards can streamline trade, ensure product quality, and promote equitable market access.

6.9 ROLE OF WHO GUIDELINES

Concerns about the safety and quality of completed herbal medical goods and medicinal plant materials have increased due to the global upsurge in the use of herbal medicines and the large market for these products. Varying nations have varying national laws and licensing requirements for herbal medicines, which causes serious problems for the pharmaceutical industry, health authorities, and the general public [10]. Herbal medicines can be classified as either prescription or over-the-counter in areas where they are governed. Beyond medications and meals, there is one more category of herbal goods that are distinct from the others. Although these herbal remedies that fall under the nonmedicinal category are becoming more and more popular, there are risks associated with them because of lax regulation, unreliable quality control, and less strict routes of distribution such mail orders and online sales. The World Health Assembly's resolution WHA56.31, which addressed traditional medicine at its 56th session in May 2003, exhorts member states to give top priority to guaranteeing the efficacy, safety, and caliber of herbal remedies. It exhorts nations to publish monographs or national standards for herbal raw materials and traditional medicine formulations, when appropriate [11]. The Director-General of the WHO was asked to provide technical support to establish procedures for monitoring and guaranteeing the efficacy, safety, and quality of herbal products. The WHO was also entrusted with creating rules and promoting information sharing in this field. The ongoing development and updates of technical guidelines regarding the quality, safety, and efficacy of herbal medicines have been called for at several conferences, including the Meeting of National Centres in the WHO Drug Monitoring Programme and the ICDRA. A detailed evaluation of the full production process of herbal medicines, from raw materials to distribution, was conducted during the

July 2001 WHO informal meeting in Ottawa, Canada, on quality control procedures for finished herbal products. The meeting's recommendations led to the creation of broad guidelines that are primarily focused on safety and quality, with a special emphasis on toxins and residues in herbal medicines. However, national agencies and parties involved in the distribution of herbal medicines have a number of difficulties in guaranteeing the quality and safety of these medications. These difficulties include creating and implementing quality standards as well as the procedures that follow for oversight and enforcement [12]. Local and particular needs should be taken into account when developing national policies and laws that are based on WHO principles. This document offers both broad and detailed guidelines for setting norms and principles. Traditional herbal remedies run the risk of becoming unavailable to their traditional users and possibly even to new users in the lack of pertinent national standards. The inability to comply with trade, registration, import, and export regulations; lowered confidence as a result of perceived health hazards; and an increase in reported adverse events linked to these medications are possible causes of this. There have been cases reported worldwide wherein herbal remedies or medical plants were found to include undesired or unwanted ingredients. These materials included heavy metals, arsenic, viruses, mycotoxins, pesticides, and radioactive particles, among other microorganisms [13]. The WHO is committed to developing a new set of technical guidelines that center on the safety and quality control of herbal medicines in order to reduce the possibility of unfavorable occurrences associated with these products. The group also plans to update current technical documentation in this field. These initiatives are in line with the WHO's 2002–2005 Traditional Medicine Strategy. The WHO has developed extensive worldwide guidelines that are a component of the larger quality control framework for herbal medicines. These guidelines particularly address the evaluation of safety with regard to potentially hazardous components in herbal medicines, with a focus on pesticide residues and biological, chemical, and radioactive pollutants.

6.10 CONCLUSION

Many attempts have been made to produce herbal monographs that set standards for identification and quality as a result of the growing usage of herbal medications. Nevertheless, the monographs created and released in various nations do not adhere to international standards, especially those established by organizations such as the WHO (1997) or the European Scientific Cooperative on Phytotherapy. The ICDRA set rules for evaluating herbal medicines, which the WHO has followed with the development of 116 monographs for specific medicinal plants. These monographs, however, do not provide a single, comprehensive source of information regarding medicinal plants. Specifically, they do not include the botany, agronomy, quality control, safety, efficacy, and regulatory aspects of herbal medicine that are required for regulation. An uniform monograph template is required in order to organize the current body of knowledge on medicinal plants. This material should include general details, cultivation, quality control, safety, efficacy, market data, regulatory considerations, and references, in addition to botanical and pharmacognostic authentication, culture, and quality control. To incorporate new information about the safety, efficacy, and quality of herbal products from a variety of literature sources, periodic supplementation and updates of these monographs are required. Furthermore, greater research efforts are required in order to produce thorough, educational monographs. These monographs ought to be vital resources for knowledge about medicinal plants; they should include quality control tests for herbal and synthetic medications as well as guarantee the security of herbal formulations used in pharmaceutical compounding.

KEYWORDS

- **herbal monographs**
- **pharmacognosy**
- **medicinal plants**
- **herbal medicine regulation**
- **pharmacopeia standards**
- **safety evaluation**

REFERENCES

1. Alamgir, A. N. M. Pharmacopoeia and herbal monograph, the aim and use of WO's herbal monograph, WHO's guide lines for herbal monograph, pharmacognostical research and monographs of organized, unorganized drugs and drugs from animal sources. In: *Therapeutic Use of Medicinal Plants and Their Extracts: Volume 1. Progress in Drug Research*. Springer: Cham, 2017, vol 73. https://doi.org/10.1007/978-3-319-63862-1_7
2. Good pharmacopoeial practices. In: *WHO Expert Committee on Specifications for Pharmaceutical Preparations: Fiftieth Report*. World Health Organization: Geneva, 2016: Annex 1 (WHO Technical Report Series, No. 996).
3. Kim, N. C. Need for pharmacopeial quality standards for botanical dietary supplements and herbal medicines. *Food Suppl Biomater Health* 2021, 1(1), e10. https://doi.org/10.52361/fsbh.2021.1.e10
4. Länger, R., Stöger, E., Kubelka, W., & Helliwell, K. Quality standards for herbal drugs and herbal drug preparations—Appropriate or improvements necessary? *Planta Med* 2018, 84(6-07), 350–360.
5. World Health Organization (WHO). *Good Pharmacopoeial Practices: Draft Chapter on Monographs on Herbal Medicines*. WHO: Geneva, 2017.
6. https://www.ipc.gov.in/
7. http://www.pharmacopoeia.co.uk/
8. http://www.pheur.org
9. http://www.usp.org/
10. Bandaranayake, W. M. *Quality Control, Screening, Toxicity, and Regulation of Herbal Drugs. Modern Phytomedicine: Turning Medicinal Plants into Drugs*. WILEY-VCH Press: Weinheim, 2006, pp. 25–57.
11. World Health Organization. *Medicinal Plants in China, WHO Regional Publications, WesternPaci®cSeriesNo.2*. WHO: Geneva, Switzerland, 1989.
12. World Health Organization—Traditional Medicine. *Regulatory Situation of Herbal Medicines. A Worldwide Review*. WHO: Geneva, Switzerland, 1998, pp. 1±5.
13. World Health Organization—Traditional Medicine. *WHO Monographs on Selected Medicinal Plants*. WHO: Geneva, Switzerland, 1999, Vol. I.

CHAPTER 7

Testing of Natural Products and Drugs

JAYA NARHIRE[1], GANESH ASABE[1], NITIN WADATE[1], CHANTIBABU KATTA[1], DEEPANKAR BAHUGUNA[1], SOHAM LOHARKAR[1], GOPAL BAJAD[1], JITENDER MADAN[1,*], SRINIVAS NANDURI[2], SAMANTHULA GANANADHAMU[3], ASHISH BALDI[4], SNIGDHA SINGH[5], RAMESH CHANDRA[5,6,7,8]

[1]*Department of Pharmaceutics, National Institute of Pharmaceutical Education and Research, Hyderabad, Telangana, India*

[2]*Department of Chemical Sciences, National Institute of Pharmaceutical Education and Research, Hyderabad, Telangana, India*

[3]*Department of Analytical Sciences, National Institute of Pharmaceutical Education and Research, Hyderabad, Telangana, India*

[4]*Department of Pharmaceutical Sciences and Technology, Maharaja Ranjit Singh Punjab Technical University, Punjab, India*

[5]*Department of Chemistry, University of Delhi, Delhi, India*

[6]*Dr B.R Ambedkar Centre for Biomedical Research, University of Delhi, Delhi, India*

[7]*Institute of Nano Medical Sciences, University of Delhi, Delhi, India*

[8]*Maharaja Surajmal Brij University, Bharatpur, Rajasthan, India*

*Corresponding author

ABSTRACT

Testing of natural products plays a vital role in ensuring the quality of products and has made considerable trends in recent years. The efficacy

Herbal Drug Industry: From Cultivation to Innovation and Global Impact.
Abhishek Tiwari, Varsha Tiwari, and Ajay Sharma (Eds.)

DOI: 10.1201/9781779640994-7

and safety of natural products need to be established, which requires a set of stringent quality control tests and optimization of analytical parameters. Qualitative as well as quantitative methods of analysis are used for the development and standardization of natural products. To ensure the quality characteristics of the natural products, numerous sophisticated instruments are employed for the quality assurance of natural products. Various spectral and analytical techniques such as high-pressure thin-layer chromatography, column chromatography (CC), high-pressure liquid chromatography, supercritical fluid chromatography, thermal analysis, inductively coupled plasma-mass spectroscopy, and liquid chromatography-mass spectroscopy have been reported for the testing of natural therapeutic entities. In addition, macroscopic and microscopic techniques such as organoleptic properties, determination of foreign matter, ash value, heavy metals, microbial contaminant and aflatoxins, swelling index, pesticide residues, and radioactive contaminants are primarily used for the qualitative features.

7.1 INTRODUCTION

Almost 75% of the worldwide population relies on natural products for prime healthcare, as per the World Health Organization (WHO) [1]. Natural products represent a rich source of novel therapeutics. Approximately 80% of commercial drugs originate from natural sources. They either contain bioactive components or provide a foundation for new product development [2, 3]. They exhibit an almost limitless range of structural diversity in terms of both their quantity and variety. The use of natural compounds for treating diseases and promoting human health indeed has a long history, dating back to ancient civilizations. Natural products, particularly from plant sources, offer a rich pool of novel therapeutic agents for the reason that of their diverse structural and chemical properties. Despite their potential, these compounds have received limited attention from major pharmaceutical industries. This chapter focuses on the analysis of natural products and emphasizes their significance for the topic of testing natural products.

The demand for natural products with potential health benefits has driven the need for more advanced analytical approaches. Environmental concerns have shaped recent analytical developments, emphasizing the importance of understanding the principles, benefits, and limitations of these methods. The future of natural product analysis is envisioned to involve automated, sophisticated, and nanoscale techniques, focusing on reducing analysis time, minimizing solvent usage, and enhancing resolution and sensitivity. This trend toward adopting unconventional, environmentally friendly methods, and hybrid approaches reflects the ongoing evolution in the domain of natural product analysis.

However, the process of extracting, separating, isolating, and purifying natural products is laborious and problematic because they are often complex in matrix; the active compounds typically are present in low concentrations of active compound, thermally stable, sensitive to oxygen, prone to degradation, and influenced by various environmental factors. For these reasons, the choice of suitable techniques and approaches is crucial for obtaining the board compounds in high quantities. Over the past few decades, various types of innovative extraction, isolation, and purification techniques have been developed. These include supercritical fluid extraction (SFE), ultrasonic-assisted extraction (UAE), microwave-assisted extraction (MAE), pulsed electric field extraction (PLE), enzyme-assisted extraction (EAE), pressurized liquid extraction (PLE), capillary electrophoresis (CE), thin layer chromatography (TLC), preparative high-pressure liquid chromatography (prep-HPLC), gas chromatography (GC), ultraviolet–visible spectroscopy (UV–Vis spectroscopy), Fourier transform-infrared spectroscopy (FTIR), nuclear magnetic resonance spectroscopy (NMR), mass spectroscopy (MS), matrix-assisted laser desorption/ionization (MALDI), and time-of-flight (TOF) MS [4], electrospray ionization-mass spectroscopy and integrated approaches like HPLC-SPE-NMR have been introduced and extensively investigated. These techniques contribute to more efficient and precise analyses in scientific fields. However, it must be emphasized that none of these techniques provides on its own a comprehensive solution to all separation complications, and the best approach is usually to employ a combination of different techniques. However, the extraction, separation, isolation, and purification of natural therapeutic molecules from natural sources remain a great challenge to scientists [5].

Hence, in this chapter, the importance and challenges associated with the extraction, isolation, purification, and its characterization of natural compounds from various sources were discussed. Importantly, the testing and characterization of natural products and contaminants in natural products were discussed in detail in the following sections (Figure 7.1).

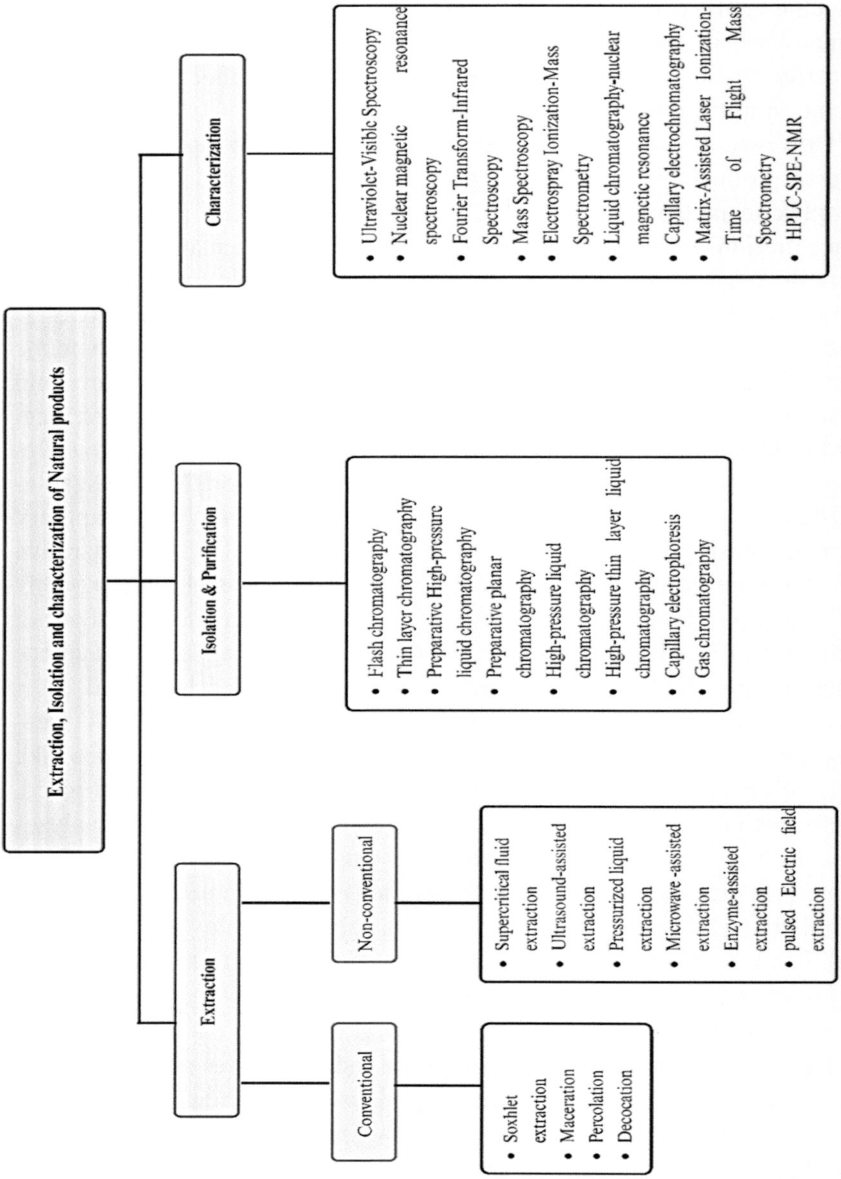

FIGURE 7.1 Flow representation of extraction, isolation, and purification and characterization of natural products.

7.2 EXTRACTION OF NATURAL PRODUCTS

The analysis of natural products involves a comprehensive approach, starting from the identification of plant materials through microscopic examination to the extraction of biologically effective compounds using various techniques. This multistep process is crucial for obtaining valuable components from both plant and animal tissues [6, 7].

Microscopic identification serves as an initial step, employing organoleptic properties such as odor, color, taste, shape, size, fracture characteristics, surface properties, and texture. This method is particularly useful for distinguishing closely related medicinal plants. The use of a light microscope and occasionally polarized or fluorescence microscopes, allows for the examination of structural features at tissue and cellular levels, aiding in accurate plant identification [8].

As soon as the plant substantial is identified, the extraction process becomes paramount. The primary goal is to isolate target compounds from complex matrices. Various extraction methods are available, including solvent extraction (SE), supercritical fluid extraction, solid-phase extraction, ultrasonic-assisted extraction [9], microwave-assisted extraction, and more. Prior to extraction, sample preparation involves drying and milling to produce finely powdered material, enhancing the extraction efficiency [10]. Recent developed advance techniques and the general aids of this parting technique most pertinent and fascinating supercritical fluid extraction applications for natural products analysis, predominantly concentrating on compounds from plants (medicinal) such as alkaloids, glycoside, carotenoids, essential oils, flavonoids, terpene, steroids, and vitamins [11].

The early and vital step in the examination of medicinally important plants is extraction. Extraction is a method used to separate two or more different compounds, such as solids, liquids, or in perspective of their solubilities in binary immiscible liquids. The extraction process plays a decisive role in isolating and recovering bioactive compounds from various sample matrices, especially bioactive compounds with significant benefits for human health. It is vital to follow the appropriate extraction process to obtain the anticipated chemical components of plant materials, facilitating further isolation along with characterization [12].

The competences of extraction are greatly prejudiced by factors, for instance, the nature of the raw materials, particle size, extraction solvent, occurrence of interfering substances, extraction temperature, extraction time, and solvent-to-solid ratio [13]. The technique involves soaking the plant or plant parts in a solvent that dissolves the medicinally active constituents while leaving the inactive matter undissolved. The solvent used is called Menstrum and the solid residue remaining after extraction is called marc. For example, the antioxidant properties of *Tinospora crispa* and *Andrographis paniculate* extracts were associated with their phenolic along with supplementary phytochemical components. The process of extracting natural products frequently includes the use of solvents that are polar (e.g., water, ethanol, methanol, etc.), intermediate-polar (e.g., ethyl acetate, acetone, methylene chloride), and nonpolar (e.g., *n*-hexane, ether, and chloroform) [14].

Acquiring quality bioactive molecules involves key stages: selecting a suitable solvent, employing abstraction methods, conducting phytochemical screening, utilizing fractionation techniques, and employing identification methods. The prime of the methods hinges on the research design. Scientists analyzed the impact of solvents (methanol, hexane, and ethyl alcohol) on antioxidant extraction from plant parts (leaves, seeds). Researcher Anokwuru et al. found that acetone and dimethylformamide are highly effective for antioxidant extraction, whereas Koffi et al. discovered methanol to be more effective for the extraction of large phenolic content in walnuts compared to ethanol [15].

The tissues of both plants and animals are efficient in producing a broad range of bioactive extracts, which can be prepared by means of various methods like extraction. While orthodox techniques include Soxhlet extraction, decoction, percolation, then maceration have been traditionally used, they are often time-consuming, solvent-intensive, and energy-intensive [5]. In response to these limitations, a variety of nonconventional extraction techniques have been developed, including UAE, PLE, MAE, SFE, EAE, PEF extraction, all of which have been used in natural product extraction and offer benefits such as reduced use of organic solvents, quicker selectivity, and longer extraction times [14, 16].

Newer techniques, such as supercritical fluid extraction, UAE that provide the benefits involving convenient operation, time-saving, and a high extract yield, are widely used for ingredient extraction. For instance, Conde–Hernandez extracted rosemary essential oil using S-CO_2, hydrodistillation, and steam distillation. The S-CO_2 method, enhanced by 2% ethanol at pressure (300 bar) and temperature (40°C), showed higher yields and antioxidant activity than the other two techniques. This modified S-CO_2 method was 92% more effectual for the extraction of vinblastine from *Catharanthus roseus* as compared to traditional methods. Additionally, Jovanovic et al. proposed that accomplished a higher polyphenol yield from *Tymus serpyllum* L. using UAE [17].

Nina Djapic proposed that extraction of *Taxodium distichum* needle uses supercritical carbon dioxide and hydrodistillation. Distinct temperature and pressure are used in SCO_2 as well as in hydrodistillation methods. In addition to this, optimal supercritical CO_2 extraction conditions (3.97% yield) were found at 17.79 MPa, 62.70°C; low oil content source will not require high temperature and pressure 22.07 MPa and 64°C, respectively [18].

SFE employs supercritical fluids, such as carbon dioxide, for eco-friendly extraction with high efficiency. It utilizes a dense fluid state between gas and liquid, offering advantages in pharmaceutical, food, and environmental applications [10, 14]. This purification method offers advantages such as reproducibility and high recovery efficiency. It is commonly employed for recovering and cleaning essential oil before GC analysis, as well as for less polar constituents like ginkgo terpenes and kavalactones from kava–kava, and other oils [19].

Ultrasound, with frequencies exceeding 20 kHz, is employed for natural product extraction, typically ranging from 20 to 100 kHz with 10–1000 W/power density. UAE uses ultrasonic waves to induce cavitation effects, enhancing mass transfer without high temperatures. UAE reduces solvent usage, energy consumption, and extraction time, proving effective for extracting bioactive substances [20]. UAE has proven highly effective in extracting biologically active matters from plants and various environments. It is noteworthy that ultrasound enhances the efficiency of extracting genistin, daidzin, malonyl genistin, isoflavones, and glycitin-from soybean, with outcomes depending on the choice of solvent [10, 21]. To extract alkaloids as of kratom leaves, particularly mitragynine and its diastereomers, the UAE approach could be considered a crucial way [22].

PLE, better known as pressurized fluid extraction (PFE), employs SE at high pressures (from 35 to 200 bar) and temperatures (to 200°C), requiring minimal solvent and offering advantages in time, yields, and reproducibility [1]. Water-based extraction, termed hot-water extraction (HWE), is also referred as pressured hot-water extraction (PHWE), supercritical water extraction, and high-temperature water extraction [23]. However, these methods are not appropriate for thermal sensitive compounds due to the high extraction temperature [5]. PLE offers an alternative to traditional methods with faster processes and lower solvent usage. MAE utilizes microwaves (frequency ranges from 300 MHz to 300 GHz) [22] and solvents to extract natural products, offering benefits in reduced extraction time, enhanced precision, and suitability for thermolabile compounds [24, 25]. EAE employs enzymes like cellulase to rupture cell walls, hydrolyze polysaccharides, and enhance extract yield, making it effective to extract bioactive elements from plant materials. In the past decade, PEF has proven valuable for enhancing drying, pressing, extraction, and diffusion processes [26]. PEF serves as a pretreatment for formerly conventional extraction methods, minimizing extraction efforts. These extraction techniques offer diverse benefits, addressing challenges posed by conventional methods; hence contributing to efficient and sustainable bioactive compound extraction from natural sources by enhancing cell membrane permeability and ultimately resulting in an increase in extraction yield [27]. Therefore, these advanced extraction techniques offer diverse approaches for extracting bioactive compounds from natural sources. Each technique has its unique benefits, making them appropriate for specific applications in food, medicinal, and environmental industries. The continuous development and integration of these techniques contribute to the efficient and sustainable extraction of valuable natural products (Figure 7.2).

7.3 ISOLATON AND PURIFICATION OF NATURAL PRODUCTS

The extracts obtained from the aforementioned methods constitute a complex mixture containing diverse natural products of varying polarities. Achieving pure bioactive compounds necessitates subsequent stages of isolation and purification [28]. The key stages for isolating and characterizing phytochemicals involve selecting and collecting various parts of plants. The components in the extract obtained from the abovementioned methods are intricate, comprising diverse natural products. To attain the active element or pure natural products, more separation and purification are necessary. This separation relies on the chemical or physical distinctions among individual natural products. The most accessible and adaptable separation method is chromatography. Chromatography is a manner of separating a mixture or component into its constituent parts by

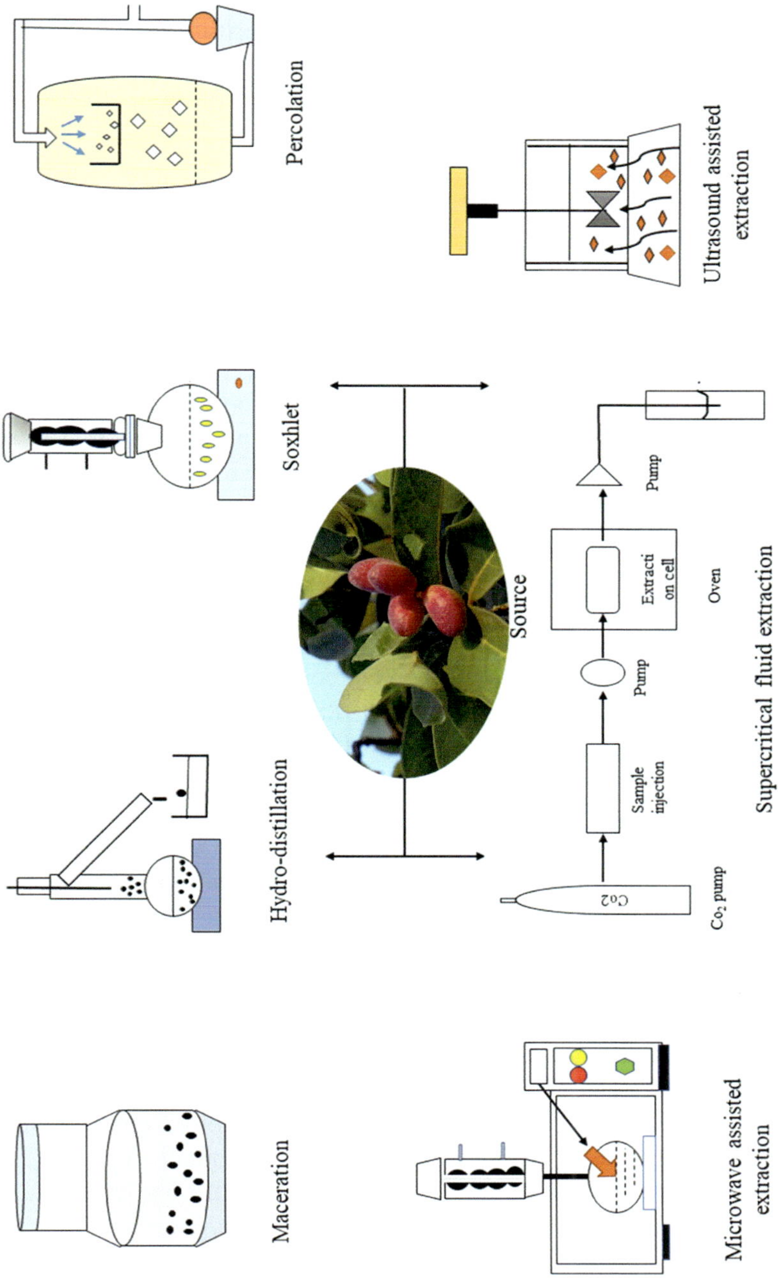

FIGURE 7.2 Diagrammatic representation of extraction techniques of natural products.

employing a mobile phase along with a stationary phase. Different chromatographic processes are used to separate and purify plant components. The separation and analysis of natural products primarily involves the use of chromatography due to its availability in several stationary phases, convenience, and economy. Chromatographic techniques, including flash chromatography, HPLC, HPTLC, TLC, and CE, particularly column chromatography, stands as the primary method employed to isolate pure natural products from complex mixtures [29].

Romeilah et al. isolated 20 compounds from *Cuminum cyminum* (seeds) oil, including α-pinene, α-phellandrene, α-terpinene, α-terpinolene, sabinene, β-pinene, β-myrcene, *p*-cymene, limonene, camphor, terpinen-4-ol, geranyl acetate, α-terpineol, geraniol, β-caryophyllene, cuminaldehyde, thymol, β-farnesene, and caryophyllene oxide [30]. Cuminaldehyde and *p*-menta-1,4-dien-7-al were positively isolated and purified from the essential oil of *Cuminum cyminum* L. by using high-speed counter-current chromatography (HSCCC) in a semipreparative scale. A binary solvent system, namely, *n*-hexane–methanol-water having ratio (5:4:1 in v/v/v) was operated for the isolation process of the compounds, which were targeted, collected, and purified through HSCCC method in the head-tail mode [31]. Various chromatographic techniques play pivotal roles in isolating and analyzing bioactive compounds. Flash chromatography, a rapid preparative column method, utilizes prepacked columns with high-flow solvent pumping. It employs isocratic and gradient systems, optimizing flow rates based on particle size. Normal and reverse-phase flash chromatography uses polar and nonpolar solvents, respectively, for efficient compound retention [32]. TLC densitometry is a simple method for qualitative and quantitative analysis, limited to substances detectable under UV light [33]. Prep-HPLC, a high-performance liquid chromatography, is valuable for isolating diverse active compounds, such as phenolic as well as flavonoid compounds. It is extensively used in phytochemical and analytical chemistry for purifying, identifying, and measuring individual components [34]. It helps to identify known compounds by evaluating the UV spectra and retention time of the known compounds.

Nowadays, high-performance liquid chromatography technique works as the main choice for research scientists due to its precision and versatility in handling a wide range of samples, making it a preferred choice in modern research for its robust capabilities in compound analysis and separation [35, 36]. Preparative planar chromatography is employed for efficiently purifying bioactive compounds in small sample sizes. HPTLC is a robust and effective implement for quantitative analysis, screening adulterations, and monitoring cultivation and extraction processes [37]. CE offers high resolution, low sample requirements, and minimal operating costs, making it versatile for biomedical and pharmaceutical analysis [38]. GC is another analytical technique for isolating and separating compounds based on volatilities, commonly used in natural product studies [39]. Mahesh Kumar and colleagues conducted a study related to the isolation of bioactive compounds from *Millingtonia hortensis* leaves using numerous chromatographic methods involving silica gel column chromatography, TLC as well as HPLC [40]. Additionally, the bioactive complexes of the methanolic extract wightii has been screened and subjected to underwent silica gel column chromatography using a glass column with silica gel (mesh size of 230–400), suspended in *n*-hexane. A total of 5 mL (milliliter) of methanolic extract was loaded into the column, and solvent combination of variable polar nature, (counting *n*-hexane, chloroform, and ethyl acetate) were sequentially used for elution by keeping a flow rate 1 mL/min [41].

HPLC remains widely recognized as the optimal analytical separation technique for the qualitative as well as quantitative analysis of natural products, particularly those derived from plant samples or herbal preparations [42]. This robust method is particularly suited for the analysis of nonvolatile compounds such as alkaloids, phenolics, and terpenoids [43]. The results of the qualitative analysis are determined based on the uniformity in the retention time of the reference values and the compounds in the analyzed sample. Quantitative assessment is performed using a standard curve created by injecting reference standards at unalike concentrations. Sample derivatization is not obligatory prior to analysis using this method [44]. Reverse-phase (RP) columns are commonly used in HPLC for the analysis of various phytoconstituents [45]. Routine HPLC methods typically employ RP octadecyl silica columns for phenolic compounds [46]. C18 columns with free silanols, water, aliphatic ligands, and a mobile phase modifier are commonly used in RP-HPLC for the parting of phenol group containing compounds [47]. UV detectors, photodiode array detectors, and diode array detectors (DAD) are commonly used to detect phenolic compounds in plant samples [48]. Various organic solvents like methanol and acetonitrile and minor concentrations of ethanoic acid, formic acid, and organofluorides compound like tri-fluoro acetic acid are mostly used in RP-HPLC for the separation of phenolic compounds from plant extract [49]. As stated by Kumar et al., HPLC analysis was directed successfully, affirming the homogeneity of vinblastine and vincristine. The homogeneity of purified compound vinblastine and vincristine was done and confirmed by HPLC analysis. The resulting single proportioned peak at retention time for 36.6 and 34.9 min was observed for vinblastine and vincristine, respectively, on a C18 symmetry column [50]. The absorbance of vinblastine and vincristine occurred maximum at 220 nm and 254 nm, respectively. A total of 76 mg of vinblastine and 67 mg of vincristine were isolated from 1 L of culture filtrate, yielding vinca alkaloids [50, 51].

7.4 CHARACTERIZATION OF NATURAL PRODUCT

Chromatography techniques, such as GC, CE, and HPLC, play crucial roles in the qualitative as well as quantitative analysis of natural products. HPLC often coupled with MS plays a vital role in detection and analysis of natural products, offering heightened sensitivity and precision in identifying and measuring compounds. In case like, HPLC has been hyphenated with mass spectrometry (HPLC-MS) and ultraviolet-photodiode array detection (HPLC-DAD) [52] is expansively used for phytochemicals characterization, offering the ability to investigate various classes of plant metabolites. Other picks such as SFC and capillary electrochromatography (CEC), offer more tools for specific applications [53].

Spectroscopic techniques like infrared (IR), NMR, UV, and MS are schooled clarify chemical structures. While UV and IR absorption expose exact functional groups of extracted natural compound, NMR provides comprehensive structural data. HPLC-NMR hyphenation, conjugation postcolumn capillary separations with NMR detection, and solid-phase extraction (HPLC-SPE-NMR), it consents meant for the identification of natural products in plant extracts [54, 55].

7.4.1 UV–VIS SPECTROSCOPY

UV–Vis spectrometry is an advantageous tool for quantitatively evaluating samples for molecules with strong chromophores in the UV range [56]. UV–Vis spectroscopy is a technique that employs absorption spectroscopy to identify and characterize molecule by measuring the absorption of light in ultraviolet and visible wavelength ranges, which is typically between 200–400 nm and 400–800 nm. It measures the known compound concentration by absorbance or transmission of UV light, using number of photons reach to detector indicate intensity of the light. This is one of the most basic techniques that need to be led while detecting a compound [57]. This technique is hasty and reduced cost compared to other techniques. Phenolic compounds such as tannins, phenols, anthocyanins, and polymer dye, form iron complexes and are detected by UV–Vis spectroscopy [15]. However, this technique is less discerning. The absorption peaks for various compounds can be found at different wavelengths, such as 520 nm for anthocyanins, 360 for phenolic acid, 320 nm for flavones, and 280 nm for phenolic extracts. Compared to other methods, UV-VIS spectroscopy is a speedy and lucrative technique [58] (Figure 7.3).

Joshi et al. stated experimental view regarding phenolic extracted natural products and their derivatives. He focused on flavonoids and phenolic compound which are physio-pharmacological beneficial to health. Usually, it is found in natural sources like fruits, cereals and leaves. Spectrometry study of flavonoids shown (below figure) absorption wavelength of flavones and relevant glycosides observed two strong spectra band I (300–380 nm) and II (240–280), respectively.

7.4.2 NUCLEAR MAGNETIC RESONANCE

NMR spectroscopy is a valued instrument for studying the structures of complex organic molecules found in plants. It has been used to identify and characterize pure natural products, and offers several advantages in the quantitative analysis of substances, including its nondestructive nature, high flux, and short analysis time [59]. Chauthe et al. utilized NMR spectroscopy on natural medicinal plants such as *Eugenia jambolana, Aegle marmelos,* and *Withania somnifera* as well as their herbal products by using internal reference standards like 1,3,5-trimethoxybenzene. Samples were dissolved in deuterated solvents. Quantitative NMR is a reliable routine analytical technique that provides several benefits, including sensitivity, universality, precision, and the ability to reduce or replace other quantitation tools. Its nondestructive nature is particularly noteworthy [60]. NMR technology is broadly used in various arenas, including medicine and health, organic chemistry, metabolomics, animal and plant microorganisms, food science, and natural products, etc. NMR spectroscopy is an authoritative method for determining the structure of

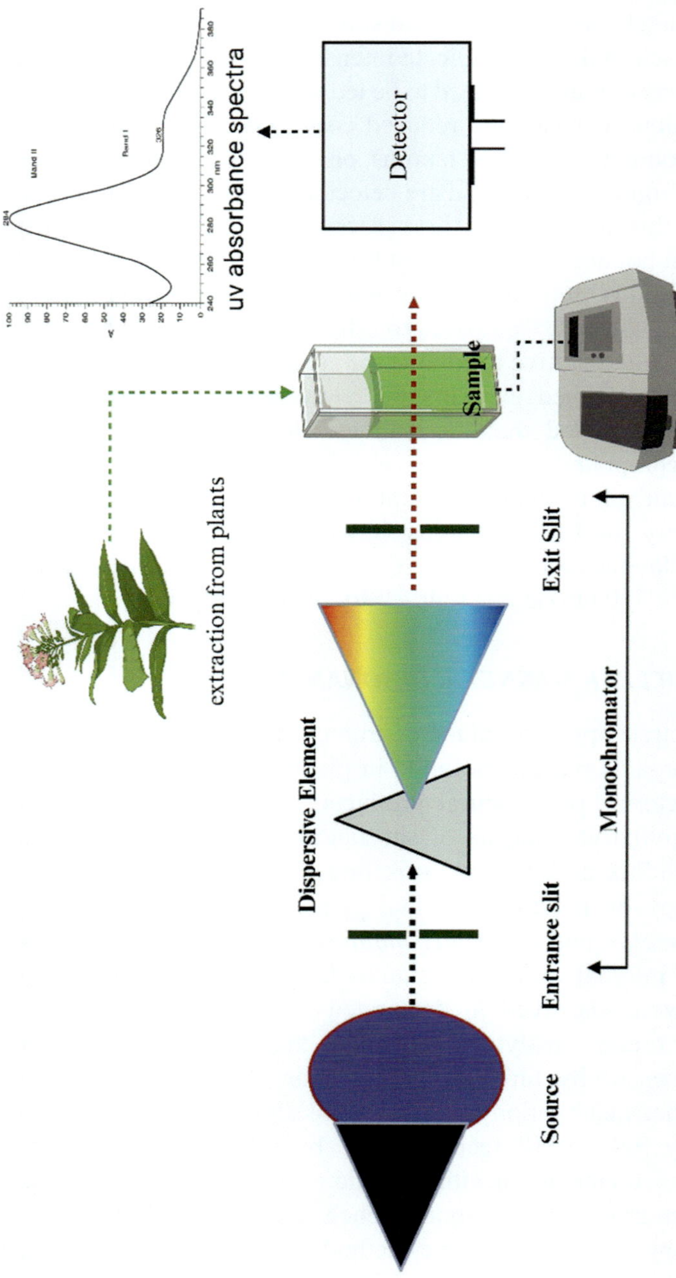

FIGURE 7.3 Schematic representation of UV–Vis spectroscopy.

new terpenoids, alkaloids, or flavonoids, as well as for the identifying or investigation of glycosides and the linkage between sugar moieties and their configuration [61].

Inclusive, NMR spectroscopy is a prevailing and most time-reserving technique for the separation and structural elucidation of unidentified components and their mixtures, predominantly for the structural elucidation of herbal plant extracts.

7.4.3 FOURIER TRANSFORM-INFRARED SPECTROSCOPY

FTIR is an appreciated tool for obtaining noteworthy evidence about the composition and structure of plants [62]. FTIR is based on the element that molecules absorb light in the infrared region of the electromagnetic spectrum. Compounds are measured over the range of 400–4000 cm^{-} of frequency [63]. This technique is specially used for the identification and characterization of functional groups, which exist in isolates from plant extracts and also for determining their chemical composition and purity [64]. Compound properties are well-defined by functional groups, and the being of single, double, or multiple bonds is identified through this data [65]. FTIR proposes a swift and nondestructive detailed inspection of plant extracts. IR spectroscopy is awfully helpful for the determination of a new synthesized molecules and the confirmation of a compound identity. As demonstrated by Dhivya et al., FTIR method has been shown to be operative in the analysis of plants like *Sarcostemma brevistigma*. It exposed appearance of flavonoids and phenolic complexes, which are known to contribute to the plant's abundant medicinal properties [66].

7.4.4 MASS SPECTROMETRY

Mass spectrometry is an essential analytical technique in support of the identification of unknown compounds as well as the quantifying known one while also elucidating the structure with the whole chemical properties of molecules. For determining a substance's fragmentation pattern, molecular mass, and formula MS is one of the crucial central techniques [67]. Through the MS spectrum, the molecular mass or concentrations of molecules or compound scan be determined. The primary technique of MS utilizes the generation of positively or negatively charged gaseous ions, which are then separated and identified depending on their mass-to-charge (m/z) ratio. Mass spectrometry has advantages in sensitivity, specificity, and speed [68]. Thermospray, ionspray, and electrospray ionization techniques are recent developments offering the special benefits of high detection specificity as well as sensitivity. Mass spectrometry has been over a widely intended for analysis of phenolic compounds. This technique is mostly active for the structural clarification of organic compounds, peptide sequencing or oligonucleotide for monitoring the existence of earlier characterised compounds in composite mixtures with high specificity by defining the molecular weight as well as diagnostic fragment of the molecule concurrently [69].

7.4.5 ELECTROSPRAY IONIZATION-MASS SPECTROMETRY

ESI-MS is a technique that is used for the chemical characterization of extracts besides compounds isolated from natural sources [70]. ESI-MS produces ions which, in the application of an electric potential to a smooth flowing fluid, it generates a liquid to get charged and then sprayed. This electro-spray forms very tiny droplets of solvent comprising the analytes. Presently, a broad range of nonvolatile and thermolabile samples, in addition to complex biological structures, are studied qualitatively and quantitatively using ESI-MS [71]. Using this method, high-molecular-weight and thermolabile materials like proteins and biopolymers may be ionized and moved into the gas phase, opening up new possibilities in the sector of medicine, plant metabolomics, and molecular biology [72].

Nowadays, liquid-phase separation methods like LC may be coupled online with MS using ESI, which is the most significant ionization technique [73]. The ESI-MS spectrum range of pure fungal vinblastine displayed product ions at 355, 522, 542, 734, 750, 793, and 811, conforming to the (M^{+H}) ion with m/z 811. Likewise, purified fungal vincristine ESI-MS exhibited a chief/major ion at m/z 825, with fragment ions at m/z 766, 807, and 825 experientials in ESI-MS [74, 75].

7.4.6 LIQUID CHROMATOGRAPHY-NUCLEAR MAGNETIC RESONANCE

LC-NMR is a method that combines the separating and analyzing capabilities of HPLC and NMR to study molecules. This technique is crucial for natural product druggists to isolate and regulate the structural chemistry of molecules. Current advances in technology have further expanded the applications of LC-NMR, as demonstrated by numerous articles on hyphenated techniques [76]. Researchers first used LC-NMR to study natural products by characterizing mixtures, enabling simultaneous liquid chromatography separation and nuclear magnetic resonance analysis. The technique has been employed to identify the structure of the bioinsecticides azadirachtin, which is a product of photoisomerization, and to analyze the geometric isomers of vitamin acetate formed upon exposure to heat [77, 78]. Liquid chromatography nuclear magnetic resonance has also been used to classify prenylated flavanones from *Monotes*, including anglers, naphthoquinones from *Cordia linnaei,* and monoterpene dimers from *Lisianthus seemanni.* Additionally, pyrrolizidine and naphthylquinolinealkaloids, glycosides, phenylphenalenones, sesquiterpene, lactones, and other compounds have been identified using LC-NMR data. A number of these descriptions involve the characterization of identified members of these structural classes using LC-NMR [79], but in a few cases, the technique has been employed to determine the structures of new correspondents of known compounds [76, 77, 80].

7.4.7 MALDI-TOF MASS SPECTROMETRY

MALDI is a gentle ionization method that is extensively used for the identification and analysis of large molecular weight compounds [70]. It has been confirmed to be a useful tool in the analysis of natural products, for example, carbohydrates and glycoconjugates. MALDI is also employed in quality control and safety assessment of natural products [81, 82]. Matrix-assisted laser desorption/ionization-time-of flight is a prevailing technique designed for confirming the identity of isolated compounds, which are derivatives of natural products such as alkaloids, flavonoids, terpenoids, carotenoids, anthocyanins, sesquiterpene lactones, steroids, diterpenes, and lipids, even including glycosylated and nonglycosylated compounds [83]. MALDI-TOF MS determines the mass of ions by separating them in time as said by their mass/charge (m/z) ratio [84, 85]. Peptides/proteins, lipids, polymers, oligonucleotides, and oligosaccharides are some of the high molecular weight compounds identified using MALDI-TOF [86]. Gottardo et al. used MALDI-TOF MSin the quick relating direct analysis of herbal blend formulated preparation for synthetic cannabinoids.

The sample preparation involved finely ground herbal blend leaves loaded onto a MALDI plate and subsequently adding a matrix or surfactant blend [α-cyano-4-hydroxy-cinnamic acid/cetyltrimethylammonium bromide (CTAB)]. The MALDI-TOF conditions included analyzing mass spectra range of m/z 150–550 by being an average of data from 50 laser shots and consuming a fast-tracking electrical energy of 20 kV. These characteristics of MALDI-TOF MS are mainly significant because traditional immunochemical or chemical techniques currently used for preliminary screening are unable to detect synthetic cannabinoids such as JWH-018 [87].

7.4.8 CAPILLARY ELECTROCHROMATOGRAPHY

CEC is crucial characterization techniques for analyzing complex mixtures like natural products. It has latent to be superior because of combination of high-pressure liquid chromatography and CE. Selecting an appropriate stationary phase is vital, considering surface chemistry and electrophoretic mobility. Sample introduction ensures through port injector. CEC offers enhanced separation efficiency, especially with polymeric monoliths, and is economically viable. However, challenges include methodological vulnerabilities, difficulties in predicting separation mechanisms and bubbles formation. Pressure-assisted CEC (p-CEC) addresses some issues by controlling the mobile phase flow. Pressure diminished bubbles or any void formation in capillary column. It involves pressurized flow as well as electro-osmotic flow [88]. Fabricating columns requires expertise, limiting reported applications. Despite limited commercial availability, CEC holds untapped potential for high-performance microscale separation in natural product analysis, promising novel insights into various analyte types (Figure 7.4).

Angelica dahurica roots, valued in traditional Chinese medicine for diaphoretic and analgesic properties, contain coumarins as active components. In 2006, Chen introduced a p-CEC method for coumarin analysis. The method utilized a capillary packed with a mixture of C18 and bare silica particles, connected to an HPLC pump. A 15 mM phosphate buffer having pH 4.8 and a methanol–acetonitrile mixture served as the mobile phase. With only 4 mL injection, the method achieved sensitive detection (LOD 0.63–0.96 g/mL) of five foremost coumarins in just 25 min,

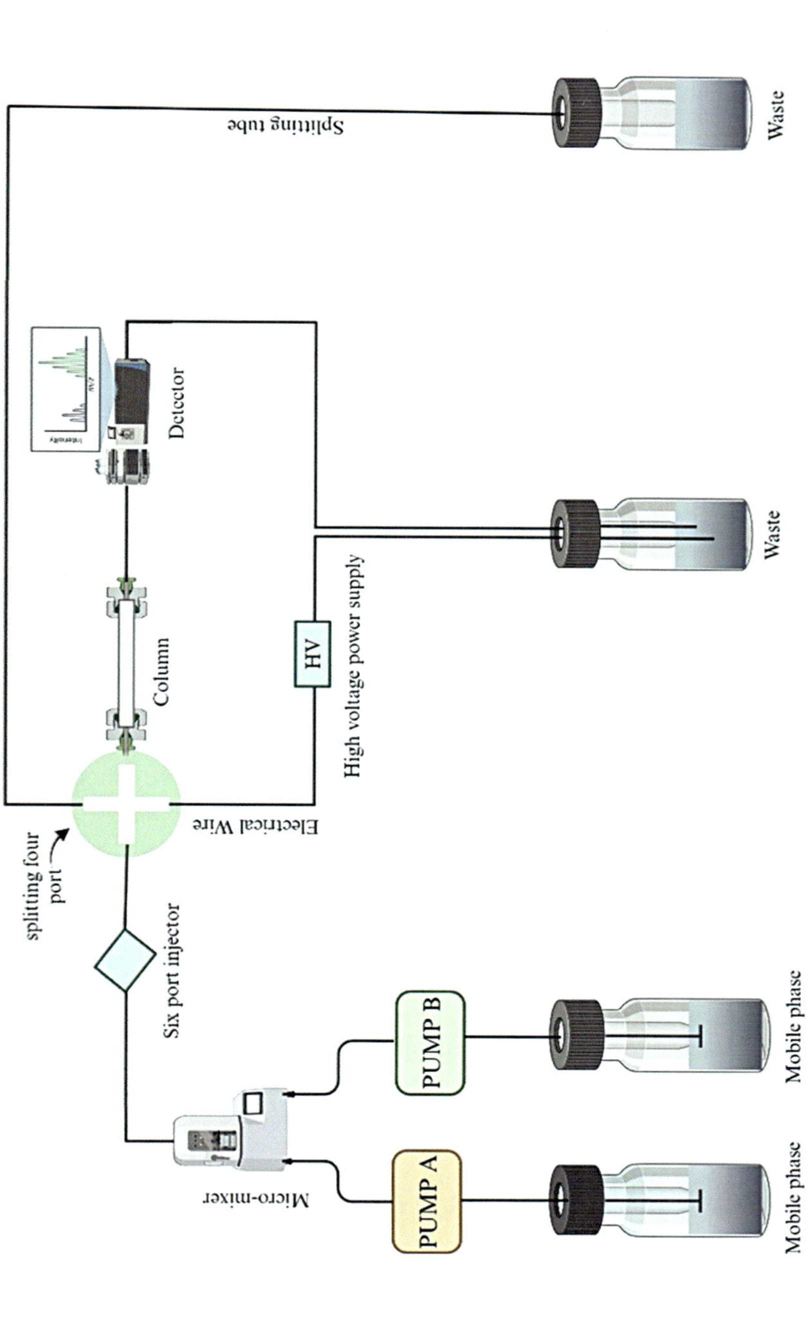

FIGURE 7.4 Schematic representation of experimental apparatus used for separation by pressure-assisted capillary electrochromatography (p-CES).

outperforming conventional HPLC. The p-CEC approach demonstrated superior plate numbers (N/m 100,000) and significantly reduced separation time [89].

7.4.9 HPLC-SPE-NMR

A technique evolving about 15 years ago, integrates high-pressure liquid chromatography along with solid-phase extraction and nuclear magnetic resonance spectroscopy. The approach involves trapping analytes post-HPLC on a guard column, eliminating the HPLC mobile phase, and transferring analytes to the NMR flow probe with an appropriate NMR solvent. The method enhances sensitivity by concentrating analytes close to the flow cell volume, enabling optimal signal-to-noise ratios.

The commercially available HPLC-SPE-NMR system offers comparable sensitivity to capillary NMR in routine natural product analysis. Approximately 2 mg of analyte per millilitre of NMR solvent is required for high-quality 2D NMR spectra overnight, while only 10 nmol of substance is needed for ^{1}H-NMR spectra within about an hour. The technique's advantages include cost reduction, spectral information preservation, and the ability to compare data recorded in solvents of identical polarity. However, challenges arise when dealing with very polar metabolites, which may require alternative SPE materials or Cap NMR approaches. Multiple SPE trapping allows users to bring semipreparative amount of analyte to the NMR detector using analytical HPLC equipment [55].

Liu et al. proposed that triterpenoid having family Ericaceae isolated from *Rhododendron latoucheae* plants. Characterization of these plant extract has been used to through hyphenated HPLC-SPE-NMR techniques. NMR and MS provide the information regarding the structural chemistry of natural products [90]. Norquinone methide is the first triterpenoid isolated from the plant, along with several other compounds including flavonoids, phenolic acids, sterols, and lignans. These compounds collectively contribute to the plant's pharmacological properties such as anti-inflammatory, antioxidant, and anticancer activities.

7.5 CONTAMINANTS IN NATURAL PRODUCTS

Contamination is the presence of an impurity, any constituent, or some other undesirable element that may cause unsuitable and harmful effect.

Most often, contaminants are accidentally or inadvertently introduced to natural products [91].

The most predictable contaminants originate in medicinal natural product and natural product are biological (bacteria and their spores, molds, yeasts, viruses; fungi and protozoa) and chemicals (heavy metals, aflatoxin, pesticide, fumigants, and radioactive substances) [92, 93]. In order to ensure high-quality natural components, it is important to eliminate contaminants such as animal matter, pests, and excrement. While it may be impossible to completely eliminate all contaminants, specifications can be established to limit their presence. These specifications can include factors such as ash values, foreign organic matter, microbial contamination, and aflatoxins, as well as contamination with heavy metals. Purity is also thoroughly related with the safe use of medication, and it is important to consider influences like values and contaminants such as other herbs in the form of foreign matter, heavy metals, and pesticides. With the use of improved analytical method, current purity evaluation includes the examination of microbial contamination, heavy metal, radioactivity, and pesticide residues. A variety of analytical techniques have been active for the examination of contaminants like microbial organisms, aflatoxin, mycotoxins, and pesticide. These techniques include gas chromatography-mass spectrometry (GC-MS), atomic absorption spectroscopy, TLC, atomic fluorescence spectrometry, high-performance liquid chromatography-mass spectroscopy (HPLC-MS), fluorescent aptasensor pico-green-based strategy, inductively coupled plasma-MS (ICP-MS), instrumental neutron activation analysis, HPLC, ICPS, and ultra-performance liquid chromatography-MS [94].

7.5.1 FOREIGN ORGANIC MATTER

Foreign organic matter involves removal of matter other than the parent source plant to get drug in purified form [95]. It is not possible to collect an herbal ingredient without small amounts of relevant part of plant or other plants. This involves removing matter that is not from the source plant to obtain a pure form of the drug. Standard should be established in order to limit the percentage of such undesirable plant impurities. Regarding the maximum quantitative limitations of foreign matter in natural raw materials, the American Herbal Products Association offers the following guidelines: Other than those specified in the specifications, part of plant of the same natural raw material species should not exceed 5% (by weight), and any other foreign matter (e.g., grass clipping in mint leaves) should not exceed 2% (by weight) [96, 97].

7.5.2 ASH VALUE

The ash content refers to the inorganic residue left after incinerating a crude drug. The determination of the ash value is a crucial parameter for assessing the purity of crude drugs in powdered form. This comprises the calculation of the total (entire) ash value, acid insoluble ash value, and water-soluble ash value, which were determined according to the conventions set forth by the Indian Pharmacopoeia [98, 99]. Acid-insoluble ash, which is obtained by treating the ash with hydrochloric acid, is mainly composed of silica and can be used as a measure of soil content.

Ash value can be determined by three different ways such as total ash, water-soluble ash, and acid-soluble ash.

1. **Total ash**: It measures the entire amount of material left over after incineration.

   %Total ash value=ash weight/weight of sample *100

2. **Acid insoluble ash**: It is residue obtained after boiling the total ash with dilute HCL and exploding remaining insoluble matter.

   % Acid insoluble ash= Acid insoluble ash weight/weight of sample *100

3. **Water soluble ash**: It is difference in weight between total ash and residue after treatment of total ash with water [100].
   %Water soluble ash=Total ash weight−water insoluble residue in total ash /weight of sample *100 [101].

7.5.3 MOISTURE CONTENT

Moisture content is a measure of the water content in a substance or material [102]. Accurate determination of moisture content is important in order to avoid mistakes in the estimation of the real weight of medication material. A low moisture contraction is indicative of improved steadiness against degradation of the product. Several methods are available for determining moisture content, such as, measurement of moisture and separation, loss on drying, chemical methods, spectroscopic methods, and electrometric methods as per IP [103]. These include loss of drying, azeotropic distillation, Karl Fischer spectroscopic, chemical, conductivity, and thermogravimetric analysis [104]. Rohmah used electric oven drying method for determining moisture content of Mekai leaf (*Pycnarrhena tumefacta* Miers) and the moisture content of dried Mekai leaves ranged from 6.95 ±0.09 to 9.30±0.60% (w/w) [104].

7.5.4 MICROBIAL CONTAMINATION AND AFLATOXIN

Microbial contamination is the presence of living microorganism in an environment, commonly including the bacteria, fungi, and virus. The bacterial species comprised *Acinetobacter species*, *Acinetobacter baumannii, Acinetobacter calcoaceticus,* Aerobic bacteria such as *Bacillus* species, *Bacillus amyloliquefaciens, Bacillus cereus, Bacillus lentus, Bacillus megaterium, Bacillus subtilis, Citrobacter diversus, Citrobacter intermidius, Klebsiella ozaena*, *Clostridium* species, *Coliforms, Enterobacteria species* and fungi namely *Aspergillus niger, Alternaria* species, *Aspergillus flavus, Aspergillus fumigatus, ctinomadura madurae, Staphylococcus epidermidis*, *Candida albicans, Candida tropicalis, Candida pseudotropicalis, Curvularia species, Serratia marcescens, Pseudomonas aeruginosa,* fungi species like *Fusarium species, Hansenula anomala, Madurella mycetomatis, Streptococcus pyogenes, Mucor species, Saccharomyces cerevisiae*, *Penicillium* species, *Trichosporon cutaneum* and *Rhizopus species, Mucor* species, *mold, Aspergillus niger*, and *Geotricum* species, are typically present in plant material and may increase due to defective mounting, harvesting, stowage or processing. While *Aspergillus, Penicillium*, and *Fusarium* are among the fungus species that are capable of producing aflatoxins, *A. flavus* and *A. parasiticus* are the most prevalent species [105]. Natural ingredients containing high starch concentration may be susceptible to increased microbial growth. Pathogenic organisms such as *Clostridium, Enterobacter, Enterococcus, Pseudomonas, Shigella,* and *Streptococcus*, have been known to contaminate such ingredients. It is crucial to establish limits for microbial contamination. Barnes et al. improperly dried or stored medicinal herbs and plants used in natural products can lead to aflatoxin contamination. The European Pharmacopoeia now provides voluntary guidance on adequate limits. The World Health Organization (WHO) sets microbial contamination limits for medicinal plant materials meant for internal use, with colony total not exceeding 10^5 CFU/g (WHO, 2007). For plant products meant for topical use or pretreated with boiling water, the colony count should not more than 10^7 CFU/g [106]. Mycotoxins and microbial contamination were analyzed primarily using microbial culture and HPLC, respectively. Microbial contamination also has adverse effects such as immune suppression and microbial infection.

7.5.5 AFLATOXIN

Aflatoxins are mainly produced by several fungal species including *Fusarium*, *Penicillium*, *Candida*, *S. cerevisiae*, and *Aspergillus*. Among these, *A. flavus* and *A. parasiticus* are the most commonly identified varieties [107]. There is a potential risk of aflatoxin contamination in herbal products if their components such as medicinal herbs and plants are not thoroughly dried or are improperly stored after preparation. Consuming even small amounts of aflatoxins present in plant material can pose significant health risks [108]. Therefore, it is crucial to determine their presence after applying a suitable clean-up procedure. Aflatoxins are the most harmful of all mycotoxins and have been the subject of widespread research [109]. Their presence in natural medicinal products can pose serious and long-lasting health risks. Aflatoxins are toxic, carcinogenic, teratogenic, and mutagenic compounds [110]. It is widely recognized that the analysis of aflatoxin in natural products is of paramount importance, as evidenced by the inclusion of methods for determining aflatoxin levels in international pharmacopoeias such as the United State Pharmacopeia, European Pharmacopeia and British Pharmacopeia. The International Agency for Research on Cancer (IARC) has likewise determined that aflatoxin is a cause of hepatic cancer, further underscoring the significance of aflatoxin contamination in natural products. Given that natural products are often taken for extended periods of time, the potential for prolonged exposure to aflatoxin among consumers makes it imperative to confirm the safety of these products. A variety of analytical techniques for aflatoxin including enzyme-linked immunosorbent, gas chromatography, liquid chromatography, lateral flow immunoassay, aptamer-based lateral flow assay, and cytometric bead array [111]. However, high-pressure liquid chromatography united with MS is the furthermost suitable test technique for determining aflatoxin levels in herbal products.

7.5.6 PESTICIDES

Pesticides are substances that are designed to regulate pests that directly harm cultivated plants [112]. Exposure to these substances, either directly and indirectly through consumption in water, fish, food and natural remedies can result in a range adverse health effect including neurological effects, respiratory diseases, birth defects, cancer, diabetes, and human genetic disorders [113]. It is essential to conduct limit tests to determine the acceptable levels of pesticide contamination by natural elements, predominantly those grown as cultivated produces, which may be filthy with harmful chemicals such as dichlorodiphenyltrichloroethane or organochlorine include DDT (dichlorodiphenyl trichloroethane), dicofol, aldrin, dieldrin, benzene hexachlorides [114, 115]. organophosphates include parathion, malathion, and methyl parathion, tetrachlorvinphos and carbamates or polychlorinated biphenyl (Table 7.1). As per WHO guidelines, various approaches are available for identification pesticides, the analytical method for determining pesticide residues is chromatography (GC and HPLC) [106]. GC or GC-MS was the primary method used for pesticides and residual solvents [116, 117]. A maximum of 1% of the total intake from all sources should come from the consumption of leftovers derived from natural materials.

TABLE 7.1 Examples of National and Regional Limits Set for Several Kinds of Pesticide Residues in Naturally Occurring Plant Materials [118]

Substance	Limit	
	European pharmacopoeia (mg/kg)	Farmacopea Argentina (FA), United States pharmacopeia (USA) (mg/kg)
Dichlorodiphenyl trichloroethane	1.0	–
Dicofol	0.5	–
Aldrin	0.05	0.05
Dieldrin	0.05	0.05
Benzene hexachlorides		
Parathion	–	0.5
Malathion	–	1.0
Methyl parathion	0.2	–

7.5.7 FUMIGANTS

Fumigants such as methyl bromide, ethylene oxide, and phosphine which have traditionally used to control pest that can contaminant natural constituents, should be used with caution. The utilization of a fumigant like ethylene oxide from natural medication is prohibited in Europe because of worries about residues that are reprotoxic, mutagenic, and carcinogenic [119].

7.5.8 HEAVY METALS

Lead, cadmium, arsenic, mercury, chromium, zinc, copper, iron, cobalt, strontium, nickel, and thallium have been reported to be contaminants of some natural substances [120]. Therefore, assessments for such noxious metals are crucial necessary to ensure the safety natural ingredients. Heavy metal exposure, when prolonged, can result in detrimental health consequences (Table 7.2). This is because these metals have the capacity to accumulate within the body and interfere with the proper functioning of critical organs, including the brain, kidneys, and liver [121].

The most common techniques used for determining metal contaminants are atomic absorption spectroscopy, neutron activation analysis, differential pulse polarography, X-ray fluorescence spectroscopy, and inductively coupled plasma optical emission spectroscopy or mass spectroscopy [117, 122].

TABLE 7.2 Limits for Heavy Metal as per WHO and FDA [123]

Sr. No	Metal	Limit (ppm)
1	Lead	10
2	Cadmium	0.3
3	Arsenic	5
4	Mercury	1
5	Chromium	2
6	Zinc	0.50

7.5.9 RADIOACTIVE CONTAMINATION

The inescapable exposure to ionizing radiation from sources like radionuclides is present in the environment. However, the utilization of irradiation can help prevent the proliferation of microorganisms in natural ingredients. This process not only sterilizes the plant material, but it also necessitates consideration of the potential radioactivity hazard. To guarantee safety, it is crucial to adhere to the recommendation of the WHO and International Atomic Energy Agency when evaluating the radioactivity of plant samples [124]. The levels of naturally occurring radionuclides were assessed using a germanium detector. According to the European Pharmacopoeia's alpha-particle spectrometry, beta particle-spectroscopy, and gamma-ray spectrometry, as methods for determining radioactive contamination [125]. Gamma-ray spectrometry was utilized to measure the activity concentrations of ^{40}K, ^{232}Th, and ^{238}U in *Alstonia boonei*, *Blighia sapida, Bridelia ferruginea, Cassia sieberiana, Lippia multiflora, Khaya ivorensis, Mondia whitei*, and *Croton membranaceus*. The highest concentrations of ^{232}Th and ^{238}U were found in *K. ivorensis*, while *L. multiflora* exhibited the highest levels of ^{40}K [126].

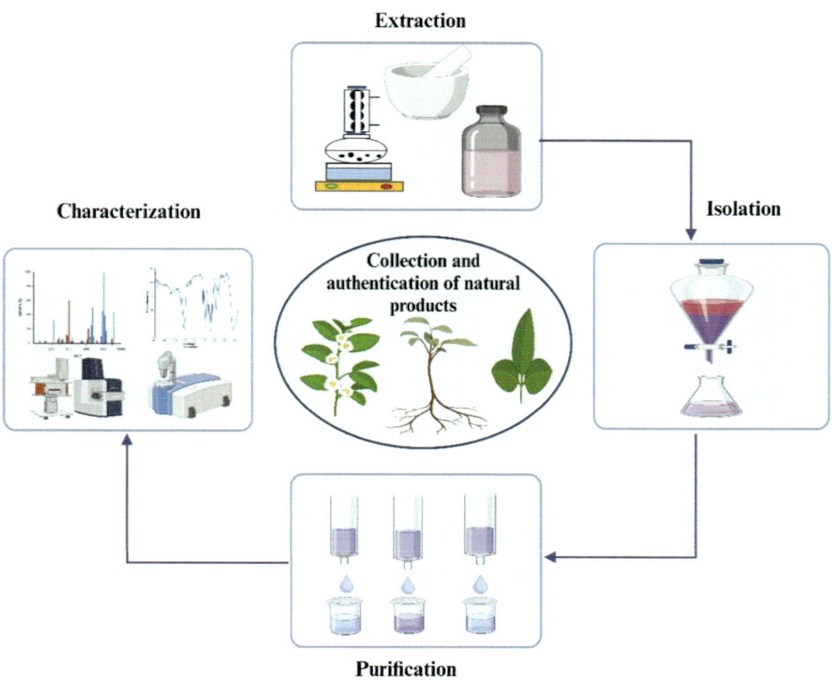

FIGURE 7.5 Representation of collection and authentication of natural products.

7.7 CONCLUSION

The analysis and extraction of natural products from diverse sources are integral to healthcare and pharmaceutical development. Traditional methods have been supplemented by advanced extraction techniques like SFE, UAE, MAE, PLE, EAE, and PEF, addressing limitations in time, solvent usage, and energy intensity while promoting sustainability. Chromatographic methods such as flash chromatography, HPLC, HPTLC, TLC, and CE play essential roles in isolating pure natural products, offering precision and versatility in separation and analysis. HPLC, especially when coupled with MS, enables sensitive and precise qualitative and quantitative analysis, essential for phytochemical characterization. Spectroscopic techniques like UV–Vis, IR, NMR, and MS make available complementary visions into chemical structures and compositions, with NMR easing comprehensive structural elucidation. Mass spectrometry techniques like ESI-MS assistance in compound identification and quantification, even in complex mixtures. Liquid-phase separation methods like LC with MS advance analytical competences, contribute to a comprehensive approach for studying natural product.

Recent advancements in analytical techniques have transfigured the characterization and safety valuation of natural extract. LC-NMR empowers concurrent separation and nuclear magnetic resonance analysis, additional in the identification of various compounds. MALDI and CEC supplementary improve analytical competences, offering insights into bulky molecular weight compounds and well-organized separation of complex mixtures. Moreover, HPLC-SPE-NMR leases for sensitive and cost-effective analysis of natural product elements. Though, safeguarding the purity and safety of natural products remains supreme. Microbial organisms, aflatoxins, heavy metals, pesticides, and radioactive substances are contaminants which pose significant health risks and must be carefully supervised. Analytical techniques, such as counting chromatography, MS, and spectroscopy, play central roles in identifying and quantifying these contaminants, ensuring the safety and efficacy of natural products for consumers. Concerted efforts guided by international standards and regulations are vital to establish and maintain quality control measures for natural products worldwide; thus revealing their vast potential in healthcare and beyond.

KEYWORDS

- **natural products**
- **analytical testing**
- **spectroscopy techniques**
- **chromatographic techniques**
- **qualitative and quantitative methods**

REFERENCES

1. Reddy, A. V. B., Moniruzzaman, M., Madhavi, V., & Jaafar, J. *Recent Improvements in the Extraction, Cleanup and Quantification of Bioactive Flavonoids*. 2020, pp. 197–223.
2. Bauer, A., & Brönstrup, M. Industrial natural product chemistry for drug discovery and development. *Nat Prod Rep* 2014, 31(1), 35–60.
3. Lachance, H., Wetzel, S., Kumar, K., & Waldmann, H. Charting, navigating, and populating natural product chemical space for drug discovery. *J Med Chem* 2012, 55(13), 5989–6001.
4. Chmelík, J., Planeta, J., Řehulka, P., & Chmelík, J. Determination of molecular mass distribution of silicone oils by supercritical fluid chromatography, matrix-assisted laser desorption ionization time-of-flight mass spectrometry and their off-line combination. *J Mass Spectrom* 2001, 36(7), 760–770.
5. Zhang, Q. W., Lin, L. G., & Ye, W. C. Techniques for extraction and isolation of natural products: A comprehensive review. *Chin Med* 2018, 13(1), 20.
6. Najmi, A., Javed, S. A., Al Bratty, M., & Alhazmi, H. A. Modern approaches in the discovery and development of plant-based natural products and their analogues as potential therapeutic agents. *Molecules* 2022, 27(2), 349.
7. Alam, F., & Najum us Saqib, Q. Pharmacognostic standardization and preliminary phytochemical studies of *Gaultheria trichophylla*. *Pharm Biol* 2015, 53(12), 1711–1718.
8. Arya, V., & Thakur, R. Organoleptic and Microscopic Analysis of Gentiana regeliana. *J Pharmacogn Phytochem* 2012, 1(2). Available from: www.phytojournal.comwww.phytojournal.com
9. Mojerlou, Z., & Elhamirad, A. Optimization of ultrasound-assisted extraction (UAE) of phenolic compounds from olive cake. *J Food Sci Technol* 2018, 55(3), 977–984.
10. Rehman, M. U., Abdullah, Khan, F., & Niaz, K. Introduction to natural products analysis. In: *Recent Advances in Natural Products Analysis*. Elsevier, 2020, pp. 3–15.
11. Ganzera, M., & Murauer, A. Separation of natural products. In: *Supercritical Fluid Chromatography*. Elsevier, 2017, pp. 439–460.

12. Thomas, E., Stewart, L. E., Darley, B. A., Pham, A. M., Esteban, I., & Panda, S. S. Plant-based natural products and extracts: Potential source to develop new antiviral drug candidates. *Molecules* 2021, 26(20), 6197.
13. Sharma, V., & Janmeda, P. Extraction, isolation and identification of flavonoid from Euphorbia neriifolia leaves. *Arab J Chem* 2017, 10(4), 509–514.
14. Ponphaiboon, J., Krongrawa, W., Aung, W. W., Chinatangkul, N., Limmatvapirat, S., & Limmatvapirat, C. Advances in natural product extraction techniques, electrospun fiber fabrication, and the integration of experimental design: A comprehensive review. *Molecules* 2023, 28(13), 5163.
15. Altemimi, A., Lakhssassi, N., Baharlouei, A., Watson, D., & Lightfoot, D. Phytochemicals: Extraction, isolation, and identification of bioactive compounds from plant extracts. *Plants* 2017, 6(4), 42.
16. Fomo, G., Madzimbamuto, T. N., & Ojumu, T. V. Applications of nonconventional green extraction technologies in process industries: Challenges, limitations and perspectives. *Sustainability* 2020, 12(13), 5244.
17. Falcão, M. A., Scopel, R., Almeida, R. N., do Espirito Santo, A. T., Franceschini, G., Garcez, J. J., et al., Supercritical fluid extraction of vinblastine from *Catharanthus roseus*. *J Supercrit Fluids* 2017, 129, 9–15.
18. Djapic, N. Essential oils of Taxodium distichum winter leaves obtained by supercritical carbon dioxide extraction method and hydrodistillation. *Separations* 2022, 9(12), 436.
19. Bilia, A. R. Pharmaceutical analysis: plant extracts ☆. In: *Reference Module in Chemistry, Molecular Sciences and Chemical Engineering*. Elsevier, 2018.
20. Chemat, F., Tomao, V., & Virot, M. Ultrasound-assisted extraction in food analysis. *Handbook of Food Analysis Instruments*, CRC Press: Boca Raton, FL, USA, 2008, 11, 85–103.
21. Rostagno, M. A., Palma, M., & Barroso, C. G. Ultrasound-assisted extraction of soy isoflavones. *J Chromatogr, A* 2003, 1012(2), 119–128.
22. Karunakaran, T., Goh, Y. S., Santhanam, R., Murugaiyah, V., Abu Bakar, M. H., & Ramanathan, S. RP-HPLC-DAD analysis of mitragynine content in *Mitragyna speciosa* Korth. (Ketum) leaf extracts prepared using ultrasound assisted extraction technique and their cytotoxicity. *Separations* 2022, 9(11), 345.
23. Ko, M. J., Nam, H. H., & Chung, M. S. Subcritical water extraction of bioactive compounds from *Orostachys japonicus*, A. Berger (Crassulaceae). *Sci Rep* 2020, 10(1), 10890.
24. Pharmacognosy Reviews | An Open Access, peer reviewed journal in the field of pharmacognosy [Internet]. [cited 2024 Feb 16]. Available from: https://www.phcogrev.com/
25. Chan, C. H., Yusoff, R., Ngoh, G. C., & Kung, F. W. L. Microwave-assisted extractions of active ingredients from plants. *J Chromatogr, A* 2011, 1218(37), 6213–6225.
26. Vorobiev, E., & Lebovka, N. I. Extraction of intercellular components by pulsed electric fields. In: Raso, J., & Heinz, V., (Eds.), *Pulsed Electric Fields Technology for the Food Industry: Fundamentals and Applications*. Springer US: Boston, MA, 2006, pp. 153–193. Available from: https://doi.org/10.1007/978-0-387-31122-7_6

27. Toepfl, S., Mathys, A., Heinz, V., & Knorr, D. Review: Potential of high hydrostatic pressure and pulsed electric fields for energy efficient and environmentally friendly food processing. *Food Rev Int* 2006, 22(4), 405–423.
28. Sasidharan, S., Chen, Y., Saravanan, D., Sundram, K., & Latha, L. Extraction, isolation and characterization of bioactive compounds from plants' extracts. *Afr J Tradit Complement Alternat Med* 2010, 8(1), 1–10.
29. Ram, M., Abdin, M. Z., Khan, M. A., & Jha, P. HPTLC fingerprint analysis: A quality control for authentication of herbal phytochemicals. In: *High-Performance Thin-Layer Chromatography (HPTLC)*. Springer Berlin Heidelberg: Berlin, Heidelberg, 2011, pp. 105–116.
30. Ramya, S., Loganathan, T., Chandran, M., Priyanka, R., Kavipriya, K., Grace Lydial Pushpalatha, G., et al., Phytochemical screening, GCMS, FTIR profile of bioactive natural products in the methanolic extracts of *Cuminum cyminum* seeds and oil. *J Drug Deliv Ther* 2022, 12(2-S), 110–118.
31. Chen, Q., Hu, X., Li, J., Liu, P., Yang, Y., & Ni, Y. Preparative isolation and purification of cuminaldehyde and p-menta-1,4-dien-7-al from the essential oil of *Cuminum cyminum* L. by high-speed counter-current chromatography. *Anal Chim Acta* 2011, 689(1), 149–154.
32. Handa, S. S., Khanuja, S., Longo, G., & Rakesh, D. D. Extraction technologies for medicinal and aromatic plants. *International Centre for Science and High Technology*. 2008, pp. 21–25.
33. Wilson, I. D., & Poole, C. F. Planar chromatography—Current practice and future prospects. *J Chromatogr B* 2023, 1214, 123553.
34. Aravind, S. G., Arimboor, R., Rangan, M., Madhavan, S. N., & Arumughan, C. Semi-preparative HPLC preparation and HPTLC quantification of tetrahydroamentoflavone as marker in *Semecarpus anacardium* and its polyherbal formulations. *J Pharm Biomed Anal* 2008, 48(3), 808–813.
35. Amit Koparde, A., Chandrashekar Doijad, R., & Shripal Magdum, C. Natural products in drug discovery. In: *Pharmacognosy—Medicinal Plants*. IntechOpen, 2019.
36. Latif, Z., & Sarker, S. D. *Isolation of Natural Products by Preparative High Performance Liquid Chromatography (Prep-HPLC)*. In: 2012, pp. 255–274.
37. Hostettmann, K., Hostettmann, M., & Marston, A. Introduction. In: Hostettmann, K., Hostettmann, M., & Marston, A., (Eds.), *Preparative Chromatography Techniques: Applications in Natural Product Isolation*, Springer Berlin Heidelberg: Berlin, Heidelberg, 1986, p. 1. Available from: https://doi.org/10.1007/978-3-662-02492-8_1
38. Xiang, Q., Gao, Y., & Yang, S. W. Recent advances of application of capillary electrophoresis in traditional Chinese medicine analysis. *Adv Mat Res* 2013, 634–638, 1388–1391.
39. Pratap Singh, A., Fathordoobady, F., Guo, Y., Singh, A., & Kitts, D. D. Antioxidants help favorably regulate the kinetics of lipid peroxidation, polyunsaturated fatty acids degradation and acidic cannabinoids decarboxylation in hempseed oil. *Sci Rep* 2020, 10(1), 10567.
40. Kumar, M. V. S., Talluri, V. P., & Rajagopal, S. V. Purification and characterization of bioactive compound from the methanolic leaf extract of *Millingtonia hortensis* Linn. *Int J Pharma Bio Sci* 2015, 6, P348–P358.

41. Bharadwaj, S., & Leela, S. (Print) www.rjptonline.org 0974-360X (Online) Research Article 1 H NMR Analysis and Bioautography Screening of Methanol Extract of Sargassum wightii by Chromatographic Separation. 2017, 10.
42. Steinmann, D., & Ganzera, M. Recent advances on HPLC/MS in medicinal plant analysis. *J Pharm Biomed Anal* 2011, 55(4), 744–757.
43. Harborne, A. J. *Phytochemical Methods a Guide to Modern Techniques of Plant Analysis*. Springer Science & Business Media, 1998.
44. Huang, Z., Wang, B., Eaves, D. H., Shikany, J. M., & Pace, R. D. Phenolic compound profile of selected vegetables frequently consumed by African Americans in the southeast United States. *Food Chem* 2007, 103(4), 1395–1402.
45. Patel, R. K., Patel, V. R., & Patel, M. G. Development and validation of a RP-HPLC method for the simultaneous determination of Embelin, Rottlerin and Ellagic acid in Vidangadi churna. *J Pharm Anal* 2012, 2(5), 366–371.
46. Robards, K. Strategies for the determination of bioactive phenols in plants, fruit and vegetables. *J Chromatogr A* 2003, 1000(1–2), 657–691.
47. Klimek-Turek, A., & Dzido, T. H. Separation selectivity of some phenolic acids in RP HPLC systems with binary mobile phase comprised various modifiers. *Adsorption* 2010, 16, 287–294.
48. Khoddami, A., Wilkes, M., & Roberts, T. Techniques for analysis of plant phenolic compounds. *Molecules* 2013, 18(2), 2328–2375.
49. Kumar, B. R. Application of HPLC and ESI-MS techniques in the analysis of phenolic acids and flavonoids from green leafy vegetables (GLVs). *J Pharm Anal* 2017, 7(6), 349–364.
50. van Tellingen, O., Beijnen, J. H., & Nooyen, W. J. Analytical methods for the determination of vinca alkaloids in biological specimens: A survey of the literature. *J Pharm Biomed Anal* 1991, 9(10–12), 1077–1082.
51. Kumar, A., Patil, D., Rajamohanan, P. R., & Ahmad, A. Isolation, purification and characterization of vinblastine and vincristine from endophytic fungus Fusarium oxysporum isolated from *Catharanthus roseus*. *PLoS One* 2013, 8(9), e71805.
52. Cieśla, Ł., & Moaddel, R. Comparison of analytical techniques for the identification of bioactive compounds from natural products. *Nat Prod Rep* 2016, 33(10), 1131–1145.
53. Serrano, J., Puupponen-Pimiä, R., Dauer, A., Aura, A., & Saura-Calixto, F. Tannins: Current knowledge of food sources, intake, bioavailability and biological effects. *Mol Nutr Food Res* 2009, 53(S2).
54. Silva, A. S., & Nabavi, S. M. Future perspectives in natural products analysis. In: *Recent Advances in Natural Products Analysis*. Elsevier, 2020, pp. 825–833.
55. Lambert, M., Wolfender, J. L., Stærk, D., Christensen, S. B., Hostettmann, K., & Jaroszewski, J. W. Identification of natural products using HPLC-SPE combined with CapNMR. *Anal Chem* 2007, 79(2), 727–735.
56. Lange, R., & Balny, C. UV-visible derivative spectroscopy under high pressure. *Biochim Biophys Acta* 2002, 1595(1–2), 80–93.
57. Rakhee, Mishra, J., Sharma, R. K., & Misra, K. Characterization techniques for herbal products. In: *Management of High Altitude Pathophysiology*. Elsevier, 2018, pp. 171–202.

58. Urbano, M., Luque de Castro, M. D., Pérez, P. M., García-Olmo, J., & Gómez-Nieto, M. A. Ultraviolet–visible spectroscopy and pattern recognition methods for differentiation and classification of wines. *Food Chem* 2006, 97(1), 166–175.
59. NMR Spectroscopy in development of herbal medicines | bruker [Internet]. [cited 2024 Feb 18]. Available from: https://www.bruker.com/es/news-and-events/webinars/2021/zh/NMR-Spectroscopy-in-Development-of-Herbal-Medicines.html
60. Chauthe, S. K., Sharma, R. J., Aqil, F., Gupta, R. C., & Singh, I. P. Quantitative NMR: An applicable method for quantitative analysis of medicinal plant extracts and herbal products. *Phytochem Anal* 2012, 23(6), 689–696.
61. Liu, Q., & Liu, Y. [Application of 13CNMR to structural identification of the flavonoid glycosides]. *Zhongguo Yi Xue Ke Xue Yuan Xue Bao* 1990, 12(5), 359–364.
62. Sm, D., & Kalaichelvi, K. UV-VIS spectroscopic and FTIR Analysis of *Sarcostemma brevistigma*, wight. and arn. *Int J Curr Pharm Res* 2017, 9, 46–49.
63. Huck, C. W. Advances of infrared spectroscopy in natural product research. *Phytochem Lett* 2015, 11, 384–393.
64. Koparde, A. A., Doijad, R. C., & Magdum, C. S. Natural products in drug discovery. In: Perveen, S., & Al-Taweel, A., (Eds.), *Pharmacognosy*, IntechOpen: Rijeka, 2019. Available from: https://doi.org/10.5772/intechopen.82860
65. Hashimoto, A., & Kameoka, T. Applications of infrared spectroscopy to biochemical, food, and agricultural processes. *Appl Spectrosc Rev* 2008, 43, 416–451.
66. Dhivya, S. M., Kalaichelvi, K., & Sharmila, S. Pharmacognostical studies on *Sarcostemma brevistigma*, Wight. and Arn.—An ethnomedicinal plant. *Int J Pharm Phytochem Res* 2017, 9(5), 657–662.
67. Ur Rehman, I., Malik, L., Zaheer, S., & Abdullah, M. A brief study of mass spectrometry of natural products. *Plant Biotechnol Persa* 2022, 4(1), 50–55.
68. Přichystal, J., Schug, K. A., Lemr, K., Novák, J., & Havlíček, V. Structural analysis of natural products. *Anal Chem* 2016, 88(21), 10338–10346.
69. Ingle, K. P., & Deshmukh, A. G. Phytochemicals: Extraction methods, identification and detection of bioactive compounds from plant extracts. *J Pharmacogn Phytochem* 2017, 6(1), 32–36.
70. Alvarez-Rivera, G., Ballesteros-Vivas, D., Parada-Alfonso, F., Ibañez, E., & Cifuentes, A. Recent applications of high resolution mass spectrometry for the characterization of plant natural products. *TrAC Trend Anal Chem* 2019, 112, 87–101.
71. Pramanik, B. N., Ganguly, A. K., & Gross, M. L., (Eds.), *Applied Electrospray Mass Spectrometry*. CRC Press, 2002.
72. Demarque, D. P., Crotti, A. E. M., Vessecchi, R., Lopes, J. L. C, & Lopes, N. P. Fragmentation reactions using electrospray ionization mass spectrometry: An important tool for the structural elucidation and characterization of synthetic and natural products. *Nat Prod Rep* 2016, 33(3), 432–455.
73. Smyth, W. F., McClean, S., Hack, C. J., Ramachandran, V. N., Doherty, B., Joyce, C., et al., The characterisation of synthetic and natural-product pharmaceuticals by electrospray ionisation-mass spectrometry (ESI-MS) and liquid chromatography (LC)-ESI-MS. *TrAC Trend Anal Chem* 2006, 25(6), 572–582.
74. Zhou, H., Tai, Y., Sun, C., & Pan, Y. Rapid identification of vinca alkaloids by direct-injection electrospray ionisation tandem mass spectrometry and confirmation by

high-performance liquid chromatography-mass spectrometry. *Phytochem Anal* 2005, 16(5), 328–333.
75. Favretto, D., Piovan, A., Filippini, R., & Caniato, R. Monitoring the production yields of vincristine and vinblastine in *Catharanthus roseus* from somatic embryogenesis. Semiquantitative determination by flow-injection electrospray ionization mass spectrometry. *Rapid Commun Mass Spectrom* 2001, 15(5), 364–369.
76. Gebretsadik, T., Linert, W., Thomas, M., Berhanu, T., & Frew, R. LC–NMR for natural product analysis: A journey from an academic curiosity to a robust analytical tool. *Science* 2021, 3(1), 6.
77. Bobzin, S. C., Yang, S., & Kasten, T. P. Application of liquid chromatography-nuclear magnetic resonance spectroscopy to the identification of natural products. *J Chromatography B* 2000, 748, 259–267. Available from: www.elsevier.com/locate/chromb
78. Castola, V., Bighelli, A., & Casanova, J. Direct qualitative and quantitative analysis of triterpenes using ^{13}C NMR spectroscopy exemplified by dichloromethanic extracts of cork. *Appl Spectrosc* 1999, 53(3), 344–350.
79. Patel, K., Patel, J., Patel, M., Rajput, G., & Patel, H. Introduction to hyphenated techniques and their applications in pharmacy. *Pharm Methods* 2010, 1(1), 2.
80. Niessen, W. M. A. *Chapter 10 Combined Techniques*. 2004, pp. 403–430.
81. Jiménez-González, A., Quispe, C., Bórquez, J., Sepúlveda, B., Riveros, F., Areche, C., et al., UHPLC-ESI-ORBITRAP-MS analysis of the native Mapuche medicinal plant palo negro (*Leptocarpha rivularis* DC.—Asteraceae) and evaluation of its antioxidant and cholinesterase inhibitory properties. *J Enzyme Inhib Med Chem* 2018, 33(1), 936–944.
82. Chagas-Paula, D., Zhang, T., Da Costa, F., & Edrada-Ebel, R. A metabolomic approach to target compounds from the asteraceae family for dual COX and LOX inhibition. *Metabolites* 2015, 5(3), 404–430.
83. Silva, R., Lopes, N., & Silva, D. Application of MALDI mass spectrometry in natural products analysis. *Planta Med* 2016, 82(08), 671–689.
84. Clark, A. E., Kaleta, E. J., Arora, A., & Wolk, D. M. Matrix-assisted laser desorption ionization–time of flight mass spectrometry: A fundamental shift in the routine practice of clinical microbiology. *Clin Microbiol Rev* 2013, 26(3), 547–603.
85. Fang, H., Chen, Y., Wu, H. L., Chen, Y., Wang, T., Yang, J., et al., Matrix-assisted laser desorption/ionization time-of-flight mass spectrometry combined with chemometrics to identify the origin of Chinese medicinal materials. *RSC Adv* 2022, 12(26), 16886–16892.
86. Lu, M., & Cai, Z. *Advances of MALDI-TOF MS in the Analysis of Traditional Chinese Medicines*. 2012, pp. 143–164.
87. Gottardo, R., Chiarini, A., Dal Prà, I., Seri, C., Rimondo, C., Serpelloni, G., et al., Direct screening of herbal blends for new synthetic cannabinoids by MALDI-TOF MS. *J Mass Spectrom* 2012, 47(1), 141–146.
88. Jorgenson, J. W., & Lukacs, K. D. Free-zone electrophoresis in glass capillaries. *Clin Chem* 1981, 27(9), 1551–1553.
89. Chen, Y., Fan, G., Chen, B., Xie, Y., Wu, H., Wu, Y., et al., Separation and quantitative analysis of coumarin compounds from *Angelica dahurica* (*Fisch. ex Hoffm*) *Benth. et*

Hook.f by pressurized capillary electrochromatography. *J Pharm Biomed Anal* 2006, 41(1), 105–116.

90. Liu, F., Wang, Y. N., Li, Y., Ma, S. G., Qu, J., Liu, Y. B., et al., Triterpenoids from the twigs and leaves of Rhododendron latoucheae by HPLC–MS–SPE–NMR. *Tetrahedron* 2019, 75(2), 296–307.
91. Crossley, S., & Baines, J. Public health measures: Monitoring of contaminants. In: *Encyclopedia of Food Safety*. Elsevier, 2014, pp. 55–61.
92. Kosalec, I., Cvek, J., & Tomic, S. Contaminants of medicinal herbs and herbal products. *Arh Hig Rada Toksikol* 2009, 60(4), 485.
93. Kosalec, I., Cvek, J., & Tomić, S. Contaminants of Medicinal Herbs and Herbal Products. *Archives of Industrial Hygiene and Toxicology* 2009, 60(4), 485–501.
94. Muyumba, N. W., Mutombo, S. C., Sheridan, H., Nachtergael, A., & Duez, P. Quality control of herbal drugs and preparations: The methods of analysis, their relevance and applications. *Talanta Open* 2021, 4, 100070.
95. Kunle, O. F., Egharevba, H. O., & Ahmadu, P. O. Standardization of herbal medicines-A review. *Int J Biodivers Conserv* 2012, 4(3), 101–112.
96. AHPA releases guidance on foreign matter limits in herbal ingredients [Internet]. [cited 2024 Feb 19]. Available from: https://www.nutraingredients-usa.com/Article/2017/10/31/AHPA-releases-guidance-on-foreign-matter-limits-in-herbal-ingredients
97. AHPA guidance policies [Internet]. [cited 2024 Feb 21]. Available from: https://www.ahpa.org/ahpa_guidance_policies
98. https://pubmed.ncbi.nlm.nih.gov/?term=TATSUTA%20K%5BAuthor%5D. Total synthesis and development of bioactive natural products.
99. Jayaraman, J. Laboratory manual in biochemistry/J. Jayaraman. *Laboratory Manual in Biochemistry [Internet]*. 1988 [cited 2024 Feb 21]; Available from: https://books.google.com/books/about/Laboratory_Manual_in_Biochemistry.html?id=UMMZugEACAAJ
100. Ahmed, S., & Hasan, M. Standardization of crude drugs: A precise review. *World J Pharm Res* 2015, 4, 155–174.
101. Yadav, V. K., Irchhiaya, R., & Ghosh, A. K. Phytochemical and pharmacognostical studies of anogeissus acuminata. *J Drug Deliv Ther.* 2019, 9(4-A), 450–457.
102. Moisture analysis techniques [Internet]. [cited 2024 Feb 19]. Available from: https://www.news-medical.net/life-sciences/Moisture-Analysis-Techniques.aspx
103. Balekundri, A., & Mannur, V. Quality control of the traditional herbs and herbal products: A review. *Futur J Pharm Sci* 2020, 6(1), 67.
104. Rohmah, M., Saragih, B., Amaliah, N., Kristopal, K., Putra, Y. H. E., & Rahmadi, A. Determination of Moisture, ash, protein, polyphenolic, flavonoids, and amino acid contents and antioxidant capacity of dried mekai (*Pycnarrhena tumefacta* Miers) leaf as potential herbal flavor enhancers. In: *Proc Int Conf Trop Agrifood, Feed Fuel (ICTAFF 2022)*.
105. Opuni K. F. M., Kretchy J. P., Agyabeng, K., Boadu, J. A., Adanu, T., Ankamah, S., Appiah, A., Amoah, G. B., Baidoo, M., Kretchy, IA. Contamination of herbal medicinal products in low-and-middle-income countries: A systematic review. *Heliyon*. 2023, 9(9), e19370. doi: 10.1016/j.heliyon.2023.e19370

106. World Health Organization. WHO Guidelines for Assessing Quality of Herbal Medicines with Reference to Contaminants and Residues. 2007, 105.
107. Shabeer, S. Aflatoxin contamination, its impact and management strategies: An updated review.
108. Sarma, U. P., Bhetaria, P. J., Devi, P., & Varma, A. Aflatoxins: Implications on health. *Indian J Clin Biochem* 2017, 32(2), 124–133. Available from: https://link.springer.com/article/10.1007/s12291-017-0649-2
109. Kumar, P. Aflatoxins: A global concern for food safety, human health and their management.
110. Wild, C. P., Miller, J. D., & Groopman, J. D. Mycotoxin control in low-and middle-income countries. 2015.
111. Zhang, L., Dou, X. W., Zhang, C., Logrieco, A., & Yang, M. H. A review of current methods for analysis of mycotoxins in herbal medicines. *Toxins (Basel)* 2018, 10(2), 65.
112. Rajmohan, K. S., Chandrasekaran, R., & Varjani, S. A review on occurrence of pesticides in environment and current technologies for their remediation and management. *Indian J Microbiol* 2020, 60(2), 125–138.
113. Ntow, W. J., Tagoe, L. M., Drechsel, P., Kelderman, P., Nyarko, E., & Gijzen, H. J. Occupational exposure to pesticides: Blood cholinesterase activity in a farming community in Ghana. *Arch Environ Contam Toxicol* 2009, 56(3), 623–630. Available from: https://doi.org/10.1007/s00244-007-9077-2
114. Hassaan, M. A., & El Nemr, A. Pesticides pollution: Classifications, human health impact, extraction and treatment techniques. *Egypt J Aquat Res* 2020, 46(3), 207–220.
115. Jayaraj, R., Megha, P., & Sreedev, P. Review Article. Organochlorine pesticides, their toxic effects on living organisms and their fate in the environment. *Interdiscip Toxicol* 2016, 9(3–4), 90–100.
116. Kellogg, J. J., Paine, M. F., McCune, J. S., Oberlies, N. H., & Cech, N. B. Selection and characterization of botanical natural products for research studies: A NaPDI center recommended approach. *Nat Prod Rep* 2019, 36(8), 1196–1221.
117. Hernández-Mesa, M., & Moreno-González, D. Current role of mass spectrometry in the determination of pesticide residues in food. *Separations* 2022, 9(6), 148.
118. WHO Guidelines for Assessing Quality of Herbal Medicines with Reference to Contaminants and Residues. 2007.
119. Barnes, J., Anderson, L. A., & Phillipson, J. D. *Herbal Medicine.* 3rd edn, Pharmaceutical Press: London, 2007, pp. 1–23.
120. Luo, L., Wang, B., Jiang, J., Fitzgerald, M., Huang, Q., Yu, Z., et al., Heavy metal contaminations in herbal medicines: Determination, comprehensive risk assessments, and solutions. *Front Pharmacol* 2021, 11, 595335.
121. Street, R. A. Heavy metals in medicinal plant products—An African perspective. *South African Journal of Botany* 2012, 82, 67–74.
122. Yuan, X., Chapman, R. L., & Wu, Z. Analytical methods for heavy metals in herbal medicines. *Phytochem Anal* 2011, 22(3), 189–198.
123. National policy on traditional medicine and regulation of herbal medicines : Report of a WHO global survey [Internet]. [cited 2024 Feb 21]. Available from: https://www.who.int/publications/i/item/9241593237

124. Suschny, O. Analytical quality control services of the International Atomic Energy Agency. *Fresenius' Zeitschrift für analytische Chemie* 1986, 323(6), 560–562.
125. Vi, N. Naturally occurring radioactive material.
126. Mukne, A., Momin, M., Betkar, P., & Joshi, V. Standardization of herbal biomolecules. In: *Herbal Biomolecules in Healthcare Applications*, Elsevier, 2022, pp. 643–667.

CHAPTER 8

Patents and Intellectual Property in Herbal Industry: The Outlook

KAVITA MUNJAL[1], ARUSHI SHARMA[2], KARAN SHARMA[3], ROHIT THAKUR[2], ASHISH BALDI[4], and VINOD KUMAR GAUTTAM[5*]

[1]*Amity Institute of Pharmacy, Amity University, Noida, Uttar Pradesh, India*

[2]*Department of Pharmaceutics, Shiva Institute of Pharmacy, Bilaspur, Himachal Pradesh, India*

[3]*Department of Pharmacology, Shiva Institute of Pharmacy, Bilaspur, Himachal Pradesh, India*

[4]*Department of Pharmaceutical Sciences and Technology, Maharaja Ranjit Singh Punjab Technical University, Punjab, India*

[5]*SGT College of Pharmacy, SGT University, Gurugram, India*

*Corresponding author

ABSTRACT

The herbal therapeutic and cosmetic ingredients are gaining popularity and recognition throughout the world due to their certain unique advantages. This motivates drug and pharmaceutical companies to examine herbs for new drug discovery and invest in traditional medicine herbs for certain conditions. This led to green chemistry and scientifically confirmed natural compounds. Global herbal medication producers are flooding these bazaars to sell their products. To promote herbal products, including medicine,

Herbal Drug Industry: From Cultivation to Innovation and Global Impact.
Abhishek Tiwari, Varsha Tiwari, and Ajay Sharma (Eds.)

DOI: 10.1201/9781779640994-8

worldwide, research centers were formed. Herbal companies started patenting their innovations to preserve their IP and money. Intellectual property rights become more relevant as herbal medicine increases. Plant and herbal medicine intellectual property protection is a hotly debated, fast changing issue that has influenced many national economies. A new global economic order has emerged from developing patent rules. The Trade-Related Aspects of Intellectual Property Rights and the Convention on Biological Diversity support plant patent law reform and plant-based pharmaceutical restrictions to protect rich and developing nations. The most frequent IP insurance for domestic pharmaceuticals is trademarks and transferring secrets. Analysts and professionals must earn reputation and selectivity through insurance rights. Herbal industry patent and intellectual property advancements and revenue contributions are highlighted in the this chapter.

8.1 INTRODUCTION

Owing to its extensive legacy of rare fauna, India is considered a "treasure house" of invaluable medicinal and aromatic plant species [1]. The Indian Ministry of Environment and Forests has identified and cataloged over 9500 plant species because of their importance to the pharmaceutical industry. Of these, about 65 plants are in high demand worldwide and are traded on a regular basis. An essential component of India's healthcare system is the generation-old practice of using plants as medicine. India is home to 45,000 distinct plant species, 15,000 of which are medicinal, and 16 agroclimatic zones. Approximately 500 species of the 1500 medicinal plants recognized by Indian systems of medicine are used primarily in the production of pharmaceuticals. Ayurveda, Siddha, Unani, and homoeopathy are just a few of the Indian medical systems that use materials primarily derived from plants, minerals, metals, marine life, and animal products. Our old writings had recorded the use of many plants for medicinal purposes [2]. These herbs have been used to make medicines for millennia. But a recent trend suggests that foreign countries are starting to show more interest in the medicinal plants that are available in India and whose intended uses are thoroughly described in our books. International patents protect a wide range of medicinal plants and their uses. The growing practice of patenting our medicinal plants and their uses has drawn criticism from the public. Many well-known plants, such as Kala Zeera, Amaltas, Indian Mustared, Karela, Brinjal, Neem, and Gudmar, are patent holders [3].

India has successfully challenged a few of the patents. Even when compared to our neighbor China, India lags behind the others in terms of patents, both quantitatively and qualitatively. The persistent ignorance and misunderstanding regarding patents is a significant problem. Our pool of patents covers a relatively small amount of information, even in areas where we have an advantage over competitors. Think about the field of herbal products, where a lot of feelings have been shared [4]. Our pool of patents covers a relatively small amount of information, even in areas where we have an advantage over competitors. Think about the field of herbal products, where a lot of feelings have been shared. There were 1889 herbal patents between 1995 and 1998, of which China possessed 889; the Indian portion was insignificant.

This chapter looks at the need to document indigenous knowledge about Indian herbs and plants, as well as their medicinal and other uses, and turn it into an easily navigable computerized database for quick access and patenting rights in order to stop other countries from patenting Indian heritage [5].

Table 8.1 lists some herbal drugs those origin country is other but their use patented by some other countries.

Table 8.1 indicates that there is a need to protect traditional medicines through legal procedures to ensure their protection from piracy.

During corona pandemic, herbal-based drug formulations treatment gained popularity due to their affordability and availability to treat physiological anomalies. Thus, the demand for traditional plant-based medicines is increasing, emphasizing their commercial value [18].

Traditional medicine often relies on natural resources and the knowledge of local and indigenous communities and healers. It is interconnected with biodiversity preservation and the rights of indigenous people over their knowledge and resources [19]. There is a risk of theft or unauthorized use of newly designed or novel medications derived from natural products. To ensure the safety of research outcomes or products, it is mandatory to protect them using legal means. The protective laws include patents and trade secrets [20].

Customary knowledge is crucially important in the drug discovery department of pharmaceutical industry. The economic value of herbal

TABLE 8.1 List of Traditional Herbal Medicines, Granted with Patent, and Copyrights

Serial Number	Herbal Medicine	Origin Country	Part Use	Medicinal Use	Copyright Claiming Country	Year
1.	Indian Head	North America	Entire plant	Immuno-modulatory	European country [6]	–
2.	*Aloe vera*	Sri Lanka	Leaves	Skin care and treatment	USA	1979 [7]
3.	Coffee	Africa	Seeds	Brain tonic	France	1881 [8]
4.	Pare	Sri Lanka and India	Seeds	Antidiabetic	United States	1999
5.	Jamaica	India	Seeds	Antidiabetic	United States	1999
6.	Ratna	India	Fruits	Antidiabetic	United states	1999 [9]
7.	Manjal	India	Whole plant	Wound healing	United States	1995 [10]
8.	Neem	India	Bark	Antifungal	USA	1983 [11]
9.	Latjira	India	Whole plant	As swelling reducing agent and a blood flow regulator	United States	1997 [12]
10.	Bach	India	Rhizome	Head lice treatment	Australia	1998 [13]
11.	Bitter melon	Sri Lanka and India	Seed, fruit	Anti-HIV	USA [14]	–
12.	Saptaragni	Sri Lanka	Root and stem	Bone and joint disorders	Japan and USA	2007 and 2017 [15]
13.	Punku	Sri Lanka	Seed oil	Biopesticides	Japan [16]	–
14.	Adigam	India and Africa	Whole plant	Anti-diabetic	WIPO (PCT)	2015 [17]

medicines and the need for addressing issues related to intellectual property, recognition, and compensation for the communities, contributing to this knowledge are listed as [21]:

1. **Abundance of plant species in traditional medicine**

   It is estimated that a significant number of plant species, ranging from 25,000 to 75,000, are used in traditional medicine [22].

2. **Limited acceptance in science and business**

   Scientists only know and accept 1% of these plant species for use in commerce. This suggests disconnect between conventional wisdom and widely accepted scientific validation. [23].

3. **The herbal medicine market worldwide**

   The value of the herbal drug market is estimated to be in the range of 60 billion USD worldwide. This highlights the economic importance of herbal remedies worldwide. [24].

4. **Contribution of local communities and indigenous people**

   Indigenous populations and local communities provide a significant contribution in the development of the modern pharmaceutical industry. Many medicinal plants discovered by these groups have formed the basis of pharmaceutical products [25].

5. **Unacknowledged contributions and inadequate remuneration**

   Indigenous populations and local communities have made significant contributions to the development of medicinal plant-based pharmaceuticals, but their knowledge and contributions are not adequately acknowledged or compensated. Pharmaceutical companies continue to receive the majority of the economic benefits.

6. **Intellectual property and ownership**

   Intellectual property rights (IPR) is defined as an exclusive privilege for intangible human creations, and it acts as a tool to protect intellect against copying of his/her creativity and knowledge. For this concept of patenting, registration of trademarks, trade secrets, publicity style, moral and other rights against unfair competition. It recognizes and defends the elusive expressions of human intelligence [26]. Thus, knowledge, data, concepts, and other "matters of the mind" that are not readily apparent or known to others without disclosure or access are referred to as intellectual property. Ownership of intellectual property can be shared or exclusive by companies, governments, associations, groups, and individuals. The passage notes that exclusive owners of intellectual property can choose various courses of action, such as keeping it unused, using it themselves, giving it away, trading it, or selling it [27].

8.1.1 ETHICAL AND LEGAL IMPLICATIONS

The lack of recognition or compensation for traditional knowledge raises ethical concerns. It implies a potential imbalance in the distribution of benefits derived from traditional medicine [28]. Thus, the traditional knowledge and indigenous peoples might not be adequately protected by the current intellectual property rights mechanisms. Communities in the area may feel that they are being victimized by "bio-piracy," the term for unauthorized use of biological resources or traditional knowledge [29].

8.1.2 CONDITIONS AND OBSTACLES FOR PATENTING

A patent is a legally recognized right that the government grants to the person who discovers or invents new intellectual property. The inventor may use this right to stop others from developing, using, or commercializing their invention for a restricted period of time.

8.1.2.1 CONDITIONS FOR GRANTING PATENTS

When claimed intellectual property is judged to be new, useful, and not readily apparent to people with the necessary expertise in the field, a patent is awarded.

8.1.2.2 PROCEDURE FOR APPLYING A PATENT

A written document called a patent application is required to fully disclose and provide a detailed description of the claimed invention. The invention should be sufficient for someone with the necessary skills to use or practice. Applications for patents must be filed in every nation where protection is desired and accessible.

8.1.2.3 OBSTACLES FOR PATENTING

A large number of patent applications are never granted because they do not satisfy the requirements of novelty, utility, and nonobviousness. Some granted patents may prove to have little or no actual value for their holders, especially when it comes to the development of novel drugs where there is uncertainty regarding the product's ultimate success [30]. Although certain facets of conventional medicine might be safeguarded by current intellectual property laws, such as sui generis systems, might be necessary [31].

8.1.3 PATENT DISTRIBUTION WORLDWIDE

The distribution of patent around the globe is nonuniform and the capabilities of filing and evaluation of patent cases requires financial and technical forces. Hence, currently, developed nations own about 95% of all patents worldwide.

8.1.4 INAPPLICABILITY OF CURRENT PATENT LAWS

The bulk of national and international conventional patent laws do not seem to be suitable or applicable for protecting biodiversity and traditional knowledge, with their requirements for inventive steps and novelty.

8.1.5 NEED FOR MODIFICATIONS IN INTELLECTUAL PROPERTY OWNERSHIP

There is a need for changing the existing intellectual property laws and creating new ones that better serve the interests of people defending conventional medical practices.

8.1.6 ROLE OF IPR IN INDIAN HERBAL INDUSTRIES

Strong intellectual property protection is required due to the burgeoning herbal industry and the substantial research and development in the field. For the protection of herbal products and processes, patents, copyrights, designs, trademarks, and geographical indications are considered essential [32].

It is true that the popularity of herbal remedies for a range of ailments has increased. This covers dietary supplements and medications for ailments like obesity, diabetes, rheumatoid arthritis, hypertension, and neurological disorders. The preference for herbal products in the global market is the reason for this trend [33].

The Indian herbal product industry's IPR landscape is as follows:

8.1.6.1 TRIPS COMPLIANCE

The TRIPS Agreement, which addresses IPR related to trade, has set uniform standards for intellectual property ever since it was created. But there has been a lot of discussion about it because of worries that if it were implemented, drug prices would rise and people would find it more difficult to afford the necessary medications, particularly in developing countries. The majority of the conversation has so far centered on contemporary medications. Examining the issue of IPR for "modern" or "allopathic" medications from the perspective of a developing country. Although their actual application may be challenging, the goals are well-defined and the techniques to attain them are widely recognized. With regard to traditional medical procedures, this cannot be said. The availability of biogenetic resources and the information of their therapeutic qualities by regional and indigenous cultures are closely related to traditional medicine. In essence, traditional medicine involves "dealing with issues related to technology transfer, protection, preservation, and promotion of cultural heritage, as well as biodiversity conservation" [34]. Policies must strike a balance because of the intricate relationships between biological resources, contemporary technologies, and community rights. Thus, it is crucial to carefully weigh the objectives and possible outcomes of traditional medicine IPR protection at the national level. Unfortunately, disagreements over concepts and points of view can sometimes make it difficult to define the objectives that should be pursued, which hampers the discussion of potential policy decisions [21].

8.2 CONTEXT AND PHILOSOPHY

Traditional medicine is used to protect, cure, diagnose, and/or restore physical and mental health status in addition to maintaining general health.

It is sometimes referred to as “the sum total of the knowledge, skills, and practices based on the theories, beliefs, and experiences indigenous to different cultures, whether explicable or not.” Even though there is not much scientific proof to support the efficacy and safety of many traditional medicines, because they are “field-tested” since early human lives, communities have amassed a wealth of empirical knowledge that has been passed down through generations of healers.

For their primary medical care, a sizable portion of the populace in many developing nations, particularly in rural regions, exclusively uses traditional medicine. For instance, 80% of people in Africa use traditional medicines, while 65% of Indians only have access to traditional medical systems. Traditional medicine remains widely popular in most Asian countries, including in highly industrialized nations like Japan, even if allopathic medication is readily available [35]. In other developed countries, “alternative medicine” is becoming more popular; a 1993 survey in the United States found that one in three people there reported using it [36]. Thus, according to WHO estimates from 2000, the worldwide market for herbal medicines is valued at $60 billion. Herbal remedies are a good alternative for people in wealthy countries, but for people in developing countries, they are often their only option. However, while herbal medications are a choice for those in developed nations, they are frequently the only one available to those in developing nations.

8.3 PLAGIARISM AND PRESERVATION

The commercial use of goods derived from traditional knowledge without giving knowledge holders any kind of return or compensation is referred to as “bio-piracy” and is introduced. This is recognized as a significant problem in developing nations. The challenges of using traditional knowledge and medicinal plants for profit in developing nations are covered in the passage. It draws attention to the historical exploitation of intellectual property rights by multinational corporations, the principles set forth at the Convention on Biodiversity, the significance of passing laws to put these principles into practice, and the function of international agreements like TRIPs in this regard. The passage also emphasizes how important sui generis systems are to protect traditional knowledge, especially in the context of genetic resources and conventional medicine [35].

Mainly in under-developing countries with a long history of using traditional systems of medicine, recent cases of "biopiracy," or the unauthorized use and exploitation of biogenetic sources linked to conventional medical knowledge is protected by western IPRs, have raised serious concerns [36]. A prime example is the US patent for "use of turmeric as wound healing," which was granted in March 1995. But in India, where it has "been applied to the scrapes and cuts of generations of children," turmeric powder is well known for its healing properties [37]. Despite being successfully challenged by the scientific committee of CSIR, India, this patent was ultimately determined to be invalid due to a lack of novelty. However, the procedure was costly, and monitoring "biopiracy-patents" may be challenging for developing nations [38–40].

After making minor modifications, researchers, or businesses assert intellectual property rights over traditional knowledge pertaining to biological resources. Patents for barbasco, endod, kava, and neem trees are a few examples [41, 42]. These and related occurrences sparked worries and inquiries in developing nations, particularly about how to safeguard their traditional knowledge, stop such piracy, and equitably distribute the benefits of that knowledge [43].

It has also brought attention to the necessity of defining who owns biological resources and related information. Pharmaceutical corporations have expressed interest in obtaining and researching traditional remedies because they believe that "promising species" may yield valuable leads for the drug discovery of novel therapeutics. Utilizing traditional knowledge has sometimes resulted in significant financial gain for businesses; one such instance is development of anticancer phytochemicals, vincristine and vinblastine (alkaloids) from the *Vinca* plant in Madagascar [26, 35, 44]. The potential to patent derived goods influences pharmaceutical companies' interest in traditional remedies because it allows for the accumulation of benefits and, eventually, their sharing.

Governments in countries with high biodiversity can choose to either organize or prevent bioprospecting and biopiracy. In exchange for unclear future advantages, the latter necessitates significant investments and efforts to regulate and enable access as well as to negotiate trustworthy agreements. The primary approach to the alternate option, which is to stop biopiracy, is to publish traditional knowledge. However, it is important to keep in mind that while publication can stop knowledge theft, it cannot stop unauthorized use—in fact, it may even make it easier—because the term "biopiracy" is typically used to refer to both the unauthorized use and the misappropriation of biological resources and/or related knowledge.

Additionally, a lot of therapeutic plants are in danger of becoming extinct. This risk may be increased if these plants are overused in an effort to meet industrial and/or export demands [22, 26]. Therefore, it is necessary to control the trade in medicinal plants, ideally as part of a larger policy framework that addresses biological resource conservation and sustainable usage [45]. Even though economical or commercial aspects are likely to have an effect on conservation efforts, traditional access/use and conservation have a different relationship. To protect biodiversity, traditional healers and local communities must be permitted to continue using and gaining access to medicinal plants; otherwise, their knowledge will eventually vanish. Plants lose value once this knowledge is lost, and the likelihood of extinction may increase even further [46]. Traditional medicine is therefore associated with the preservation of biodiversity and the rights of indigenous peoples, in addition to the challenges posed by the trading among the community health interest in guaranteeing access to traditional drugs and the possible economic gains from its industrial development. The Convention on Biological Diversity (CBD) and the TRIPS are two important agreements, pertinent international agreements that must also be taken into consideration when analyzing this problem.

8.3.1 CBD AND TRIPS'S RELATIONSHIP TO TRADITIONAL KNOWLEDGE

TRIPs and the CBD are two significant conventions of international level that affect IPR on the contents of indigenous systems of traditional knowledge.

The CBD is introduced first time in December 1993, in order to support and providing broad coverage that direct the sustainable use and protection of biological resource against ruthless destruction. Beyond conservation in the conventional sense, it also tackles issues like burden-and benefit-sharing between nations that commonly shares and uses the biological resources, along with the exchange amongst indigenous or colonized populations and users of the modern society. The paragraph emphasizes the connection between the TRIPS Agreement and the CBD, particularly as it relates to traditional knowledge. It implies that one of the main problems in developing nations is the exploitation of traditional knowledge without providing enough compensation.

The fundamental element of the Convention is covered under Article 3 that clearly mentioned about recognition of each State's sovereign right to use its own bio and genetic sources. This is a change from the prior belief that these resources are a shared human inheritance that everyone can access [35, 46]. Additionally, Article 8(j) of the CBD, which specifically recognizes the role that local and indigenous communities have played to conserve the biodiversity, affirms to the rights of local communities over the information they possess. Article 8(j) of the CBD emphasizes how important it is to protect, honor, secure, and innovate the information, customs, and innovations of indigenous and local communities. The creation and utilization of technologies, particularly indigenous and traditional, are encouraged by Article 18.4.

It also demands that their knowledge, inventions, and customs be respected and upheld. In addition, the CBD insists that any profits made up of the use of demographic biogenetic sources and related information be distributed equally, fairly, and on mutually agreeable terms. The CBD is a foundational contract with specific goals and directives. It is anticipated that countries will set up guidelines for genetic resource access and will use their respective legal frameworks to put the ideas into practice of CBD about the preservation and application of genetic resources. The CBD only permits other countries to enact their own laws in this area; it does not impose any norms. Although acknowledging communities' rights over their knowledge and States' sovereign rights over their biogenetic resources. It appears that only a small number of nations have recognized the value of traditional knowledge and passed laws to preserve it [20]. In a similar vein, the majority of nations have not yet passed laws controlling who has access to their genetic and biological resources.

8.3.2 MAJOR OUTCOMES OF CBD

The 1992 Rio de Janeiro Convention on Biodiversity recognized that bioresources belong exclusively to sovereign states. But a lot of developing nations have not passed laws to put the Convention's resolutions into effect.

8.3.3 THE TRIPS ACCORD

The TRIPS Agreement serves as the foundation for the WTO Agreements, which subject Member States to obligations on a global scale. As a result, it is enforceable against WTO Member States and governed by the WTO's dispute settlement process. As a last option, this dispute resolution mechanism may permit trade sanctions against noncompliant Member Countries, guaranteeing the WTO's agreements and regulations are followed.

The national laws of all participating countries must incorporate several specific requirements specified in the TRIPS Agreement for the protection of intellectual property rights. Consequently, TRIPS deals with clearly defined private rights, whereas the CBD primarily focuses on ambiguous public rights. In addition, TRIPS requires nations to make sure that IPRs are effectively protected. One of the main tenets of TRIPS is that, subject to certain requirements being met, patents must be available for inventions across all technological domains. Consequently, TRIPS requires that pharmaceutical patents be granted for a minimum of 20 years. Given that many developing nations only seldom or never granted medicine patents before TRIPS, these new regulations significantly boost the protection offered to (modern) pharmaceuticals. As a result, it is predicted that those nations' pharmaceutical prices will rise [47, 48], which helps in restricting the access. However, it soon becomes clear that the existing laws do not match needs and reality when attempting to apply IPR on traditional treasure for which TRIPS establishes standards to an information field (traditional health care practice) for which they were not intended. For instance, a significant shortcoming that affects the majority of IPR forms is the absence of protocols for managing jointly held intellectual property.

8.3.4 ROLE OF TRIPS IN PROTECTION

TRIPs stipulate that patents will be granted for inventions that satisfy specific requirements and works to harmonize national intellectual property regimes.

8.3.5 ADDITIONAL LEGAL INSTRUMENTS

One law that protects plant varieties, promotes the expansion of the seed industry, and guarantees farmers have access to high-quality seeds is the Protection of Plant Varieties and Farmers' Rights Act, 2001. Discussed in terms of preserving biological diversity, sustainable resource use, and equitable benefit sharing is the Biodiversity Act, 2002, which established the National Biodiversity Authority for efficient oversight.

One important thing to note is that the Biodiversity Act prohibits anyone from requesting IPRs for any innovative outcome obtained from the data or research from biological sources in India, both domestically and internationally, unless they have written permission as per the proforma provided by the National Biodiversity Authority for the said purpose. To protect biological resources and traditional knowledge, India has passed laws. According to the Biological Diversity Bill, 2000, obtaining IPRs based on biological resources found in India requires prior approval from the National Biodiversity Authority [49].

8.3.6 REGULATORY FRAMEWORK

The application of intellectual property rights to innovations in herbal medicine, unique act provisions and guidelines, and associated regulatory requirements are all covered in this chapter. In conclusion, the integration of various legal instruments and regulatory frameworks in India reflects a holistic approach to protecting intellectual property in the herbal industry while ensuring sustainable practices and fair benefit-sharing in line with biodiversity conservation [50].

8.3.7 CALLS FOR SUI GENERIS SYSTEMS

The inability to protect traditional knowledge through conventional intellectual property mechanisms has led to calls for the creation of a sui generis system. Sui generis refers to a unique or special system tailored to address specific needs [51]. The difficulties in preserving customs, discoveries, and methods pertaining to biological resources point to the necessity of a sui generis framework. It also discusses how patents are currently distributed, how little traditional knowledge can be protected by current international and national patent laws, and how the TRIPS Agreement and the CBD relate to one another. In certain nations, national laws and some sui generis laws are viewed as tools for protecting traditional knowledge holders and providing them with useful advantages. To safeguard the knowledge, inventions, and practices related to biological resources, some experts suggest developing a sui generis system that is distinct from the current IPR framework. But the particulars and specifications of such a system are still being worked out [52].

8.3.8 EXPLOITATIONS OF MEDICINAL PLANTS FOR PROFIT IN UNDERDEVELOPED NATIONS

Resources for medicinal plants abound in developing nations, but in the past, multinational firms have taken advantage of these resources without paying the knowledge holders.

8.3.9 SIGNIFICANCE OF BILATERAL AND MULTILATERAL AGREEMENTS

The transfer of indigenous resources used for development, research, or commercial production requires bilateral and multilateral agreements based on established norms. When it comes to safeguarding traditional knowledge related to genetic resource access, there is a propensity to establish sui generis systems. Article 27.3 of TRIPs contemplates this system.

8.3.10 EQUITY CONSIDERATIONS

Equity considerations, which highlight the need for justice and compensation for traditional knowledge holders, are frequently the foundation of proposals for preserving traditional knowledge.

8.3.11 COSTS OF DEVELOPING NEW MEDICINES

The cost of developing new medication from scientific a new chemical medication's development can cost anywhere from USD 80 million to several billions.

8.3.12 ROLE OF PATENTS

Ideas and how they are incorporated into new goods and procedures are protected by patents. They grant inventors a 20-year exclusive monopoly for the commercial exploitation of their innovations.

8.3.13 PROTECTABLE SUBJECT MATTERS FOR PHARMACEUTICAL PRODUCTS

For pharmaceutical products, there are three main protectable subjects that need to be covered by patents:

- A patent for the discovery of novel chemical elements.
- A patent covering the production know-how.
- Trademark patent.

8.3.14 CONVENTION ON EUROPEAN PATENT

Article 53(b) of the European Patent Convention does not provide protection for plant and animal varieties or essential biological processes utilized in the production of plants or animals. However, this clause does not apply to microbiological processes or their byproducts [53].

8.3.15 CHALLENGES FACED BY HERBAL INDUSTRIES IN IPR PROTECTION

The Ayurvedic sector, which has its roots in ancient Indian wisdom, is at a pivotal point in its development, with many opportunities and problems to be faced. The growing interest in natural treatments and holistic health care around the world presents a special opportunity for the Ayurvedic industry to grow and impact the global health care system. The principles of Ayurveda have enormous potential for growth because they are in perfect harmony with the increasing demand for traditional and customized therapeutic systems. Furthermore, technological and scientific developments present important opportunities to confirm the efficacy of Ayurvedic treatments and products, strengthening their credibility in mainstream medicine. Notwithstanding these prospects, the sector must contend with issues related to regulation compliance, quality control, and standardization [54]. Ayurveda must strike a careful balance between embracing modernity and maintaining its fundamental traditions as it evolves to meet current demands. Ayurveda, Yoga, Unani, Siddha, and Homeopathy are just a few of the many traditional Indian health care systems that are included in the Ayush sector. This industry, which is expanding quickly, is focused on natural healing techniques and overall wellness. The Ayush sector has grown in popularity due to the growing interest in complementary and alternative medicine throughout the world and its tried-and-true methods and healing properties (Figure 8.1). The Ayush industry is a major player in the health care sector, contributing significantly to the promotion of general well-being and providing a range of therapeutic alternatives for those who want a more individualized and integrated approach to their health [54].

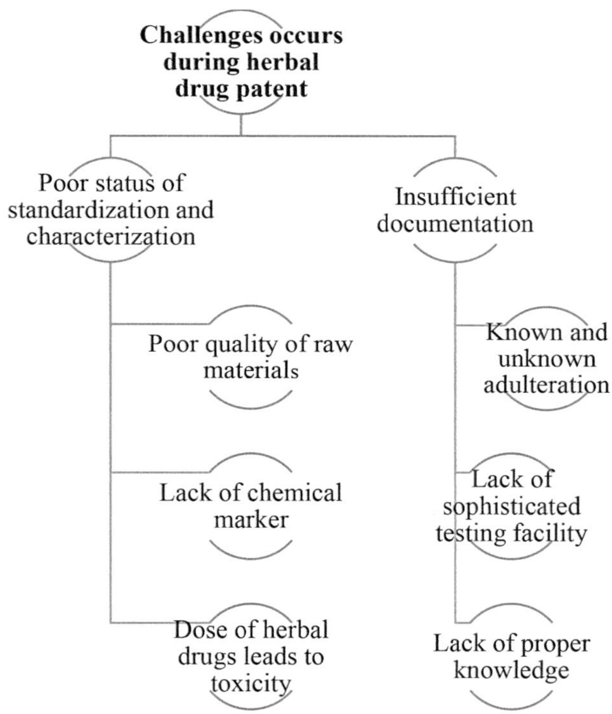

FIGURE 8.1 Challenges faced by herbal drug industries for grant of the patents on herbal drugs/medicines.

Between 2014 and 2020, the Ayush sector's sales grew by more than 17%. India is rapidly moving up the value chain of the global herbal industry. In 2020, the top 81 Ayush companies in India exported goods worth a total of INR 5400 crores, while imports were only INR 600 crores. In 2020, the two largest exporters of aromatic and medicinal plants worldwide were China and India, who together represented for roughly 30% and 11% of the overall value of exports [55]. The Ayush sector research states that from INR 85.5 billion in 2010 to INR 280.4 billion in 2019, the sample 81 enterprises' turnover increased by three times. As to a report by the World Health Organization, 98 nations in 2019 have implemented National Policies for Traditional Medicine, compared to 25 countries in 1999 when the topic was first introduced [56].

Activities such as the production and distribution of traditional medicine-based medications, the cultivation of medicinal plants, and the examination of natural products for potential therapeutic benefits can all contribute to the commercial value of traditional medicines. Safety and efficacy testing conducted by scientists can be supplemented by traditional medicine. Herbal medicines are challenging to protect under existing patent laws due to the lack of databases and the widespread use of the same medicinal plants across countries. The majority of dosage forms used in traditional herbal medicines, such as tinctures, powdered herbal materials, and fatty oils, are directly derived from herbal preparations. The production processes are often simple, with limited know-how [57].

8.3.16 PROCESS PATENTS VIEWED AS LESS VALUABLE

Because they are harder to police, "process" patents are typically thought to have less economic value than "product" patents. Nonetheless, profitable monopoly rights may be obtained through "product-by-process" patent claims [58].

8.3.17 INTELLECTUAL PROPERTY RIGHTS OVER BIOLOGICAL RESOURCES

By making minor modifications, researchers and businesses can assert their intellectual property rights over biological resources and traditional knowledge. One way to use traditional knowledge to develop useful products is through biotechnology [59].

8.3.18 CATEGORIES OF PATENTABLE HERBAL MEDICINE INVENTIONS

The passage divides patentable innovations pertaining to herbal medicine into four categories:

1. Formulation patents on herbal medicine.
2. Combination patents on herbal medicine.
3. Process patents on herbal medicine.
4. New indication of herbal drug and herbal medicine.

8.3.19 PROCESS PATENT IN HERBAL MEDICINES

Creating pharmaceutical preparations, extracting active ingredients, preparing herbal medications, and other processes can all be considered creative contributions in the development of herbal medicines.

8.3.20 IMPORTANCE OF NEW INDICATION

A new indication for a known herbal drug, such as discovering its effectiveness in preventing or treating specific diseases, can be protected by patent law.

8.3.21 LEGISLATION AND PROTECTION OF TRADITIONAL KNOWLEDGE

The passage points out that many nations lack laws governing access to their biological and genetic resources, while only a small number of nations have passed laws to preserve traditional knowledge.

8.3.22 STRATEGIES FOR SAFEGUARDING NATURAL GOODS, CONVENTIONAL HERBAL REMEDIES, AND HERBAL PHARMACEUTICALS

- New chemical component patents derived from natural products.
- Patents for substances known to exist in natural products.

1. **New chemical component patents derived from natural products:** Numerous novel therapeutic compounds can be found in nature, and a large number of medications are derived from plants. In this field, inventiveness can emerge at several

critical stages, such as separation, refinement, clarification of structure, identification of new biological characteristics, and creation of practical analogs or derivatives.

2. **Patents for substances known to exist in natural product:** The biological activity of a known compound must be connected to it for patentability. One can patent novel applications for well-known goods and materials.

3. **Biodiversity contribution to modern industry:** Particularly in the pharmaceutical industry, some pharmaceutical companies have benefited greatly from traditional knowledge related to biodiversity [60].

4. **The Digital Library of Traditional Knowledge (TKDL):** India has made great strides in preserving traditional knowledge, especially when it comes to medicinal plants. Patent examiners worldwide can readily access information about traditional knowledge by using the TKDL, which functions as an electronic database. This lessens the possibility of patents being incorrectly granted based on information that is already publicly known [61].

The Indian government is committed to ensuring that this traditional knowledge is acknowledged as nonpatent literature, as evidenced by its efforts to promote the TKDL internationally, especially within the World Intellectual Property Organization (WIPO). This highlights how crucial it is to include traditional knowledge in the international system of IPR and to stop patents from being used to misappropriate it. The proposal for the preservation of traditional knowledge is essential for safeguarding India's biological resources and recognizing the rights of local and indigenous communities. It also includes the drafting of appropriate legislation. This is consistent with initiatives in other nations, like the Philippines and Australia, where robust national laws have been passed to protect indigenous genetic resources and acknowledge communities' rights over their biological resources [62]. A proactive step would be to compile indigenous knowledge about Indian plants and herbs, including their medical and other applications, and to turn that knowledge into an accessible database. The creation of a National Bio-resource Register serves multiple purposes. First, it acts as a data bank for those seeking information, providing easy access to valuable knowledge. Second, it can generate revenue through fees for access, while also establishing conditions for the responsible use of this information. All things considered, these programs show a thorough approach to protecting and using traditional knowledge for the good of nearby communities, opposing the unwarranted patenting of Indian heritage, and making sure that the advantages of such knowledge are distributed fairly [63, 64].

8.4 CONCLUSION

The specific points of interest of herbal drugs are contributing to an overall noticeable quality increase. Developing countries are looking into the ethnopharmacological approach to medication disclosure and are recording patents for herbal remedies. Herbal medicine producers from all over the world are gathering at these bazaars in an attempt to secure a clamp for their goods. In an effort to introduce herbal goods, including herbal medicine, to the global arcade, numerous research institutes were established. The importance of IPR in the herbal drug market is growing as it expands. Analysts and specialists need to gain recognition and take a step forward in the direction of selective use of insurance rights. IP includes copyrights, trademarks, exchanges of privileged information, and licenses. Many people might agree that there is no IP guarantee for over-the-counter herbal medications, to be honest, this is not true. Trademarks and exchange mysteries are the most prevalent forms of assurance of Intellectual Properties for domestically produced medications. Herbal medicines' particular areas of emphasis are clearly improving overall quality. Developing nations have started to keep track of patents for herbal remedies and have been studying the ethnopharmacological approach to medication disclosure. At these bazaars, manufacturers of herbal medicines from all over the world gather in an attempt to get a clamp for their goods. In an effort to introduce herbal items, including herbal medicine, to the global market, numerous research centers were established. The significance of IPR protections in the herbal medication sector is growing as it expands. Analysts and specialists need to become well-known and take a step forward in the direction of selectivity by using insurance rights. Intellectual property includes copyrights, trademarks, licenses, and exchange-privileged information. Many people would agree that there is no IP guarantee for herbal remedies made at home or related products, to be honest, this is not true. Trademark and exchange mysteries are the most well-known forms of intellectual property insurance for domestically manufactured pharmaceuticals.

KEYWORDS

- **herbal drugs patent**
- **intellectual property**
- **drug discovery**
- **herbal industries**

REFERENCES

1. Rates, S. M. Plants as source of drugs. *Toxicon* 2001, 39(5), 603–613. https://doi.org/10.1016/s0041-0101(00)00154-9.
2. Sharma, A., Shanker, C., Tyagi, L. K., Singh, M., & Rao, C. V. Herbal medicine for market potential in India: An overview. *Acad J Plant Sci* 2008, 1(2), 26–36.
3. Kartal, M. Intellectual property protection in the natural product drug discovery, traditional herbal medicine and herbal medicinal products. *Phytother Res* 2007, 21(2), 113–119. https://doi.org/10.1002/ptr.2036.
4. Sahoo, N., Manchikanti, P., & Dey, S. H. Herbal drug patenting in India: IP potential. *J Ethnopharmacol* 2011, 137(1), 289–297. https://doi.org/10.1016/j.jep.2011.05.022.
5. Ashtari, G. The challenges of protecting traditional knowledge through an IP regimen with regard to particular problems posed by traditional medicine. *Iran J Med Law* 2012, 1(2), 61–68.
6. Hudson, J. B. Applications of the phytomedicine Echinacea purpurea (Purple Coneflower) in infectious diseases. *J Biomed Biotechnol* 2012, 2012, 769896. https://doi.org/10.1155/2012/769896.
7. Dutt, B. A study of patenting activity in Aloe vera. *J Intellect Prop Rights* 2002, 7, 330–341.
8. Malik, K. A., & Zafar, Y. Intellectual property rights in plant biotechnology: A contribution to crop biosecurity. *Asian Biotechnol Dev Rev* 2005, 8, 7–42.
9. SWAMTtTATHAN, M. S., & Howard, H. Two techniques were tried, namely, smearing the stigmatio exudation from the pollen parent on the stigma of the pistillate parent, before pollination, and applying a suitable artificial medium for pollen germination on the cut surface of the style after. *Sci Sustain Food Security: Selected Papers of MS Swaminathan* 2010, 3, 275.

10. https://www.wipo.int/export/sites/www/tk/en/docs/use-of-turmeric-in-wound-healing-e.pdf
11. Hellerer, U., & Jarayaman, K. S. Greens persuade Europe to revoke patent on neem tree. *Nature* 2000, 405(6784), 266–267. https://doi.org/10.1038/35012778.
12. Verma, S. A review study on Achyranthes aspera (Amaranthaceae)-A valuable medicinal herb. *J Med Plant Stud* 2016, 4(3), 6–7.
13. https://patents.google.com/patent/US6103248A/en.
14. Lee-Huang, S., Kung, H. F., Huang, P. L., Huang, P. L., Li, B. Q., Huang, P., Huang, H. I., & Chen, H. C. A new class of anti-HIV agents: GAP31, DAPs 30 and 32. *FEBS Lett* 1991, 291(1), 139–144. https://doi.org/10.1016/0014-5793(91)81122-o
15. Sekiguchi, Y., Mano, H., Nakatani, S., Shimizu, J., & Wada, M. Effects of the Sri Lankan medicinal plant, Salacia reticulata, in rheumatoid arthritis. *Gen Nutrit* 2010, 5(1), 89–96. https://doi.org/10.1007/s12263-009-0144-3
16. Amarasinghe, K. Bio-piracy and its impact on Biodiversity: A special review on Sri Lankan context. *J Environ Protect Sci* 2018, 269. https://patents.google.com/patent/WO2015189858A1/en.
17. Bhatia, P., & Chugh, A. Role of marine bioprospecting contracts in developing access and benefit sharing mechanism for marine traditional knowledge holders in the pharmaceutical industry. *Glob Ecol Conserv* 2015, 3, 176–187.
18. Aguilar, G. Access to genetic resources and protection of traditional knowledge in the territories of indigenous peoples. *Environ Sci Policy* 2001, 4(4–5), 241–256.
19. Rivera, J. O., Loya, A. M., & Ceballos, R. Use of herbal medicines and implications for conventional drug therapy medical sciences. *Alter Integr Med* 2013, 2(6), 1–6. http://dx.doi.org/10.4172/2327-5162.1000130.
20. Jadhav, C. A., Vikhe, D. N., & Jadhav, R. S. Global and domestic market of herbal medicines: A review. *Res J Sci Technol* 2020, 12(4), 327–330. https://doi.org/10.5958/2349-2988.2020.00049.2
21. Veer, V., & Gopalakrishnan, R. (Eds.). *Herbal Insecticides, Repellents and Biomedicines: Effectiveness and Commercialization*. Springer, 2016, pp. 1–264. http://dx.doi.org/10.1007/978-81-322-2704-5
22. Patil, K., & Wadekar, R. Herbal drug patenting. In: Mandal, S. C., Chakraborty, R., & Sen, S. (Eds.), *Evidence Based Validation of Traditional Medicines*. Springer: Singapore, 2021. https://doi.org/10.1007/978-981-15-8127-4_27.
23. Cohen, I. G., Gerke, S., & Kramer, D. B. Ethical and legal implications of remote monitoring of medical devices. *Milbank Q* 2020, 98(4), 1257–1289.
24. Wang, X., & Chan, A. W. K. Challenges and patenting strategies for Chinese herbal medicine. *Chin Med* 2010, 5(1), 1–4.
25. Zhang, X. Traditional medicine: Its importance and protection. *Protecting and Promoting Traditional Knowledge: Systems, National Experiences and International Dimensions* 2004, Part, 1, 3–6.
26. Mugabe, J. Intellectual property protection and traditional knowledge. In: *World Intellectual Property Organization. Intellectual Property and Human Rights*. WIPO: Geneva, 1999, pp. 97–125.
27. Papageorgiadis, N., & Sharma, A. Intellectual property rights and innovation: A panel analysis. *Econ Lett* 2016, 141, 70–72.

28. Sam, S. Importance and effectiveness of herbal medicines. *J Pharmacog Phytochem* 2019, 8(2), 354–357.
29. Alves, R. R., & Rosa, I. M. Biodiversity, traditional medicine and public health: Where do they meet? *J Ethnobiol Ethnomed* 2007, 3, 1–9.
30. Du, J., & Tang, X. L. Natural products against cancer: A comprehensive bibliometric study of the research projects, publications, patents and drugs. *J Cancer Res Therapeut* 2014, 10(Suppl 1), 27–37. https://doi.org/10.4103/0973-1482.139750.
31. Peria, E. V. (2001, February). The community protocol in the AEAN Framework Agreement on access to genetic resources. In: *ASEAN Workshop on the TRIPS Agreement and Traditional Medicine, Jakarta*, pp. 13–15.
32. Singh, H. (2003, October). Intellectual property rights (IPR) issues in horticulture: An Indian scenario with particular reference to medicinal plants. In: *VII International Symposium on Temperate Zone Fruits in the Tropics and Subtropics 662*, pp. 465–470.
33. World Health Organization. Traditional Medicine 2008, Fact sheet No. 134.Available from URL: http://www.who.int/mediacentre/factsheets/fs134/en/(accessed 30.09.10)
34. Eisenberg, D. M., Kessler, R. C., Foster, C., Norlock, F. E., Calkins, D. R., & Delbanco, T. L. Unconventional medicine in the United States-Prevalence, costs, and patterns of use. *N Engl J Med* 1993, 328(4), 246–252.
35. Timmermans, K. Intellectual property rights and traditional medicine: Policy dilemmas at the interface. *Soc Sci Med (1982)* 2003, 57(4), 745–756. https://doi.org/10.1016/s0277-9536(02)00425-2.
36. Mashelkar, R. A. Intellectual property rights and the Third World. *Curr Sci* 2001, 81(8), 955–965. http://www.jstor.org/stable/24106520
37. Agarwal, A. & Narain, S. Pirates in the garden of India. *New Sci* 1996, 152(2053), 14–15.
38. Government of India Protection of biodiversity and traditional knowledge—the Indian experience. Document no. WT/CTE/W/156. 2000.
39. Sampat, P. Judgement protects indigenous knowledge. *World Watch* 1998, 11(1), 8–8.
40. Wiser, G. M., & Downes, D. R. Comments on improving identification of prior art. In: *Recommendations on Traditional Knowledge Relating to Biological Diversity Submitted to the United States Patent and Trademark Office*. Center for International Environmental Law: Washington, DC, 1999, pp. 1–18.
41. Posey, D. A. Protecting indigenous peoples' rights to biodiversity. *Environment* 1996, 38(8), 6–18.
42. Posey, D., & Dutfield, G. Beyond intellectual property: Toward traditional resource rights for indigenous peoples and local communities. *J Aboriginal Health,* January 2004, 115.
43. Douglas, D. J. The restructuring of local government in rural regions: A rural development perspective. *J Rural Stud* 2005, 21(2), 231–246.
44. Kadidal, S. Plants, poverty, and pharmaceutical patents. *Yale Law J* 1993, 103, 223–258.
45. Nairobi: African Centre for Technology Studies. Newman, E. B. Earth's vanishing medicine cabinet: Rain forest destruction and its impact on the pharmaceutical industry. *Am J Law Med* 1994, 20(4), 479–501

46. Correa, C. M. Protection of traditional systems of medicine, patenting and promotion of medicinal plants. In: Chaudhury, R. R., & Rafei, U. M. (Eds.), *Traditional Medicine in Asia*. WHO South East Asia Regional Office: New Delhi, 2002, pp. 227–245.
47. Gupta, A. K. Rewarding local communities for conserving biodiversity: The case of the honey bee. In: Guruswamy, L. D., & McNeely, J. A. (Eds.), *Protection of Global Biodiversity: Converging Strategies*. Duke University Press: Durham/London, 1998, pp. 180–198.
48. Velasquez, G., & Boulet, P. *Globalization and Access to Drugs: Perspectives on the WTO/TRIPS Agreement*. World Health Organization: Geneva, 1999.
49. Boyd, M. R. The position of intellectual property rights in drug discovery and development from natural products. *J Ethnopharmacol* 1996, 51, 17–27.
50. Cullet, P., & Raja, J. Intellectual property rights and biodiversity management: The case of India. *Global Environ Polit* 2004, 4(1), 97–114.
51. Santini, A., Cammarata, S. M., Capone, G., Ianaro, A., Tenore, G. C., Pani, L., & Novellino, E. Nutraceuticals: Opening the debate for a regulatory framework. *Br J Clin Pharmacol* 2018, 84(4), 659–672.
52. Dhar, B. *Sui Generis Systems for Plant Variety Protection*. Quaker United Nations Office: Geneva, 2002, pp. 1–32.
53. Goel, R. Protection and conservation—TRIPs and CBD: A way forward. *J Intellect Property Law Pract* 2008, 3(5), 334–338.
54. van Dijk, T. W. P. The limits of patent protection : Essays on the economics of intellectual property rights. [Doctoral Thesis, Maastricht University]. Datawyse / Universitaire Pers Maastricht 1994. https://doi.org/10.26481/dis.19940915td.
55. Ahmad, F., Zaidi, M. A. S., Sulaiman, N., & Majid, F. A. A. Issues and challenges in the development of the herbal industry in Malaysia. *Prosiding Perkem* 2015, 10(1), 227–238.
56. Chaudhary, A., & Singh, N. Intellectual property rights and patents in perspective of Ayurveda. *AYU*, 2012, 33(1), 20–26.
57. Arya, H., & Bhatt, K. T. *Chapter 22 - Introduction of Intellectual Property Rights, The Design & Development of Novel Drugs and Vaccines*. Academic Press, 2021, pp. 275–281, https://doi.org/10.1016/B978-0-12-821471-8.00022-2.
58. Saggar, S., Mir, P. A., Kumar, N., Chawla, A., Uppal, J., & Kaur, A. Traditional and herbal medicines: Opportunities and challenges. *Pharmacogn Res* 2022, 14(2), 107–114. https://doi.org/10.5530/pres.14.2.15
59. Moore, K. A. Worthless patents. *Berkeley Technol Law J* 2005, 20(4), 1521–1552.
60. Utkarsh, G., Gadgil, M., & Rao, P. S. Intellectual property rights on biological resources: Benefiting from biodiversity and people's knowledge. *Curr Sci* 1999, 77(11), 1418–1425.
61. Miladinović, Z., Varga, S., & Radojković, M. Patent law protection of inventions in medicine and pharmaceutical industry. *Vojnosanit Pregl* 2013, 70(6), 600–605. https://doi.org/10.2298/vsp1306600m.
62. Thomas, P. N. Traditional knowledge and the traditional knowledge digital library: Digital quandaries and other concerns. *Int Commun Gaz* 2010, 72(8), 659–673.
63. Gupta, V. K. *An Approach for Establishing a Traditional Knowledge Digital Library*. NISCAIR-CSIR: India, 2000, pp. 307–319.

64. Sen, S., & Chakraborty, R. Traditional Knowledge Digital Library: A distinctive approach to protect and promote Indian indigenous medicinal treasure. *Curr Sci* 2014, 106(10), 1340–1343.

CHAPTER 9

Patent Searches and Literature Review in Herbal Science

GANA MANJUSHA K.[1], ARYA LAKSHMI MARISETTI[2], and M. V. N. L. CHAITANYA[3*]

[1]Vignan Institute of Pharmaceutical Technology, Visakhapatnam, Andhra Pradesh, India

[2]Department of Pharmacognosy & Phytochemistry, School of Pharmaceutical Sciences, Delhi Pharmaceutical Sciences & Research University, New Delhi, Delhi, India

[3]School of Pharmaceutical Sciences, Lovely Professional University, Punjab, India

*Corresponding author

ABSTRACT

Intellectual property (IP) is a crucial aspect of herbal science research, providing a framework for protecting innovation and fostering advancements. Intellectual property rights (IPRs) are closely linked to bio-larceny and the infringement of IPR schemes in the western style. In this chapter, we review the present-day status of the art of IP management in herbal science and present strategies for developing an effective IP management plan. A review of existing literature underscores the diverse applications of patent search studies, highlighting the importance of strategic planning, the identification of retrieval techniques to mitigate unpredictability, and the adoption of search procedure designed to address intricacy and vagueness. In addition, we discuss strategies for fostering a culture of IP awareness in the realm of herbal sciences while contributing to the

Herbal Drug Industry: From Cultivation to Innovation and Global Impact.
Abhishek Tiwari, Varsha Tiwari, and Ajay Sharma (Eds.)

DOI: 10.1201/9781779640994-9

advancement of the field. The cases discussed provide insights into various approaches for utilizing the advantages of the commercialization of historical information and return to its original communities.

9.1 CONDUCTING PATENT SEARCHES FOR HERBAL PRODUCTS

A patent is a legally sanctioned record issued by a government, affording an innovator's exclusive rights to produce, utilize, and distribute an invention over a designated timeframe. This legal safeguard also extends to substantial enhancements made to previously devised creations. The fundamental rationale behind the bestowal of patents is to incentivize innovators in propelling technological advancements. As stated by the United Nations's definition, a patent constitutes a legally binding entitlement bestowed by a country's government upon its inventor. Within the realm of legal frameworks, Patent Law constitutes a distinct facet of intellectual property right (IPR). Central to Patent Law is the pivotal notion of novelty and the requirement for inventions to be nonobvious. Additionally, the origination in question must possess legal utility [1]. The grant of a patent serves as a deterrent, prohibiting imitators and independent originators from utilizing the patented invention throughout the duration of its protection.

As per a survey conducted by the World Trade Organization (WTO), the amount of herbal medications traded globally has increased to US$60 billion. In the contemporary landscape, the pharmaceutical industry is undergoing significant expansion, driven by advancements stemming from the exploration of medicinal plants and their derivatives. However, a critical issue arises in the realm of intellectual property (IP), as pharmaceutical companies commonly overlook the acknowledgment and compensation of individuals contributing intellectual knowledge related to traditional medicines. Paradoxically, these pharmaceutical entities reap economic gains from the exploitation of such traditional medicinal knowledge, as highlighted by Aguilar in 2001 [2].

Consequently, there exists a compelling need to raise awareness and establish comprehensive policies and legal frameworks aimed at safeguarding the IPR of those who generate and possess traditional knowledge. This safeguarding mechanism could be achieved through the granting of patents for newly developed products or processes derived from traditional medicinal knowledge, encompassing areas such as herbal drugs/extracts, formulations, and phytoconstituents. This approach, advocated by Bayram in 2005, seeks to address the imbalance in the recognition and compensation associated with intellectual contributions in the domain of traditional medicine [3].

9.1.1 INTRODUCTION TO PATENT SEARCHES

9.1.1.1 DEFINITION AND IMPORTANCE OF PATENT SEARCHES IN HERBAL SCIENCE

A patent search primarily involves conducting research and engaging in data mining processes specific to a particular patent. Patent searches in herbal science encompass the systematic exploration of existing patents related to herbal products, formulations, and processes. These searches aim to uncover a comprehensive understanding of the IP landscape within the field of herbal science. Conducting a thorough patent search is a crucial prerequisite for inventors and innovators prior to initiating the patent filing process.

In case of herbal medicines, a patent search involves the examination of granted patents, patent applications, and related documents to identify innovations, technologies, and discoveries in the realm of herbal medicine, plant extracts, and natural remedies. It is a proactive step in navigating the vast repository of global patent databases to extract knowledge that can influence research, development, and innovation in the herbal sciences.

The importance of patent searches lies in their capacity to provide researchers with insights into prior art—existing knowledge and innovations—that may impact the novelty and inventiveness of their own work. By conducting thorough patent searches, researchers can avoid duplication of efforts, gain awareness of existing technologies, and identify gaps in the current state of herbal science. Furthermore, understanding the patent landscape allows researchers to make informed decisions regarding the direction and focus of their studies.

9.1.1.2 SIGNIFICANCE OF IDENTIFYING EXISTING PATENTS IN THE FIELD

Identifying existing patents in herbal science holds paramount importance for several reasons. First and foremost, it aids researchers in avoiding infringement on existing IPR. Knowing what has already been patented allows researchers to navigate their projects with a clear understanding of boundaries, ensuring that their work aligns with the principles of IP law.

Moreover, by identifying existing patents, researchers gain access to a wealth of knowledge that can fuel innovation and creativity. Patents often contain detailed descriptions of methodologies, formulations, and technologies, serving as valuable resources for inspiration and building upon existing ideas. This collaborative and cumulative approach fosters advancements in herbal science by leveraging the collective knowledge within the scientific community.

In the commercial sphere, understanding the existing patent landscape is critical for businesses engaged in the herbal products market. It enables companies to strategize their product development, assess potential partnerships, and make informed decisions about entering specific markets. Awareness of existing patents is also essential for IP management, helping organizations protect their own innovations and navigate the competitive landscape.

The initiation of patent searches in herbal science is a proactive and strategic step that not only safeguards researchers from legal pitfalls but also enhances the overall quality and impact of scientific endeavors in the herbal sciences. By recognizing the significance of identifying existing patents, researchers contribute to a dynamic and collaborative ecosystem that fosters innovation, knowledge exchange, and sustainable growth in herbal science.

9.1.2 METHODS OF CONDUCTING PATENT SEARCHES

In the contemporary landscape, patents have emerged as critical assets for innovative enterprises, particularly in the face of heightened global competition. To adapt to this dynamic environment, companies are increasingly integrating their business strategies with their IP strategies. The field of patent informatics is dedicated to the systematic exploration, analysis, and presentation of patent information. This discipline aims to reveal intricate relationships and discern trends that may elude observation when engaging with patent documents on an individual basis [4].

This perspective underscores the transformative impact of information and communication technology on patent searching methodologies. The traditional paradigm of manual catalog-based access has given way to a more dynamic online accessibility approach [5].

As the global patent collection continues to expand at a rapid pace, the retrieval and analysis of this extensive knowledge repository have evolved into intricate, exhaustive, and highly interactive tasks. Successfully navigating this landscape demands considerable expertise encompassing diverse search strategies [6]. The growth in the information and communication technology sector further accentuates the strategic importance of patent searching. This necessitates a shift toward sophisticated search methodologies and leveraging technological advancements for comprehensive retrieval and insightful analysis [7].

9.1.2.1 OVERVIEW OF SEARCH STRATEGIES

The exploration of patent searches assumes significant importance, warranting in-depth scrutiny, particularly in the contemporary legal landscape governing the regulatory mechanisms for accessing and utilizing biological resources, alongside benefit-sharing considerations [8]. Within this context, critical inquiries arise regarding the execution of patent searches, the dependability and effectiveness of publicly available official databases and websites, the utilization of information for patent analysis, and the necessary precautions to be observed when undertaking a patent search in the context of proposing a research project [9].

The present chapter delves into these critical questions, aligning with concerns articulated by scientists (Figure 9.1). A key focus of the study involves elucidating the attributes of an effective patent search, emphasizing the importance of strategic planning, the identification of recovery techniques to mitigate unsureness, and the adoption of search processes designed to address intricate and unclear [10].

9.1.2.2 TYPES OF PATENT SEARCH

9.1.2.2.1 State-of-the-Art Search for Herbal Products

The state-of-the-art search for herbal products represents a foundational exploration encompassing all pertinent documents within the herbal science field. It involves surveying patents filed by specific applicants, inventions attributed to particular inventors, and relevant literature such as scientific articles, theses, and "gray literature" like instruction manuals.

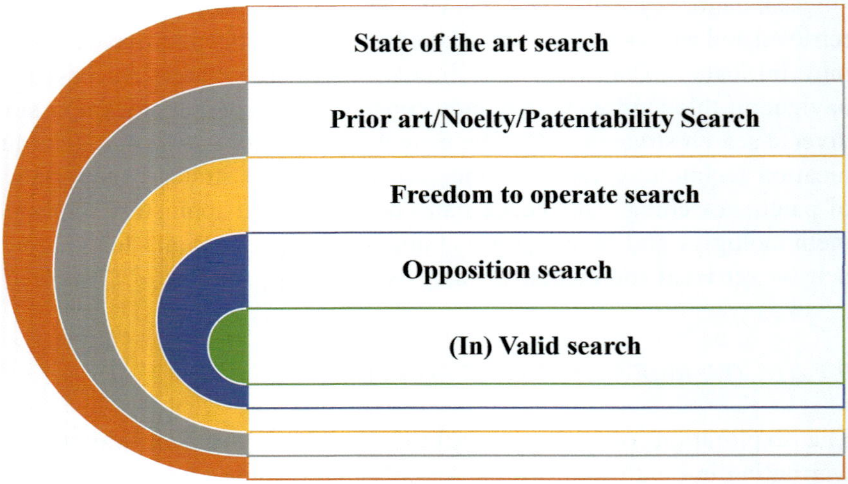

FIGURE 9.1 Patent search types.

Unlike other searches, the state-of-the-art search does not necessarily precede patent application filing still serves to establish publicly available knowledge and information concerning herbal products [11].

9.1.2.2.2 Prior Art/Novelty/Patentability Search for Herbal Products

Specific to herbal products, the Prior Art/Novelty/Patentability search is an essential precursor typically conducted in the industry before filing a patent application. This search aims to assess the novelty, inventiveness, and industrial applicability of a proposed herbal formulation or process. It scrutinizes publications, including patents and technical literature, to identify the closest prior art relevant to the herbal innovation.

9.1.2.2.3 Freedom to Operate (FTO) Search for Herbal Products

The freedom to operate (FTO) search, also known as freedom to act search, presents particular challenges in the herbal product context. Given that patents are exclusionary rights, this search is intricate and potentially costly.

FTO searches for herbal products involve identifying regions without existing patent protection, determining the duration of current patent protection, and assessing the territorial and time limitations of patents. In the scenario of inventing a unique herbal technology, an FTO search helps identify geographical areas where no patent protection exists, allowing for strategic commercial exploitation [11].

9.1.2.2.4 Opposition Search for Herbal Products

In the herbal science domain, an Opposition search involves third parties, "opponents," conducting a search to challenge the granting of a patent. This search aims to bring forward arguments against the patent's approval, typically by uncovering earlier works of art that may have been overlooked throughout the testing process.

9.1.2.2.5 (In)Validity Search for Herbal Products

An (In) Validity search, akin to an opposition search, may be initiated later in the patent's lifetime for herbal products. It seeks to find previous art that could render a patent that has been awarded void or to evaluate the current validity of a patent in force. This type of search is crucial in ensuring the robustness of a herbal product patent against potential challenges.

9.1.2.3 UTILIZING ONLINE PATENT DATABASES

The advent of digital technology has revolutionized the landscape of patent searches, with online patent databases offering a wealth of information at researchers' fingertips. Platforms such as the United States Patent and Trademark Office (USPTO), the European Patent Office (EPO), and the World Intellectual Property Organization (WIPO) issue user-friendly interfaces to access a vast repository of global patents.

Researchers can leverage advanced search functionalities on these platforms to narrow down results based on criteria such as publication date, inventor names, and patent classifications (Table 9.1). Online databases not only facilitate broader access to patent documents but also offer tools for data analysis and visualization, enhancing the efficiency of patent searches in herbal science [12].

TABLE 9.1 List of Some Patent Database Pros and Cons of the Individual Database

S.No.	Major Patent Databases
1.	**Patentscope (WIPO)** • Access: PATENTSCOPE • Search 45 million patent documents + 2.7 million published international patent applications (PCT). • Data coverage: 44,970,000 records (PCT – 2,652,401 + national offices – 42,307,897). • Sorting: Results by application date or relevance. • Features: Statistical machine translation tool, legal status information, links to national databases, full-text search capability. • Limitations: Lower data coverage compared to Espacenet and Depatisnet28. • Challenges: Retrieval issues with patent number search, no options to filter results based on publication dates/applicants. • Additional: Statistical analysis of searches, graphical representation of top patent offices, IPC, and publication dates. Enhanced patent data export capability.
2.	**PatFT—United States Patent and Trademark Office (USPTO)** • Access: PatFT • Coverage: Patents issued from 1976 to the present, PDF images for all patents from 1790 to the present. • Features: Integrated machine translation, patent legal status information, advanced search options, various tools (AppFT, GPSN, PAIR). • Limitations: Full-text searches and other tools only for US patents.
3.	**Espacenet—European Patent Office (EPO)** • Access: Espacenet • Coverage: Access to over 90 million patent documents worldwide. • Tools: Global Patent Index (GPI), Cooperative Patent Classification (CPC) search, patent legal status information, machine translation. • Limitations: Full-text search only for EP and WO documents, challenges in patent number search. • Advantages: Free patent database with extensive tools for better search results.
	Regional/National—Multinational—Free Patent Databases
4.	**JplatPat—Japan Patent Office (JPO)** • Access: [JplatPat](http://www.jpo.go.jp/ https://www.jplatpat.inpit.go.jp/web/all/top/BTmTopEnglishPage) • Platform: Japanese platform for patent information by INPIT. • Features: Tools like Patent Map Guidance (PMGS), access to Patent Abstracts of Japan (PAJ) by keywords. • Limitations: Full-text searches and other tools only for JP and PCT documents. • Additional: Information on legal status, English translations of Japanese patents, and utility models.

TABLE 9.1 *(Continued)*

S.No.	Major Patent Databases
5.	**SIPO—China** • Access: [SIPO] (http://english.sipo.gov.cn/, http://www.psssystem.gov.cn/sipopublicsearch/ensearch/searchEnHomeIndexAC.do) • Patent Documents: Various patent documents from 94 patent institutions + full-text patent descriptions published by 40 patent agencies. • Features: Chinese Patent Machine Translation System (CPMT), tools to access Chinese and PCT documents. • Limitations: Full-text searches and other tools only for Chinese and PCT documents.
6.	**INPAIRS—India** • Access: INPAIRS • Patent Documents: Access to patent documents published and applied in the Indian Patent Office. • Features: Tools and links to check published applications, application status, patent agent register, and patent fees. • Additional: Links to other international patent database websites, full-text searches, and tools for Indian patents and PCT documents.
7.	**DEPATIS—Germany** • Access: DEPATIS • Patent Publications: Searches on patent publications from around the world, including the DEPATIS electronic document archive. • Features: IPC reclassifications displayed, extensive coverage (nearly 90 million patent documents). • Advantages: Successful retrieval using patent number search, free patent database with large coverage.
8.	**AusPAT—Australia** • Access: AusPAT • Patent Records: Access to Australian patent records dating back to 1904. • Features: Quick, structured, and advanced search options. • Limitations: Limited data coverage (approximately 7% of world patenting activity), access to only Australian patents.
9.	**CPD—Canadian Patent Database** • Access: CPD • Patent Documents: Access 95 years of patent descriptions and images, updated weekly. • Features: Full text searches and other search tools for Canadian patents. • Additional: Various tools available to access Canadian patents.
10.	**Czech Republic** • Access: Czech Republic Patent Database • Patent Applications: Contains patent applications published since 1991. • Features: Quick, structured, and advanced search options, links to national and foreign patent databases.

TABLE 9.1 *(Continued)*

S.No.	Major Patent Databases
11.	**EAPATIS—Eurasian Patent Organization (EAPO)** • Access: EAPATIS • Patent Documents: 60 million descriptions of patent documents from EAPO, WIPO, EPO, USPTO, and CISPATENT. • Features: Multi-aspect patent search in several official languages, over 20 local databases constantly updated.
12.	**Finland** • Access: Finnish Patent and Registration Office • Patent Applications: Contains public patent applications since the early 1970s. • Features: Bibliography, processing, payment, and legal status data, links to Espacenet service.
13.	**Ireland** • Access: IPO Ireland. • Patent Documents: Access to patent documents published and applied in the Irish Patent Office. • Features: Tools and links to check application status, protection abroad, patent agents, and patent fees.
14.	**IPONZ—New Zealand** • Access: IPONZ • Patent Register: Online tool to search the New Zealand Patent Register, access to published patent abstracts. • Features: Retrieve information about published, granted, and unexamined New Zealand patents.
15.	• **KIPRIS—Korean Intellectual Property Rights Information Service** • Access: KIPRIS • Patent Documents: Access to over 2.1 million published applications and patents registered in Korea. • Features: Translated Korean patent abstracts, links to national and foreign patent databases.
16.	**IPOS—Singapore** • Access: IPOS Singapore. • IP Applications: Access to information related to IP applications and registrations at the Intellectual Property Office of Singapore. • Features: Tools and links to check published applications, application status, and international patent classification of Singapore patents.
17.	**Industrial Property Office of Slovak Republic** • Access: Industrial Property Office of Slovak Republic • Patent Documents: Bibliographic data of granted patents, information about published, granted, and unexamined Slovakian and foreign patents.

TABLE 9.1 *(Continued)*

S.No.	Major Patent Databases
18.	**Slovenia Intellectual Property Office (SIPO)** • Access: SIPO Slovenia • Patent documents: Retrieve information about published, granted, and unexamined Slovenian and foreign patents.
19.	**Swissreg—Switzerland** • Access: Swissreg • Patent Documents: Access Swiss and European patents, with all Swiss patents filed after January 1978 included. • Features: Online searches of published Swiss patent applications and patents.
20.	**IPSum—United Kingdom** • Access: IPSum • Patent Status: View patent status and get up-to-date information on UK patent applications. • Features: Search published patent applications and registered UK patents, links to other patent databases like Espacenet.
	IP.com • Access: IP.com • Services: Intellectual property solutions provider offering access to InnovationQ, Prior Art Database, IP Professional Services, IP Portfolio Management, and IP Analytics tools.

9.1.2.4 KEYWORDS AND CLASSIFICATION CODES FOR EFFECTIVE SEARCHES

Over the past 25 years, patent search methodologies have seen limited evolution, with Boolean logic and keyword searches, despite their enduring use, facing challenges in precision and effectiveness. The reliance on set theory and exclusion principles, inherent in Boolean searches, persists, making it the preferred method for locating patents due to its reproducibility and defensibility in decision-making by patent professionals [13].

However, the inherent limitations of Boolean searches, such as missing relevant documents and retrieving unrelated ones, have become increasingly apparent, especially in the context of the growing number of infringement suits. The consequences of missing even a single pertinent patent document can be financially significant. Consequently, there is a reluctance to rely solely on Boolean or keyword searches for patentability assessments [14, 15].

To address these issues, researchers have proposed alternative techniques leveraging the patent structure. These include the introduction of a noise elimination (NE) algorithm based on keyword-weighted distribution, aiming to eliminate noisy patent data [16]. Another study proposes a patent retrieval system architecture that exploits Change citation patterns and patent metadata to create small initial sets of patents. Complex methodologies, involving multiple indexing of patents, language-specific indexes, and the incorporation of retrieval models like language model (LM) and Okapi BM25, have demonstrated success, notably in the CLEF-IP 2010 [17].

Moreover, the fusion of text-based and citation-based scoring has shown improved results in patent retrieval. Patent structure analysis has become a focal point, with segmentation of claim parts to identify subtopics and the subsequent creation of queries for effective retrieval. The impact of various patent fields like title, claim, abstract, and background summary on retrieval effectiveness has been investigated. Learning-to-rank approaches, considering LM-based retrieval score and International Patent Classification (IPC) classification features, have outperformed previous methodologies [18].

In the realm of query formulation, the effectiveness of terms extracted from different fields, their combination, and weighting based on log(tf)idf values have been explored. Key Phrase Extraction techniques have been found to be superior to tf or tf-idf scores, particularly from the "description" section, for invalidity searches. Studies suggest that optimal queries consist of 20–30 terms. Give words taken out of the abstract, claims, and description more weight when adjusting patent information and citation structures to produce limited first sets of patents [19].

Innovative approaches like multiple query representation for prior art search, collaborative filtering algorithms, and stage-wise patent retrieval methods have been proposed, demonstrating improved precision. Simpler yet effective information retrieval techniques, such as using lists making use of patent numbers in the description area for citation purposes., have proven comparable to more advanced methods, especially when patent applications contain citations [7].

Query expansion techniques have been explored to handle term mismatches, utilizing external knowledge bases like WordNet and Wikipedia. Proximity-based frameworks, using independent claims and IPC classification, have been suggested for query expansion term selection [20, 21].

The landscape of patent searches is undergoing transformation, with a shift toward more sophisticated and multifaceted approaches. From NE algorithms to proximity-based frameworks, researchers are exploring diverse strategies to enhance the precision and effectiveness of patent retrieval.

9.1.3 EXPLORING SUCCESSFUL PATENT SEARCHES IN HERBAL SCIENCE AND LESSONS LEARNED

Patent searches in herbal science present a unique set of challenges and opportunities due to the rich diversity of natural compounds and traditional knowledge associated with herbal products. By employing advanced search techniques one can find out the prerequisites for patents of herbal products.

9.1.3.1 PATENT INFORMATION RETRIEVAL IN INDIA AND GLOBALLY

In the context of patent information retrieval, India currently relies on the Technology Information and Forecasting Council and the National Informatics Centre as the primary free online databases. Notably, the Traditional Knowledge Digital Library (TKDL) plays a crucial role, offering access to approximately 11 million pages of information related to traditional knowledge associated with medicinal plants in India. This vast repository aids patent examiners worldwide in conducting prior art searches.

Globally, the USPTO took a pioneering step in the 1970s by introducing "computerized classification searching to the public." Subsequently, the International Patent Documentation Center was established in Austria in 1972, creating a worldwide patent index database. Further advancements occurred in 1998 when the EPO launched esp@cenet®, contributing to the global accessibility of patent information.

9.1.3.2 LITERATURE REVIEW ON PATENT SEARCH STUDIES

A review of existing literature underscores the diverse applications of patent search studies:

9.1.3.2.1 Patent Overlapping Studies

Conducting cluster analysis and identifying claim overlap profiles enable the assessment of a patent's competitive potential in various technological domains [22].

9.1.3.2.2 Trends in Patenting Activity

Researchers have explored patent databases to analyze trends in patenting activity, providing insights into the focus of research in specific sectors, such as Indian agriculture [23].

9.1.3.2.3 Systematic Patent Analysis

Systematic analyses, such as the examination of phytochemicals in tea, have revealed missing information and gaps in patents related to specific enzymes [24].

9.1.3.2.4 Technology-Specific Research

Scientists have engaged in technology-specific exploratory research, crafting, drafting claims for various biosequences, addressing problems with the tools that are currently available for sequence analysis, and looking for patent information.

9.1.3.2.5 Decision Models for Patent Search

The development of deterministic and probabilistic decision models has been a focus, aiding researchers in determining what to search, where to search, how to proceed with further searches, which claims to prioritize, and how to assess legal status.

9.2 UTILIZING PATENT LITERATURE FOR RESEARCH

In the realm of scientific inquiry, patent literature serves as a valuable and often underutilized resource. This section explores the methodologies for extracting meaningful information from patents, emphasizing the comprehension of patent documents, and the identification of key data for research purposes [25].

9.2.1 EXTRACTING INFORMATION FROM PATENTS: UNDERSTANDING PATENT DOCUMENTS

Patent analysis involves managing vast volumes of structured and unstructured data, demanding intelligent tools for effective analysis. Commonly employed tools include text mining and visualization approaches, each playing a crucial role in extracting and representing valuable information from patent documents (Figure 9.2).

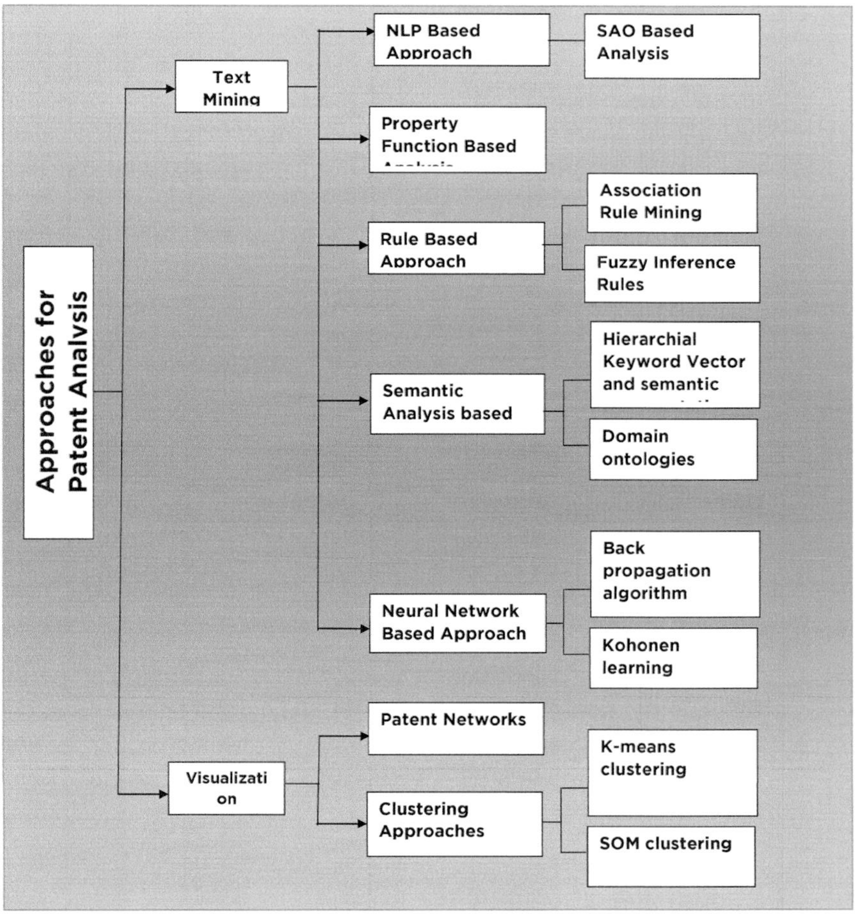

FIGURE 9.2 Approached for patent analysis.

9.2.1.1 TEXT MINING TECHNIQUES

- Text mining utilizes analytical tools to extract meaningful information from natural language text, focusing on unstructured data.
- Supports enterprise business intelligence, competitor discovery, security monitoring, sentiment analysis, and biomedical applications.
- Faces issues in accurately representing concepts and classifying synonyms within large documents.

9.2.1.1.1 NLP-Based Techniques

- Makes use of computational techniques to analyze and portray textual data.
- Natural language processing, or NLP, is used in the field of patent analysis to extract grammatical patterns from text and translate technical information into simple linguistic structures.
- Categorization: Keyword-based approaches and Subject-Action-Object based approaches.
- Challenges include lexical and grammatical ambiguities.
- Despite limitations, NLP-based approaches effectively process large documents.

9.2.1.1.2 Property-Function Based Techniques

- Involves using grammatical analysis to identify features and functionality from patent filings.
- Eliminates the need for predefined keywords or patterns.

Example Systems

1. *Trend Perceptor:* Identifies technological trends through property-function methodology and NLP, aids TRIZ trend analysis.
2. *Property-Function Based Patent Network:* Mines properties and functions, constructs a patent network, beneficial for identifying technological connotations.

9.2.1.1.3 Rule-Based Techniques

- Rely on inference rules and association rules for creating meaningful associations among structures in large datasets.

- Effective for creating associations but faces challenges with incomplete knowledge representation.

Example Systems

1. *Patent Trend Change Mining:* Captures identifies changes in patent trends via association rule mining without the need for specialist knowledge.
2. *Strategy Planning Method with FIS:* Integrates patent analysis with Fuzzy Inference System, applied in construction domain planning.

9.2.1.1.4 Semantic Analysis-Based Techniques

- Leverage domain knowledge to establish relationships among domain-specific concepts, effective in identifying similarities among patents.
- Faces challenges in parsing natural language structures.

Example Systems

1. *Semantic Analysis of Patent Claims:* Captures dependency relationships among claim elements, validated in DNA chip technology.
2. *Semantic Intellectual Property Management System:* Extracts key concepts, demonstrates effectiveness in retrieval and classification.

9.2.1.1.5 Neural Networks-Based Technique

- Utilizes backpropagation algorithm for patent classification and technology forecasting.

Example Systems

1. *Backpropagation Neural Network for Patent Quality:* Identifies patents specific to a technology, faces potential cold start problem.

9.2.1.2 VISUALIZATION TECHNIQUES

- Utilized for representing patent information visually and understanding technological trends.

- Dependency on text mining approaches for information extraction.
- Example Techniques: Technological trends identification, inventor-company-topic model, semantic network visualization, research direction identification model.
- Challenges may arise, but visualization techniques complement text mining for comprehensive analysis.

Both approaches contribute to the effective extraction and representation of valuable insights from patent documents.

9.2.1.2.1 Identifying Key Information for Research Purposes

Effectively leveraging patent literature for research necessitates the identification of key information. Researchers should adopt systematic strategies to extract relevant data:

1. **Keyword analysis:** Employing comprehensive keyword analysis is pivotal. Identifying key terms related to the research domain enables researchers to filter through extensive patent databases efficiently.

2. **Citation analysis:** Exploring citations within patents and to patents provides a network of related inventions. Researchers can trace the lineage of innovations and discern emerging trends within a particular scientific field.

3. **Legal status examination:** Assessing the legal status of a patent offers insights into its enforceability and potential expiration. Researchers can prioritize active patents or focus on expired ones, tailoring their analysis accordingly.

4. **IPC:** Utilizing IPC codes facilitates the categorization of patents based on their subject matter. Researchers can employ these codes to streamline searches and identify patents relevant to their research focus.

9.2.2 INTEGRATING PATENT FINDINGS INTO RESEARCH

The integration of patent findings into scientific research is a strategic approach that can significantly impact experimental design and spur advancements, particularly in the realm of herbal product development.

9.2.2.1 HOW PATENT LITERATURE CAN INFLUENCE EXPERIMENTAL DESIGN

1. **Identification of novel methodologies:** Patents often encapsulate inventive methodologies. Researchers can extract and incorporate these novel approaches into their experimental designs, enhancing the efficiency and innovation of their studies.
2. **Optimization strategies:** Patents frequently detail optimization strategies for processes or formulations. Researchers can leverage these insights to fine-tune their experimental parameters, leading to improved outcomes and resource efficiency.
3. **Integration of technology:** Patented technologies, when integrated into experimental setups, can elevate the precision and reproducibility of research. Researchers should explore patents to identify cutting-edge technologies applicable to their field.
4. **Avoidance of redundancy:** Thorough analysis of existing patents helps researchers avoid redundant experiments. Understanding what has already been explored can guide scientists in selecting novel avenues, contributing to the progression of knowledge.

9.2.2.2 LEVERAGING PATENTED TECHNOLOGIES FOR HERBAL PRODUCT DEVELOPMENT

Herbal product development stands to benefit significantly from the integration of patented technologies, fostering innovation in the following ways:

1. **Formulation enhancements:** Patents often disclose unique formulations and delivery systems. Researchers in herbal product development can draw inspiration from these formulations to enhance the bioavailability and efficacy of herbal products.
2. **Bioactive compound identification:** Patented technologies frequently delve into the identification and isolation of bioactive compounds. Researchers can leverage these findings to identify key compounds in herbal extracts, contributing to the development of standardized and potent herbal products.

3. **Quality control strategies:** Patented methods for quality control and authentication of herbal products provide valuable tools for developers. Integrating these strategies ensures the consistency and safety of herbal products in the market.
4. **Sustainable production practices:** Patented technologies often address sustainable and eco-friendly production methods. Researchers can adopt these practices in herbal product development to align with growing consumer preferences for environmentally conscious products.

Incorporating insights from patent literature into experimental design and herbal product development represents a symbiotic relationship between scientific research and innovation. Researchers and developers who adeptly navigate this intersection can advance their fields, bringing novel solutions to the forefront of scientific exploration and commercial application.

9.2.3 POTENTIAL PITFALLS

The integration of patent literature into research endeavors comes with inherent challenges and potential pitfalls that demand careful consideration. Addressing these challenges is paramount for ensuring the reliability and applicability of information derived from patents.

9.2.3.1 KEYWORD SEARCH

Describing an invention in layman's terms often involves using words that convey its function, construction, or even a given name, leading to a temptation to rely solely on keywords when searching. However, this approach has pitfalls to consider [26, 27].

1. **Context:** Keywords can be imprecise due to their various meanings. For instance, the word "bridge" may refer to diverse contexts such as a construction for passage, a musical instrument part, a dental insert, or an electrical circuit element. Different constructions like suspension or cantilever bridges add further complexity.

2. **Synonyms:** Chemistry introduces synonyms for compounds, where a chemical formula like CH_3COOH may be recognized by a chemist, but a layman may refer to it as "vinegar." Online services like ChemSpider assist in chemical entity searches.
3. **Language of patents:** Patent drafters often use deliberately obscure or specialized terms. Everyday items may be described differently in patents, such as a pen termed a "writing instrument." Spelling variations and invented words add to the complexity, emphasizing the importance of creativity in patent writing.
   - "More than one" may be replaced by "a plurality."
   - New adverbs like "slideably" emerge.
   - Contradictions like "detachably attached" are common.
4. **Translation challenges:** Translating patents introduces challenges, as the original term "Device for eliminating stray radiation" may lose its sense when translated into English as "Useless radiation preventer."

When conducting keyword searches in patents, it is crucial to consider these nuances, including potential spelling variations and the inventive language used by patent writers.

9.2.3.2 ADDRESSING LIMITATIONS AND BIASES IN PATENT LITERATURE

1. **Publication bias in patents:** Like scientific literature, patents may exhibit a certain degree of publication bias. Researchers should be aware that not all inventions or experimental outcomes make it into patent filings. Understanding this bias is crucial for obtaining a comprehensive view of the research landscape.
2. **Incomplete experimental details:** Patents may lack exhaustive details regarding experimental methodologies. Researchers should be cautious about incomplete information, recognizing that critical experimental nuances might not be fully disclosed.

3. **Commercial intent and overstatement:** Patents, being legal documents, may sometimes be crafted with commercial intent, leading to potential overstatement of results. Researchers must critically evaluate the claims made in patents and consider potential exaggerations.

9.2.3.3 VERIFYING AND VALIDATING INFORMATION OBTAINED FROM PATENTS

1. **Cross-verification with scientific literature:** Information extracted from patents should be cross-verified with findings in peer-reviewed scientific literature. Researchers should rely on a combination of patent data and published studies to establish the robustness of the information.
2. **Experimental reproducibility:** Researchers should approach patent-derived information with a focus on experimental reproducibility. Verifying the replicability of experimental outcomes ensures the reliability of data obtained from patents.
3. **Expert consultation:** In cases where the intricacies of patented technologies or methodologies are complex, seeking expert consultation becomes essential. Engaging with experts in the field can provide valuable insights into the feasibility and reliability of incorporating patented information into research.
4. **Legal interpretation:** Researchers should be mindful of the legal context of patents. Consulting legal professionals or patent experts can aid in the accurate interpretation of patent claims and disclosure, preventing misinterpretation that may impact research outcomes.

By addressing these potential pitfalls, researchers can enhance the robustness and credibility of their studies when incorporating insights from patent literature. A nuanced approach that considers the biases inherent in patents and employs rigorous validation measures ensures that research outcomes are built on a foundation of reliable and accurate information (Tables 9.2 and 9.3).

9.2.4 REAL-WORLD EXAMPLES

TABLE 9.2 Patent on Ayurvedic/Herbal Extracts

S. No.	Patent No.	Title	Main Herbs	References
1.	55/MUM/ 2008	Ayurvedic formula and herbal extract for the management of diabetes	*Momordica charantia*	[28]
2.	1734/KOL/ 2007	An Ayurvedic medication preparation method that effectively combats leukemia and intestinal and lung cancer Lime	Asafoetida and black jeera	[28]
3.	1938/DEL/ 2006	An Ayurvedic composition synthesis method for hepatic disease treatment	Kagzi nimbu (lemon) [*Citrus medica* (aurantifolia)], Sarjika [Salsola kali Linn., *Fagonia cretica* Linn., Barilla], and Varat (Kapard) *Cypraea moneta*	[28]
4.	1623/ MUM/ 2006	An Ayurvedic formula taken orally to treat cardiac conditions and high blood pressure	Arjuna, *Terminalia arjuna*; Ajamoda, Apium graveolens; Punarnava, *Boerhavia diffusa*; Rasona, *Allium sativum*; Shigru, *Moringa oleifera*; Draksha, *Vitis vinifera*; Pippali, *Piper longum*; Guduchi, *Tinospora cordifolia*, and Triphala	[28]
5.	228/CHE/ 2006	A method for making Ayurvedic tooth paste or powder	*Azadirachta indica* menthol thymol camphor and gall nut	[28]
6.	3207/DEL/ 2005	An Ayurvedic remedy for mending broken bones, acting as an anti-inflammatory, and preparing it	*Cissus quadrangularis*, *Pterocarpus marsupium* heartwood, buffalo/cow milk, and *Chenopodium murale* (kurund)	[28]
7.	726/CHE/ 2005	A remedy from Ayurveda that treats viral hepatitis	*Luffa cylindrica* or *Luffa acutangula* or *Luffa operculata* and seeds of *Cuminum cyminum*	[28]
8.	313/CHE/ 2005	A special blend of Ayurvedic ingredients to treat a rare kind of mulleri and ysgenesis	Asoka, Asana, and Bilwa, *Shorea robusta* Gaertn, *Pinus roxburghii* Sargent, *Cyperus rotundus* Linn., *Sida rhombifolia*, *Cyperus rotundus* Linn., *Gmelina asiatica* Linn., *Nardostachys jatamansi* DC, *Randia dumetorum* Linn., *Kaempferia galangal* Linn., *Teramnus labialis* Spreng., *Phaseolus trilobus*, *Inula racemosa* Hook. f., *Cinnamomum zeylanicum*, *Syzygium aromaticum* Merr., Parmelia (Sangejaranath), *Crocus sativus* Linn., *Cinnamomum camphora* T. Nees & Ebem	[28]

TABLE 9.2 *(Continued)*

S. No.	Patent No.	Title	Main Herbs	References
9.	146/MUM/ 2005	An Ayurvedic herbal hair oil recipe and recipe formulation	Jatamansi (*Nardostachys jatamansi* (D. Don) DC.) Amla, Brahmi (*Gratiola*) Bhringraj (*Eclipta alba*), *Thistles spicatum* and Kavath (*Feronia elephantum*)	[28]
10.	31/MUM/ 2005	Ayurvedic-based herbal formula for cancer and skin conditions, as well as the production method that goes with it.	*Murraya paniculata* (Bhutkati), *Latanacamara* (ghanera or Tantani), *Terminalia* (Kinjal), *Toalia asiatica* (Jangli Mirch) chawat or dhundari and teakwood	[28]

TABLE 9.3 Patent on 30 Medicinal Plants in India

Plant/Herb	Number of Patent Applications Published	Number of Patents Granted References	References
Lemon	65	16	[29]
Neem	173	47	[29]
Aloe vera	185	43	[29]
Erminalia bellerica	123	25	[29]
Turmeric	103	16	[29]
Ginger	86	19	[29]
Pepper	80	17	[29]
Garlic	59	13	[29]
Sandal/Chandan	50	29	[29]
Arjuna	47	16	[29]
Amla	47	12	[29]
Almond	23	12	[29]
Poppy	18	05	[29]
Camphora	14	04	[29]
Senna	06	03	[29]
Jasmine	25	07	[29]
Nutmeg	26	03	[29]
Veitver	09	04	[29]
Rose geranium	94	19	[29]
Patchouli	07	02	[29]
Chamommila	06	02	[29]
Basil/Tulsi	60	09	[29]

TABLE 9.3 *(Continued)*

Plant/Herb	Number of Patent Applications Published	Number of Patents Granted References	References
Lavender	10	01	[29]
Rosemary	15	01	[29]
Mint	57	16	[29]
Kawanch	28	06	[29]
Jamun	10	01	[29]
Celastrus	11	02	[29]
Psoralea	20	01	[29]
Musli	19	04	[29]

9.3 IP MANAGEMENT IN HERBAL SCIENCE

9.3.1 OVERVIEW OF IP IN HERBAL SCIENCE

IP plays a crucial role in the field of herbal science, providing a framework for protecting innovations and fostering advancements. This section provides an overview of the types of IP relevant to herbal products and emphasizes the importance of safeguarding innovations in this dynamic field.

9.3.1.1 TYPES OF IP RELEVANT TO HERBAL PRODUCTS

Patents associated with traditional medical knowledge, such as those based on maca and kava, face challenges in meeting patent criteria, especially regarding novelty and inventiveness. The longevity, dissemination, and public documentation of traditional medicines may hinder their eligibility for patent protection. Herbal remedies, often natural products, may struggle to demonstrate inventive steps, but alterations or purifications in pharmaceutical drugs derived from these products can qualify for patents [30].

Trade secrets, as confidential information, provide economic advantages but lose protection once disclosed. Traditional medical knowledge holders may opt for secrecy, limiting access to individual healers. Other IP tools like trademarks protect product sources, but they do not safeguard the knowledge itself [31]. Geographical indications identify origin-associated characteristics but cannot protect against unassociated use [32].

A number of countries have passed sui generis laws to protect traditional medical knowledge. One such example is the Act on Protection and

Promotion of Traditional Thai Medicinal Intelligence in Thailand. At the international level, WIPO's negotiations on traditional knowledge protection embody a sui generis approach [33].

Preserving traditional knowledge, as the TKDL in India demonstrates., aids in defensive protection against illegitimate patents. However, recording does not give the underlying knowledge legal protection. and may have unintended consequences. The TKDL, which prevents erroneous patent grants, is not publicly accessible to safeguard against misuse [34].

9.3.1.2 IMPORTANCE OF PROTECTING INNOVATIONS IN THE FIELD

1. *Encouraging research and development:* IP protection incentivizes researchers and herbal scientists to invest time and resources in exploring new formulations, extraction techniques, and therapeutic applications. The prospect of securing exclusive rights through patents fosters innovation in the herbal science domain.
2. *Market competitiveness and branding:* IP, particularly trademarks, contributes to market competitiveness by allowing herbal products to stand out in a crowded marketplace. Establishing a recognizable brand through trademark protection enhances consumer trust and loyalty.
3. *Commercialization and industry growth:* IP protection facilitates the commercialization of herbal innovations, attracting investments from industries looking to capitalize on novel discoveries. This, in turn, contributes to the overall growth and expansion of the herbal science sector.
4. *Preservation of traditional knowledge:* IP frameworks, when designed thoughtfully, can also contribute to preserving traditional knowledge associated with herbal practices. Balancing the protection of innovations with the recognition of traditional wisdom ensures a holistic approach to herbal science.

9.3.2 IP MANAGEMENT STRATEGIES

IP management is a critical aspect of herbal science research, requiring a thoughtful approach to strike a balance between the need for publication and the imperative of IP protection. This section outlines strategies for developing an effective IP management plan in the realm of herbal science.

9.3.2.1 DEVELOPING AN IP STRATEGY FOR HERBAL SCIENCE RESEARCH

9.3.2.1.1 Early Assessment of Patentability

- Make a comprehensive search of previous art to assess the patentability of herbal innovations.
- Evaluate the novelty and nonobviousness of herbal formulations, extraction methods, and bioactive compounds.

9.3.2.1.2 Strategic Filing of Patents

- Prioritize patent filings for innovations with high market potential and commercial value.
- Consider filing provisional patents to secure an early filing date while allowing time for additional research and development.

9.3.2.1.3 Collaborative IP Ventures

- Explore collaborative IP ventures and partnerships to pool resources and share risks.
- Develop clear agreements and frameworks for IP ownership and commercialization in collaborative research projects.

9.3.2.1.4 Trade Secret Protection

- Identify aspects of herbal science that can be treated as trade secrets, such as proprietary extraction methods or unique formulations.
- Implement internal protocols to maintain the confidentiality of trade secrets within research teams.

9.3.2.1.5 Customized IP Policies

- Develop customized IP policies tailored to the specific nature of herbal science research.
- Clearly define inventorship, ownership, and licensing terms within the institutional or organizational IP policy.

9.3.2.2 BALANCING THE NEED FOR PUBLICATION WITH IP PROTECTION

9.3.2.2.1 Timely Disclosures in Patent Applications

- Draft patent applications strategically to disclose essential aspects of the herbal innovation while preserving undisclosed elements.
- Leverage the patent system to provide a balance between public disclosure and IP protection.

9.3.2.2.2 Consideration of Defensive Publishing

- Explore defensive publishing for aspects of herbal research that may not be suitable for patent protection.
- Defensive publications can serve as a proactive measure to establish prior art and prevent others from obtaining patents on similar innovations.

9.3.2.2.3 Selective Data Sharing

- Be selective in data sharing and publication, particularly for innovations in the early stages of research.
- Evaluate the timing of publication concerning the IP filing process to optimize protection.

9.3.2.2.4 Strategic Use of Collaboration Agreements

- Integrate IP considerations into collaboration agreements with external partners or institutions.
- Clearly define rights and responsibilities regarding IP ownership and publication rights in collaborative research endeavors.

Effective IP management in herbal science is a multifaceted process that requires proactive planning and a nuanced understanding of the balance between knowledge dissemination and protection. By adopting tailored strategies and fostering a culture of IP awareness, researchers can navigate the complexities of IP in herbal science while contributing to the advancement of the field.

9.3.3 ETHICAL CONSIDERATIONS AND CASE STUDIES

Bio-robbery refers to the process in which the rights of indigenous societies to their resources and knowledge are eroded and replaced by IPR. Biopirates, described as privateers of life, engage in the exploitation of biodiversity and the traditional knowledge and practices of rural and indigenous communities. Biopiracy involves the misappropriation and commercialization of genetic resources and traditional knowledge of a nation and its indigenous people. Specifically, pharmaceutical biopiracy refers to the legal exploitation by pharmaceutical companies of Indigenous communities' traditional understanding of medicine. Developing countries like India, abundant in bio-resources and traditional knowledge, are often targeted by biopirates.

Joseph E. Stiglitz, a distinguished economist and Nobel Prize winner, highlights the issue of bio-robbery in the context of the WTO's Trade-Related Aspects of Intellectual Property Rights (TRIPs) Agreement. Bio-robbery involves global corporations profiting from traditional medicines and foods, suppressing Businesses in the nation that have been providing these things for a long time. Biopirates use genetic resources and materials for their own gain. They are mainly comprised of pharmaceutical, cosmetic, and agrifood companies, drawing on biodiversity hotspots to create supposedly "innovative" products and secure monopolies through the patent system.

Biopiracy often results in patents being granted to the "first-to-document" (pharmaceutical company) rather than the "first-to-design" (indigenous community). This practice involves profiting from freely available natural products using methods passed down through generations by local communities. Unfortunately, biopirates rarely provide any benefit or fair compensation to local communities and traditional knowledge holders. The issue of IPRs becomes closely linked to bio-robbery and the infringement of western-style IPR systems.

The lack of legal protection for biological and cultural heritage has left indigenous communities vulnerable to bio-robbery and IP theft, as seen in cases such as neem. Existing patent systems, based on western ideals, are criticized for favoring large transnational corporations in industries such as pharmaceuticals and agrochemicals.

To address the pervasive issue of biopiracy and provide justice to the guardians of traditional medicinal knowledge, international treaties have been proposed. Two significant treaties in this regard are:

1. Convention on Biological Diversity (CBD)
    - Originated from the Rio Earth Summit in 1992.
2. Nagoya Protocol on Biodiversity
    - Negotiated in Japan in 2010.

These international treaties aim to protect people and biodiversity from biopirates by establishing guidelines and regulations to curb unethical practices related to bio-robbery.

9.3.3.1 CBD

The CBD plays a crucial role in addressing issues related to the over-exploitation and extinction risk of medicinal plants. Many medicinal plants face extinction due to excessive harvesting driven by industrial and export demands, reminiscent of historical instances like the extinction of the contraceptive plant Silphium in the Ancient Mediterranean World. To counter this, regulating trade in medicinal plants becomes imperative, ideally within a comprehensive policy framework focused on conserving and sustainably using biological resources [35, 36].

The CBD stands out as a an international agreement recognizing indigenous populations' ownership of biodiversity and reaffirming their right to keep this knowledge safe. Despite its significance, The more potent TRIPs are in conflict with the CBD. Key articles within the CBD emphasize the importance of respecting and preserving the knowledge, inventions, and traditions of the local and indigenous people, ensuring their involvement and approval in wider applications. Equitable benefit-sharing from the utilization of such knowledge is also highlighted [37].

Article 18.4 of the CBD encourages contracting parties to foster cooperation for technology development and application, including traditional and indigenous technical methods. However, challenges arise due to insufficient protection of indigenous and traditional peoples' rights in many countries. Inadequate and ineffective national IP laws, when combined with ineffective enforcement, make it difficult for nations to protect their medical plants and related knowledge from exploitation. [38]. Addressing this issue requires strong collaborations between CBD, the WTO, the World Health Organization (WHO), and groups like the Species Survival Commission (SSC) and the International Union for Conservation of Nature (IUCN). The IUCN/SSC Medicinal and Aromatic Plants Group can be very helpful in finding solutions for the efficient preservation and long-term growth of biodiversity [39].

9.3.3.2 NAGOYA PROTOCOL ON BIODIVERSITY

The Nagoya Protocol on the Fair and Equitable Sharing of Benefits and Access to Genetic Resources represents a significant agreement developed to address the escalating loss of biodiversity on Earth. Formulated as an extension of the CBD, the Nagoya Protocol outlines mechanisms for implementing the CBD. The protocol, particularly its Access and Benefit-Sharing (ABS) provision, emphasizes establishing frameworks to control costs incurred by pharmaceutical corporations in the course of finding new drugs.

The ABS provision of the Nagoya Protocol mandates the creation of systems that necessitate pharmaceutical companies to bear the expenses associated with accessing genetic resources. However, this aspect of the Nagoya Protocol has raised concerns within the pharmaceutical industry. Many businesses believe that Benefit-Sharing and Access requirement has the potential to escalate product development costs and introduce complications in the drug discovery process. Expenses associated with product development have the potential to complicate the medication discovery process. Organizations must donate a sizable amount of their earnings and royalties to host nations and indigenous people in accordance with the protocol.

The revised patent system, introduced as a result of the It is expected that the Nagoya Protocol will raise the total cost of medication development. In adherence Following the guidelines provided by the Nagoya Protocol, institutions will need to engage in joint licensing agreements interacting with the communities that provide them with genetic resources. This shift in the operational landscape is viewed as a potential impediment by pharmaceutical companies, as it requires them to navigate more complex legal and financial arrangements, potentially impacting the efficiency and cost-effectiveness of drug development processes.

The Indian experiences outlined in various cases serve as valuable models for other countries seeking to address the challenges associated with the commercialization of traditional knowledge. These cases highlight successful initiatives that aim to protect indigenous rights and ensure fair benefit-sharing. Here is a reconstructed summary of the provided information:

1. **Honey Bee Network and Society for Research and Initiatives for Sustainable Technology and Institutions (SRISTI)**

    - The establishment of the Honey Bee Network in 1988–1989 marked a change in thinking about how to handle people's creativity, knowledge bases, and ethics surrounding conservation.
    - The establishment of SRISTI and related research programs was a consequence of the Honey Bee Network's growth [40].

2. **Cameroon—1994 Forestry Law**

    - In Cameroon, an agreement with the US National Cancer Institute (NCI) in 1994 led to the inclusion of ABS provisions for genetic resources in the new Forestry Law [41, 42].

3. **Peru—International Cooperative Biodiversity Groups (ICBG) Project**

    - The ICBG project's know-how licensing scheme had an impact on the creation of a draft law in Peru that protected indigenous groups' collective property rights [43].
    - The Peruvian process highlighted conflicts that need resolution to align measures with indigenous and local community priorities [44].

4. **Turmeric Case in India**

    - Turmeric, a plant widely used in traditional Indian Ayurvedic Medicine, became the subject of a US patent in 1995 for a wound treatment method.
    - Indian scientists challenged the patent, leading to its overturn in 1997, marking a significant case of successfully reversing a biopiracy patent.
    - This case prompted the creation of the TKDL in India to prevent the patenting of existing knowledge [45, 46].

5. San Nation in South Africa

- The San nation concluded a deal with South Africa's Council for Scientific and Industrial Research that recognized the San as the custodians of traditional knowledge. related to Hoodia plant use.
- After negotiations, an agreement was established to split the revenue from creating a medication that fights fat derived from the Hoodia plant [47].

6. Costa Rica—Merck Agreement (1991)

- In 1991, Merck and Costa Rica's Instituto Nacional de Biodiversidad (INBio) signed a contract, where Merck received plant samples and traditional use information.
- Merck agreed to pay royalties to INBio, creating a model for mutually beneficial agreements [40].

7. Neem Tree Case

- Neem tree, used traditionally in India for various purposes, faced patents in Europe and the United States.
- Public demonstrations and challenges resulted in the revocation of the European patent but not the US patent [40].

8. Shaman Pharmaceuticals

- Founded in 1990, Shaman Pharmaceuticals utilized ethnobotany for drug development, conducting studies in various countries.
- Shaman prioritizes sustainable relationships with indigenous groups, sharing benefits through the Healing Forest Conservancy [48].

9. Kani Model of Benefit Sharing in India

- The Kani community in India developed a benefit-sharing model based on the discovery of the therapeutic properties of *Trichopus zeylanicus*.
- The Kani Model involved transferring production technology to a pharmaceutical company, with a 1:1 sharing of license fees and royalties [49, 50].

These cases as mentioned above collectively demonstrate diverse strategies and successful models for protecting traditional knowledge, ensuring benefit-sharing, and fostering sustainable relationships between indigenous communities and external.

The cases discussed provide insights into various approaches for returning gains from the commercialization of traditional knowledge to the original communities. These approaches can be categorized as follows:

1. **Harmonize IPR laws ("TRIPS Solution"):**
   - This approach suggests harmonizing IPR laws across countries, essentially introducing the wealthy nation IPR policies in developing nations. The idea is to create uniform legal protections globally.
   - The implication is that uneven IPR protection contributes to unequal commercialization, and by standardizing laws, benefits could be more equitably distributed.

2. **Reform rich country IPRs**
   - An alternative perspective proposes that the problem lies in the IPR regimes of rich countries. Advocates of this view call for the elimination of patentability of plants, often expressed as "no patents on life."
   - Additionally, there is a call for the mandatory disclosure of traditional knowledge used in obtaining patents.

3. **Place ethnobotanical knowledge in the public domain**
   - Recognizing that much traditional knowledge is conveyed through oral tradition, this approach emphasizes the importance of documenting and publishing this knowledge.
   - By placing ethnobotanical knowledge in the public domain, the aim is to prevent the exclusive commercialization of traditional knowledge by ensuring it is freely accessible to all.

4. **Create knowledge-sharing contracts**
   - This approach involves introducing constructing barriers to knowledge transfer and contractual procedures.
   - The idea is to regulate the sharing of traditional knowledge through formal contracts, ensuring that communities receive fair compensation when their knowledge is commercialized.

5. Promote indigenous commercialization

- This perspective emphasizes the importance of enabling commercialization within the originating communities, irrespective of the property rights established by industrialized countries.
- Encouraging indigenous commercialization aims to empower local communities economically and ensure that they benefit directly from the commercial use of traditional knowledge.

KEYWORDS

- **patenting of herbal products**
- **patent searches**
- **intellectual property right**
- **traditional knowledge**

REFERENCES

1. Chaudhary, A., & Singh, N. Intellectual property rights and patents in perspective of Ayurveda. *Ayu* 2012, 33(1), 20. Available from: http://dx.doi.org/10.4103/0974-8520.100298
2. Aguilar, G. Access to genetic resources and protection of traditional knowledge in the territories of indigenous peoples. *Environ Sci Policy* 2001, 4(4–5), 241–256. Available from: http://dx.doi.org/10.1016/s1462-9011(01)00028-4
3. Bayram, S. Patent research on 15 medicinal plants which are significant for phytotherapy and have preparations in the European market. *J Ethnol* 2005, 51, 59–73.
4. Trippe, A. J. Patinformatics: Tasks to tools. *World Pat Inf* 2003, 25(3), 211–221. Available from: http://dx.doi.org/10.1016/s0172-2190(03)00079-6
5. Adams, S. The text, the full text and nothing but the text: Part 2-the main specification, searching challenges and survey of availability. *World Pat Inf* 2010, 32(2), 120–128.
6. Joho, H., Azzopardi, L. A., & Vanderbauwhede, W. A survey of patent users: An analysis of tasks, behavior, search functionality and system requirements. In: *Proceedings of the Third Symposium on Information Interaction in Context USA*, 2010, Crossref, pp. 13–24.
7. Khode, A., & Jambhorkar, S. A literature review on patent information retrieval techniques overview of search strategies. *Indian J Sci and Techn* 2017, 10, 1–13.

8. and the Protection of Plant Varieties and Farmers' Rights Act, 2001 ensures the use of biological resources in a manner that rights of country and communities are protected. The National Biodiversity Authority (NBA), Chennai, and Protection of Plant Varieties and Farmers' Rights Authority. In: *Various provisions of the Biological Diversity Act*. 2002.
9. Deboys, J. Decision pathways in patent searching and analysis. *World Pat Inf* 2004, 26(1), 83–90. Available from: http://dx.doi.org/10.1016/j.wpi.2003.09.001
10. Sudhir, H. B. Some reflections on patent search: A case study of medicinal plants of India. *J Intellect Prop Rights* 2006, 11, 207–213.
11. Clarke, N. S. The basics of patent searching. *World Pat Inf* 2018, 54, S4–S10. Available from: http://dx.doi.org/10.1016/j.wpi.2017.02.006
12. Singh, V., & Vincent, C. Patent database: Their importance in prior art documentation and patent search. *J Intellect Prop Rights* 2016, 21, 42–56.
13. Lee, W., Leung, C. K., & Song, J. J. Reducing noises for recalloriented patent retrieval. In: *IEEE Fourth International Conference on Big Data and Cloud Computing. BdCloud),* Australia: Crossref, 2014, pp. 579–586.
14. Benson, C. L., & Magee, C. L. A hybrid keyword and patent class methodology for selecting relevant sets of patents for a technological field. *Scientometrics* 2013, 96(1), 69–82. Available from: http://dx.doi.org/10.1007/s11192-012-0930-3
15. Blair, D. C., & Maron, M. E. An evaluation of retrieval effectiveness for a full-text document-retrieval system. *Commun ACM* 1985, 28(3), 289–299. Available from: http://dx.doi.org/10.1145/3166.3197.
16. Cao, Y., Fan, J., & Li, G. A user-friendly patent search paradigm. *IEEE Trans Knowl Data Eng* 2013, 25(6), 1439–1443. Available from: http://dx.doi.org/10.1109/tkde.2012.63.
17. Joachims, T. *Learning to Classify text Using Support Vector Machines: Methods, Theory and Algorithms*. Norwell, Crossref, 2002.
18. Meij, E., Weerkamp, W., & de Rijke, M. A query model based on normalized log-likelihood. In: *Proceedings of the 18th ACM Conference on Information and Knowledge Management*. New York, NY, USA: ACM; 2009.
19. Verma, M., & Varma, V. Applying key phrase extraction to aid invalidity search. In: *Proceedings of the 13th International Conference on Artificial Intelligence and Law*. New York, NY, USA: ACM, 2011.
20. Kwok, K. L., & Chan, M. Improving two-stage ad-hoc retrieval for short queries. In: *Proceedings of the 21st Annual International ACM SIGIR Conference on Research and Development in Information Retrieval*. New York, NY, USA: ACM, 1998.
21. Criscuolo, P., & Verspagen, B. Does it matter where patent citations come from? Inventor vs. examiner citations in European patents. *Res Policy* 2008, 37(10), 1892–1908. Available from: http://dx.doi.org/10.1016/j.respol.2008.07.011.
22. Shin, J., & Park, Y. Generation and application of patent claim map: Text mining and network analysis. *J Intellect Prop Rights* 2005, 10(3), 198–205.
23. Mittal, R., & Singh, G. Patenting activities in agriculture from India. *J Intellect Prop Rights* 2005, 10(4), 315–320.
24. Phadnis, R. Patent analysis as a tool for research planning: Case study of phytochemicals in tea. *J Intellect Prop Rights* 2005, 10(3), 221–231.

25. Abbas, A., Zhang, L., & Khan, S. U. A literature review on the state-of-the-art in patent analysis. *World Pat Inf* 2014, 37, 3–13. Available from: http://dx.doi.org/10.1016/j.wpi.2013.12.006
26. ChemSpider [Internet]. Chemspider.com. [cited 2023 Dec 17]; Available from: http://www.chemspider.com/.
27. Do you know English? The challenge of the English language for patent searchers, World Pat. *World Pat Inf* 2014, 39, 35–e40.
28. Gov.in [Internet]. [cited 2023 Dec 17]; Available from: https://ipindiaservices.gov.in/publicsearch
29. No title [Internet]. Gov.in. [cited 2023 Dec 17]; Available from: http://ipindiaservices.gov.in
30. Intellectual Property and Genetic Resources, Traditional Knowledge and Traditional Cultural Expressions: An Overview. WIPO Publication No;
31. Promoting Access to Medical Technologies and Innovation: Intersections between Public Health, Intellectual Property and Trade. WIPO Publication No;
32. Wipo.int [Internet]. [cited 2023 Dec 17]; Available from: http://www.wipo.int/edocs/pubdocs/en/wipo_pub_1049.pdf
33. Eiland, M. L. Patenting traditional medicine. In: *Patenting Traditional Medicine*, 1st edn, Nomos Verlagsgesellschaft mbH, 2018, pp. 7–46.
34. Laws and legislative measures [Internet]. Wipo.int. [cited 2023 Dec 17]; Available from: http://www.wipo.int/tk/en/legal_texts
35. Intergovernmental committee (IGC) [Internet]. Wipo.int. [cited 2023 Dec 17]; Available from: http://www.wipo.int/tk/en/igc/index.html
36. Newman, E. B. Earth's vanishing medicine cabinet: Rain forest destruction and its impact on the pharmaceutical industry. *Am J Law Med* 1994, 20(4), 479–501. Available from: http://dx.doi.org/10.1017/s0098858800006869
37. Sumner, J. *The Natural History of Medicinal Plants*. Timber Press: Portland, Oregon, 2001.
38. Bodeker, G. *Indigenous Medical Knowledge: The Law and Politics of Protection - This Study was Presented at the Oxford Intellectual Property Research Centre Seminar*. St. Peter's College: Oxford on, 2000.
39. Berniard, J., Zámboriné Németh, E., Craker, L., & Köck, O. Possibilities and limitations of medicinal and aromatic plant production in the 21st century. In: *International Conference on Medicinal and Aromatic Plants*. Budapest Hungary, 2002.
40. SRISTI [Internet]. SRISTI. [cited 2023 Dec 17]; Available from: http://www.sristi.org
41. Laird, S. A. *Biodiversity and Traditional Knowledge; Equitable Partnerships in Practice*. People and Plants Conservation Series. Earthscan Publications LTD: London, Sterling VA, 2002.
42. Laird, S. A., & Lisinge, E. E. Sustainable harvest of Prunus africana on Mount Cameroon: Benefit sharing between Plantecam company and the Village of Mapanja. In: *Case Studies on Benefit Sharing Arrangements, Secretariat, CBD, 4th Conference of the Parties (COP4)*. Bratislava, Slovakia, 1998.
43. Muller, R. Regulating bioprospecting and protecting indigenous peoples knowledge in andean community: Decision 391 and its overall impacts in the region. In: *Paper*

Presented at the UNCTAD Expert Meeting on Traditional Knowledge, Innovations and Practices, 2000.
44. Tobin, B. Redefining perspectives in the search for protection of traditional knowledge: A case study from Peru. *Rev Eur Community Int Environ Law* 2001, 10(1), 47–64. Available from: http://dx.doi.org/10.1111/1467-9388.00260.
45. Finger, J. M. *Poor People's Knowledge: Promoting Intellectual Property in Developing Countries*. World Bank: Herndon, VA, USA, 2003.
46. Rawat, R. B. S. Paper presented in: International Systems for the Protection of Traditional Knowledge, organized by Ministry of Commerce, Government of India and UNCTAD. New Delhi; 2002.
47. SA. Alive magazine [Internet]. alive. 2015 [cited 2023 Dec 17]; Available from: http://www.alive.com
48. Ernet.in [Internet]. [cited 2023 Dec 17]; Available from: http://stp.unipune.ernet.in/ipr/ipr_tm.htm
49. Idrc.ca [Internet]. [cited 2023 Dec 17]; Available from: http://archive.idrc.ca/books/reports/1996/30-02e.html.
50. Dedeurwaerdere, T., Krishna, V., & Pascual, U. *Environmental Economy and Policy Research: Biodiscovery and IPR; A Dynamic Approach to Economic Efficiency*. Discussion Paper Series, 2005

CHAPTER 10

Herbal Drug Licensing and Compliance

RAVIKIRAN VEGADA[1], JANKHANA BARAIYA[2], and SOURABH JAIN[3*]

[1]*Department of Pharmacognosy, Sharda School of Pharmacy, Pethapur, Gandhinagar, Gujarat, India*

[2]*Department of Pharmacognosy, School of Pharmacy, RK University, Rajkot, Gujarat, India*

[3]*Department of Pharmacognosy, Arihant School of Pharmacy & Bio-Research Institute, Gandhinagar, Gujarat, India*

*Corresponding author

ABSTRACT

Herbal medications or supplements are natural substances derived from plant parts, often used for their therapeutic benefits when taken as supplements. Around the world, these products are regulated according to the specific laws, guidelines, and oversight of governmental and expert bodies. Regulatory agencies, established in accordance with local laws, oversee the registration and compliance of herbal health products. In India, for instance, the Department of AYUSH regulates herbal medicines under the Drug & Cosmetic Act, requiring manufacturing licenses for production and sale. This legislation aligns with international standards set by organizations like the USFDA, the European Medicines Agency, the Therapeutic Goods Act, and the World Health Organization, ensuring quality and safety in the production and distribution of herbal products.

10.1 INTRODUCTION

Herbal medicines (HMs) are industrially prepared mixtures containing pure and natural active ingredients derived from plants, which are not

Herbal Drug Industry: From Cultivation to Innovation and Global Impact.
Abhishek Tiwari, Varsha Tiwari, and Ajay Sharma (Eds.)

DOI: 10.1201/9781779640994-10

chemically modified and contribute to the therapeutic effects of the product [1]. Many consumers turn to these plant-derived remedies under the belief that they are inherently safer than conventional medications due to their natural origin [2]. However, like traditional medicines, HMs contain various chemical compounds that can exert pharmacological actions, leading to both minor and severe side effects, such as elevated blood pressure, liver damage, renal dysfunction, and in extreme cases, death [3, 4].

Safety concerns with HMs can also arise from contamination with mold, yeast, bacteria, or interactions with conventional medications [4, 5]. Regulatory authorities, such as Drug Regulatory Authorities (DRAs), enforce rigorous quality, safety, and efficacy evaluations of medications before they are approved for marketing, ensuring they are used safely [6]. Manufacturers are required to provide evidence of toxicity screening and adhere to Good Manufacturing Practices (GMPs) to ensure product quality [6].

The complexity of HMs, which may contain numerous natural components in varying amounts, poses challenges in standardization, ethical considerations, and budget constraints for conducting clinical studies to assess their effectiveness [7, 8]. International treaties like the Convention on International Trade in Endangered Species of Wild Fauna and Flora regulate the global trade of herbal drugs to protect endangered species [9].

Globally, HMs fall under various regulatory categories, including complementary medicines, over-the-counter medicines, supplements, natural health products (NHPs), prescription medicines, and traditional HMs. Different countries enforce varying degrees of manufacturing regulations for herbal products. For example, in Germany, herbal products marketed as "phytomedicines" must meet the same rigorous standards for quality, safety, and efficacy as conventional pharmaceuticals [10]. In contrast, in the United States, many herbal products are classified as dietary supplements and do not undergo preapproval based on these factors [10].

10.2 POLICIES FOR MINIMUM REQUIREMENTS IN THE EASTERN MEDITERRANEAN REGION FOR THE HERBAL MEDICINAL PRODUCTS REGISTRATION

Over the past decade, the global market for herbal medications has experienced significant growth. In 2000, the Convention on Biological Diversity estimated the global market for HMs at approximately US$60 billion. During this period, countries like Japan witnessed a more than doubling of their herbal medicine market from 1991 to 2000. Similarly, the United States saw substantial growth, with the market expanding from US$1.6 billion in 1994 to US$5.4 billion in 2000.

In the World Health Organization Eastern Mediterranean Region, there has been a steady rise in the use of herbal remedies. Countries like Iran rely heavily on domestically produced HMs for basic healthcare, while others, such as the United Arab Emirates, import herbal products mainly from Europe, Asia, or the United States. Importantly, many imported herbal products contain multiple plant ingredients, posing challenges for testing and quality control, which are critical for evaluating these products.

One of the key challenges in the region is the varying classifications of herbal products across different countries, which include traditional medicines, nutritional supplements, and functional foods. This diversity complicates efforts for harmonizing safety and quality control standards across borders. In many countries, HMs are not adequately covered by existing safety monitoring systems, leading to gaps in information regarding their efficacy, safety, and quality assurance.

To address these issues, governments are urged to establish national regulations governing the importation and production of herbal medicines. The Eastern Mediterranean DRAs Conferences in 1999 and 2001 provided initial guidance for developing regulatory frameworks for HMs. However, specific guidelines tailored to the needs of major producers and importers of herbal medicines are necessary.

In 2002, the WHO Eastern Mediterranean Regional Committee adopted Resolution EM/RC49/R.9, which called for the development of national policies and guidelines on complementary, alternative, and traditional medicine. This resolution aimed to enhance coordination among health ministries and improve the regulation of HMs across the region.

The complexities of the HM market require collaborative efforts among countries to exchange best practices, standardize safety and quality control requirements, and enhance regulatory frameworks to ensure the safe and effective use of HMs globally.

10.2.1 CATEGORIZATION OF HERBAL MEDICINES

10.2.1.1 TRADITIONAL HERBAL MEDICINES

Herbal treatments in the Eastern Mediterranean Region are defined as therapies involving single herbs or combinations thereof, which have a well-established history of safety and efficacy or have been used within the local community for at least 15 years. This category also includes formulations from traditional medicine that have undergone minor modifications. Additionally, herbal remedies not native to the region, such as ginseng, may be included if they are widely used and sufficient information regarding their safety and effectiveness is available. These criteria aim to ensure that herbal treatments meet established standards of safety and efficacy before being recognized and utilized within the region.

10.2.1.2 NOVEL HERBAL MEDICINES

In the context of HM, substances, whether single herbs or combinations, may be categorized as "new herbal medicines" under certain conditions. This includes herbs that are not traditionally used in the community or region, are used infrequently, sparingly (in a small percentage of patients), or in novel combinations that have not been previously tested.

To facilitate a harmonized assessment, it is proposed to establish a regional list of traditional herbal substances or combinations. Nations can submit proposals to the WHO Eastern Mediterranean Regional Office for inclusion in this list. The list should include:

- Scientific botanical name (Latin binomial nomenclature) of the plant
- Common English name of the plant
- Local names of the plant in regional languages
- Part of the plant used
- Name of the HM
- Dosage form (e.g., extract, powder, and herbal tea)
- Administration method (oral, topical, inhalation, etc.)
- Safe dosage range (daily dose) as documented in literature

HMs should be classified for safety as follows:

- **Class I:** Demonstrated safety from prolonged traditional use
- **Class II:** Considered safe under specific conditions, ideally supported by well-established documentation
- **Class III:** Herbal remedies with questionable safety profiles

This classification system aims to ensure that HMs are systematically evaluated and categorized based on their safety and usage patterns, providing a framework for their regulated use within the Eastern Mediterranean Region.

10.2.1.2.1 Safety Requirements for "New Herbal Medicines"

The safety information needed to register new herbal remedies will be the same as that needed for any novel substance:

- Toxicity of single dose
- Toxicity of repeated dose
- Chronic poisoning
- Toxicity directed against organs, if required
- Hypertoxicity to the immune system
- Toxicology to fetuses and embryos, if needed
- If required, mutagenicity or genotoxicity
- Carcinogenicity, where applicable
- Local tolerance

Certain unusual cases, such as novel mixtures of well-known compounds, might not require all of these research.

A clear identification and description of the ingredients must serve as the foundation for any evaluation of traditional herbal remedies. It is essential to carry out a literature search. Included in this should be general literature, such as contemporary handbooks on phytotherapy, phytochemistry, and pharmacognosy, as well as traditional handbooks specific to each individual form of therapy. It should also include publications in scholarly journals and official monographs like national and WHO monographs, as well as additional reliable information about herbal remedies. Database searches on offline or internet databases, if available, such as the National Library of Medicine's Medline or the WHO adverse drug reaction database, should also be included. Not only should searches concentrate on the particular herbal medication mixture, but they should also cover various plant sections, allied plant species, and data derived from chemotaxonomy. It is important to evaluate the toxicological data on individual constituents in relation to herbal remedies.

In their applications to the World Health Organization Regional Office, countries in the Eastern Mediterranean Region ought to provide information about trustworthy sources of this kind of data. When evaluating this bibliographic data, special consideration should be made to the traits and kind of preparation that have been documented within the scholarly works:

- Is the herbal preparation mentioned in the literature the same one?
- Is it possible to extrapolate the results, for example, comparing an extract made with 40% ethanol to one made with 60% ethanol?
- How long and how much the herbal remedy was used for; has it produced enough experience with safety?
- Is it likely that dangers would have been identified by empirical research?

The information requirements for novel herbal medications should be taken into consideration when determining if more data or new testing are needed. Much of the testing needed for these new medications might be substituted by experience that has been reported. It is important to carefully evaluate whether the current body of knowledge on toxicology is sufficient to address all problems posed in a reasonable and suitable manner. Effects like genotoxicity that are difficult to detect experimentally should receive special consideration.

If there is insufficient knowledge to ensure safe usage in sensitive populations, such as young children and pregnant or lactating women, it should be determined by the evaluation. Information about traditional usage, such as using it as an agent to increase abortion, should be evaluated while evaluating safety during pregnancy.

10.2.1.2.2 Minimum Standards for Herbal Medicine Products' Effectiveness

- Acute diseases, which start out quickly and last for a short time
- Chronic illnesses, which develop slowly and endure for a long time
- Health-enhancing effects

The term "acute disease" usually refers to a condition that is life-threatening or for which postponing treatment will result in worsening health or incapacity to treat the illness. Examples of these conditions include severe cardiovascular, gastrointestinal, endocrine, hematological, and immune disorders and diseases.

Patients with specific medical disorders, such as menopause, hay fever, and appetite loss, occasionally recover on their own without the need for medical assistance. Data from reliable sources such as national monographs and pharmacopeias, as well as other reputable publications like WHO monographs, may be used to support the effectiveness of HMs in this field. Clinical data are necessary, although preclinical efficacy data might not be. The effectiveness and clinical data could be checked if customary usage of medications with well-established documentation indicates changes in the dose form, route of administration, or medical indication (see Tables 10.1 and 10.2). Clinical trials, preclinical data, and/or well-established documentation should be used to demonstrate the efficacy. Preclinical research is required to determine whether the modifications could affect the medication's pharmacodynamic properties.

TABLE 10.1 Different Types of Drug License and Minimum Requirement

Sr. No.	Name of License	Minimum Requirement
1	AYUSH Manufacturing License	The business that is applying must possess a manufacturing facility situated on industrial land
		A single product can only be manufactured on a plot of land measuring 1200 square feet. The land area will grow in proportion to the number of products that are to be manufactured
		A GMP-certified manufacturing facility is required
		The proposed company must employ at least two Ayurvedic pharmacists and two Ayurvedic experts
		The manufacturing facility is equipped with all the machinery needed for production and packaging
2	AYUSH Retail and Wholesale License	In order to qualify for an AYUSH Retail or Wholesale License, a store must meet the National Building Code, 2005, requirements for height and space, with a minimum of 10 square meters
		The business must be 15 square meters in size and meet the 2005 National Building Code requirements for height in order to be eligible to apply for both an AYUSH Retail and Wholesale License

TABLE 10.1 *(Continued)*

Sr. No.	Name of License	Minimum Requirement
3	AYUSH Loan License	The company lending the manufacturing facility needs to hold an AYUSH manufacturing license
		The manufacturing facility that is being lent has to be located on industrial property
		The manufacturing facility that is being lent needs to have a separate area for storing finished goods and raw materials, as well as an office where regular company operations can be conducted
		The possession of pharmacies or Ayurvedic experts is not necessary for the bearer of a loan license
		The loan license needs to be renewed on a regular basis

TABLE 10.2 Documents Required to Apply for AYUSH License [13]

Sr. No.	Documents Required for AYUSH License
1	If the applicant is producing AYUSH products, a copy of their production license
2	The manufacturing facility's site plan
3	Details of the manufacturing formula and manufacturing process
4	Completed report on product specifications
5	List of applied and approved products for COPP certification
6	Three rounds of process validation reports
7	Information on the technical team, including their titles, backgrounds, and credentials
8	List of machinery to be utilized in production
9	Water and HVAC system diagrams
10	Evidence of Safety and Efficacy in Compliance with Drugs and Cosmetics Rules, 1945, Rule 158B
11	Taking responsibility for the absence of nonherbal substances, which applies to herbal goods
12	Engaging in activities related to adherence to the Drugs and Cosmetics Act, Drugs and Cosmetic Rules, Drugs and Magic Remedies (Objectionable Advertisements) Act, 1954, and the rules that accompany it (applied exclusively to herbal items)
13	KYC details of the applicant
14	Provide proof of premises (rent agreement) address
15	Constitution document of the business

10.2.2 QUALITY CONTROL OF HERBAL MEDICINAL PRODUCTS

10.2.2.1 APPROACHES TO QUALITY ASSURANCE

Manufacturers and regulatory agencies share responsibilities for quality assurance. GMP, good laboratory practice, and good agricultural and collection practice (GACP) guidelines must be followed by manufacturers. They also need to set suitable requirements for their final goods, go-betweens, and raw materials, and assemble thorough records of pharmaceutical development and testing that are well-organized. The manufacturer must work tirelessly to advance standards and modify them in light of current understanding. It is recommended that producers work together to build master files for medicines that contain standards and quality controls.

National health regulatory agencies should create guidelines on all aspects of quality assurance, assess producer-submitted data and dossiers, and verify that goods meet producer-specified requirements once they are marketed. Regulatory bodies ought to make it easier for high-quality herbal medications to reach consumers by giving small manufacturers guidance and training, as well as monographs in pharmacopeias.

Only until the manufacturing and distribution of herbal medications are governed by a sufficient registration system will such regulations be able to be put into practice.

10.2.2.2 QUALITY CONTROL OF IMPORTED HERBAL DRUGS

All imported HMs must adhere to the quality control regulations, safety standards, and efficacy requirements of the importing nations. The following criteria need to be considered in order to regulate the quality of imported herbal medical products:

- The national health regulatory authority should grant permits to importers, dealers, and producers of imported HM items
- Dealers in imported HMs are required to apply for one or more licenses, based on the nature of their operation (manufacturing, distribution, etc.)
- It is the responsibility of the local business looking to import and sell herbal medicinal items in a country to apply for an import license

In order to bolster an import licensing application, the importing company must provide the following details:

- Company details
- Details of the applicant acting on behalf of the business
- A certificate of business registration or corporation
- The layout of the store

Importers will only be permitted to deal in goods that have been authorized in the exporting nations, and they will be obliged to furnish information on every imported herbal medicinal product that they handle. Specific specifications for every HM imported include:

- Whole product formula (in the languages of the nations that are exporting and importing)
- A collection of labels, a brochure, a carton, and an example sales pack
- Specifics on the producer and assembler(s)
- A license or certificate from the health authorities of the country or origin where the product is manufactured. In the event that the HM is imported, an export certificate

Each national health regulatory body may create its own standards for quality control of imported herbal medical goods based on the aforementioned baseline requirements.

10.2.2.3 GUIDELINES RELATED TO "GACP" AND "GMP"

The World Health Organization GACP recommendations for medicinal plants and GMP should be followed by all parties involved in the manufacture of herbal medicinal products. HM producers must get a license and be registered. A quality assurance system ought to be suitable and appropriate for the kind of production and the local conditions, such as industrial or agricultural production. The main objective should be to execute a plausible idea of quality assurance, such as locating and removing possible sources of contamination, rather than implementing every single technical detail.

Producers of botanical raw materials should be provided with incentives to promote the use of GACP methods. Incentives could take the form of providing seeds and seedlings, choosing fertilizers and pesticides, offering technical and logistical assistance in the selection of suitable places for agricultural production, or supplying or advising on technology for harvesting and primary processing. In recognition of their efforts, the government ought to award certifications to manufacturers who meet GACP requirements in accordance with national circumstances.

10.2.2.4 GUIDELINES RELATED TO QUALITY CONTROL

Setting proper standards and specifications serves as the cornerstone of quality control. Consult official monographs and pharmacopeias for information on acceptable qualifications.

The robustness and availability of the approach must be taken into account while selecting analytical techniques. If a complete validation of more complex techniques like high-performance liquid chromatography, gas chromatography, and gas chromatography/mass spectrometry is not feasible, it might be better to use straightforward techniques like microscopic identification, thin-layer chromatography, or active substance titration. A thorough validation will be required for every test if such sophisticated techniques are applied.

10.2.2.4.1 Product Information

All information required for using the product properly should be included in the product information. Typically, the information will have the following components:

- Brand name of formulation
- A quantitative list of the active components that includes plant names and the Latin name of the plant utilized
- Dosage form
- Indications
- It is necessary to specify the dosage levels for children and pregnant women, if applicable, as well as the lowest, maximum, and average values
- Administration route
- Length of usage

- Adverse consequences, where appropriate
- Information of overdose
- Cautions, warnings, and limits
- Drug interactions, if relevant
- Issue date
- Expiry date
- Lot number
- Name and complete address of the manufacturer or company

10.2.3 PHARMACOVIGILANCE OF HERBAL MEDICINAL PRODUCTS

10.2.3.1 ADVERSE DRUG REACTION (ADR) REPORTING

Pharmacovigilance units are required for the gathering and evaluation of data about herbal and traditional medicine. In cases where these units are available, information about herbal and traditional remedies ought to be included.

Every adverse drug reaction (ADR) report needs to be examined for any potential connections to complementary or alternative medicine. Health practitioners ought to be incentivized to inquire with their patients on the utilization of herbal and traditional medicines, encompassing medicinal foods, and to incorporate details on concurrent use in their ADR report.

Every herbal medication needs to be properly identified by its dosage, brand name (if any), and composition. The pharmacovigilance unit should make an effort to get complete information if such information is absent from the ADR report, for example, by contacting the reporting healthcare provider.

The evaluation is to be carried out in collaboration with a group of toxicological and pharmacognosy specialists, as well as other medical specialists, such as conventional healers.

10.2.4 REGULATING THE PROMOTION OF HERBAL MEDICINAL PRODUCTS

Every advertisement should get approval from the national authority in charge of regulating HM practices and products before it is made public.

After a thorough review of the advertisement's content, the regulatory body should grant an advertising permit to guarantee that the public is given accurate information about the product that is free of misleading or unclear statements. To guarantee that all advertisers of herbal medicinal products get an advertising authorization from the national government prior to such advertisements being circulated, notice should be given to the print and electronic media.

Cooperation and the exchange of information about advertisements for herbal medicinal products should be promoted among the member nations of the region [11].

10.3 DRUG CONTROLLING AUTHORITIES AND DIFFERENT TYPES OF DRUG LICENSE IN DIFFERENT COUNTRY

10.3.1 INDIA

The Drug and Cosmetic Act (D and C) 1940 and Rules 1945 govern herbal medications in India. They contain clear guidelines for the use of Unani, Siddha, and Ayurvedic medicine. Regulations are overseen by the Department of AYUSH, which mandates that the manufacture or distribution of HMs can only take place once a manufacturing license has been secured, if applicable.

The D and C Act increases control over export, quality, packaging, labeling, production, licensing, and formulation composition. The GMP criteria that must be followed when making herbal pharmaceuticals are outlined in Schedule "T" of the Act. You can obtain the official pharmacopeias and formularies for the drug quality standards. Any herbal product that fits into one of the two categories listed in the first schedule of the D and C Act's approved texts must be licensed in accordance with those texts:

ASU drugs

- Patent or proprietary medicines [12].

10.3.1.1 DIFFERENT TYPES OF DRUG LICENSE

- AYUSH Manufacturing License. Required if the business wants to manufacture and market its own ASU products/treatments, for which it will use its own manufacturing facility.
- AYUSH Wholesale and Retail License.
- AYUSH Loan License.
- AYUSH Third-Party Manufacturing License.

10.3.1.2 STEP-WISE PROCESS

STEP 1—Documentation: In India, the AYUSH Registration procedure is entirely application-based and conducted online. The relevant AYUSH license application form is filled out with a few supporting documents that are supplied in the correct forms and contain the most recent data. Your application could be rejected in its entirety if any of these documents are not filed correctly. As a result, we highly advise that you hold off on starting the application submission procedure until you are certain that you have all the required paperwork.

STEP 2—Apply for GMP Certificate: In order to control the quality of manufactured medications and cosmetics items as well as the manufacturing process itself, the World Health Organization has released standards for GMPs. Many countries have embraced these rules, one of them being India. Therefore, even pharmaceuticals and cosmetics made in India are required to abide by these regulations and get a GMP Certificate from the Drug Controller General of India attesting to their compliance. Nonetheless, the involved state's Drug Control Department may receive the application. One crucial document that must be supplied with the AYUSH licensing application is the GMP Certificate.

STEP 3—Apply for COPP Certificate, if applicable The World Health Organization created the Certificate of Pharmaceutical Products to verify the quality of medications being exported from one nation to another. This Certificate must be received by the exporter from its country of origin and is typically requested by the National Health Authorities of the importing country. This certificate must be provided when applying for an AYUSH license if producers of AYUSH medications and cosmetics intend to market their goods outside of India. The Drug Controller General of India issues COPP certificates, just like they do GMP certificates. Nonetheless, the involved state's Drug Control Department may receive the application.

STEP 4—Download the form for AYUSH License Certificate You can start the online application procedure for an AYUSH license as soon as you are certain you have all the required paperwork. Form 24D must be submitted for the issuance of an AYUSH production license and Form 25E for the issuance of an AYUSH financing license, according to Rule 153 of the Drugs and Cosmetics Rules, 1945. Since these licenses are state-specific, the e-Aushadhi webpage is where you can get the relevant application.

STEP 5—Fill out and submit the Application: After downloading the application, you must manually enter all relevant information. These include the specifics of the company's address or the location of the production plant, the specifics of the good that will be produced and/or sold, and the personnel that will be working there. Once the application has been completed, get a scanned copy of it and upload it to the department's website together with the scanned copies of the required paperwork and application costs.

STEP 6—Verification by AYUSH Department's Commissioner

The department will review the application in its entirety and confirm all of the information it contains after receiving it. Additionally, a commissioner from the AYUSH Department would come to your office, place of business, or industrial site to perform a physical inspection and write a report on the findings. The department will ultimately choose whether or not to approve your application based on the Commissioner's findings.

STEP 7—AYUSH license granted: The Department shall issue the applicant in Form 25D the AYUSH license if it has approved the application based on its review of the form and the main office/manufacturing facility of the firm. The Department typically needs 60 days to process the online form used to apply for an AYUSH certificate.

10.3.1.3 VALIDITY

Before the introduction of the Drugs (4th Amendment) Rules, 2021, an AYUSH license in India had a maximum validity of five years, requiring renewal before expiry. However, with the implementation of these rules on October 1, 2021, the lifetime validity of the AYUSH license has been extended. This extension is contingent upon the annual submission of an online self-compliance statement, or until the license is suspended or revoked. Additionally, every five years, the manufacturing facility must undergo inspection and confirm the GMP Certificate.

10.3.1.4 GOVERNMENT FEES

Effective October 1, 2021, the 4th Amendment to the Drug Rules in India revised the application fees for an AYUSH license. The fee increased from Rs. 1000 to Rs. 2000 for any number of Ayurvedic, Unani, and Siddha medications and cosmetics. Furthermore, the fee for the first 10 unique ASU medications is now Rs. 3000 [13].

10.3.2 UNITED STATES OF AMERICA

The US Food and Drug Administration (FDA) categorizes botanical products based on their intended use as food, drugs, or dietary supplements. Products intended to prevent, diagnose, treat, alleviate, or cure a disease are classified as drugs and must undergo marketing under a New Drug Application approved by the FDA. Dietary supplements fall under the Dietary Supplement Health and Education Act of 1994, where premarket approval is not required, and manufacturers are responsible for ensuring product safety and compliance with labeling regulations based on the FDA's regulatory criteria [14].

10.3.3 CANADA

Health Canada has regulated herbal remedies and traditional medicines, including Ayurvedic medicine, since January 1, 2004, under NHP laws. Manufacturers, packers, labelers, or importers must register with Health Canada before commencing operations. This process involves registering the product(s) and manufacturing site(s), providing comprehensive information on product composition, standardization, testing methods for stability, microbiological and chemical contaminants, safety, effectiveness, ingredient characterization, and quantification by assay or input [15]. NHPs must adhere to contaminant limits and comply with GMPs guidelines set by Health Canada [16].

10.3.4 EUROPEAN UNION

The European Medicine Agency provides two methods for registering HMs:

Full marketing authorization under Directive 2001/83/EC, requiring a dossier with data from clinical trials, pharmacological, toxicological, and physicochemical testing, as well as evidence of effectiveness, safety, and quality.

Simplified registration under Directive 2004/24/EC for traditional herbal medicinal products with longstanding use and sufficient bibliographic evidence supporting their efficacy. Products must meet quality requirements specified in the European Pharmacopoeia or member state pharmacopeias and demonstrate therapeutic use for a minimum of 30 years, including 15 years within the EU [17].

10.3.5 AUSTRALIA

Herbal products in Australia are regulated by the Therapeutic Goods Administration under complementary medicine. Traditional Chinese medicine, Ayurvedic medicine, and indigenous Australian remedies fall under this category. Complementary medicines not requiring medical supervision must be listed on the Australian Register for Therapeutic Goods (ARTG). Products for higher-risk therapeutic uses require registration on the ARTG, ensuring claims are supported by evidence [18].

10.3.6 SAUDI ARABIA

In Saudi Arabia, herbal products are classified as traditional goods, accepted if they have been traditionally used for at least 50 consecutive years. Products must adhere to traditional preparation methods and dosages. Evidence requirements vary:

- Pharmacopeial evidence for conventional products.
- Nonpharmacopeial evidence supported by at least two independent sources demonstrating safety and effectiveness [19].

10.3.7 PHILIPPINES

The Philippines regulates HMs under conventional product regulations, requiring registration with the Bureau of Food and Drugs before manufacturing, importing, or selling. Products must demonstrate customary use dating back at least 50 years, supported by literature from medicine, history, and anthropology. Imported products must provide a plant authenticity certificate from the country of origin [20].

10.3.8 MALAYSIA

In Malaysia, herbal products are controlled goods requiring registration before market release. Products are categorized as conventional goods or health supplements, with strict labeling requirements and functional claims approval by the authorities.

These regulations ensure HMs meet safety, quality, and efficacy standards in their respective markets, promoting consumer protection and public health [21].

10.4 CONCLUSION

There is a growing market for herbal products due to factors like the acceptance of these products by consumers for use in healthcare, cosmetics, and diet supplements; research and the pharmaceutical industry are focusing on the herbal sector for financial reasons; and an increasing number of countries are giving legal status to herbal products and allowing the trade of these products legally. The development of globally acceptable products, however, is being hampered by issues such as variations in the status of components and excipients and regulatory requirements pertaining to quality, safety, and efficacy data. Harmonizing laws around the world pertaining to herbal products will help give this promising market the much-needed boost.

While some jurisdictions, particularly in the USA, do not, others offer a second, less strict registration process for HMs, allowing efficacy to be conceivable as a result of traditional use. As a result, a lot of these goods manage to avoid thorough enough scrutiny because they are sold as dietary supplements. This must be taken into account when creating or updating registration systems in nations like Kuwait, which import these goods and evaluate them based on the regulations in effect in their country of origin. Kuwait must specify exactly what an HM is and mandate that all pertinent goods be examined collectively to avoid any being mistakenly classified as dietary supplements due to the variations in other nations' definitions.

KEYWORDS

- **natural substances**
- **supplements**
- **regulations**
- **herbal medications**

REFERENCES

1. Alostad, A., Steinke, D., & Schafheutle, E. International comparison of five herbal medicine registration systems to inform regulation development: United Kingdom, Germany, United States of America, United Arab Emirates and Kingdom of Bahrain. *Pharmaceut Med* 2018, 32(1), 39–49.
2. Ekor, M. The growing use of herbal medicines: Issues relating to adverse reactions and challenges in monitoring safety. *Front Pharmacol* 2014, 4, 177.
3. International Agency for Research in Cancer Working Group on the Evaluation of Carcinogenic Risks to Humans. *World Health Organization, International Agency for Research on Cancer*. World Health Organization, 2002.
4. Zheng, E. X., & Navarro, V. J. Liver injury from herbal, dietary, and weight loss supplements: A review. *J Clin Transl Hepatol* 2015, 3, 93–98.
5. Brown, A. C. Liver toxicity related to herbs and dietary supplements: Online table of case reports. *Part 2 of 5 series, Food Chem Toxicol* 2017, 107(Pt A), 472–501.
6. Yee, S., Chu, S., Xu, Y., & Choo, P. Regulatory control of Chinese proprietary medicines in Singapore. *Health Pol* 2005, 71, 133–149.
7. Sahoo, N., Manchikanti, P., & Dey, S. Herbal drugs: Standards and regulation. *Fitoterapia* 2010, 81, 462–471.
8. Parveen, A., Parveen, B., Parveen, R., & Ahmad, S. Challenges and guidelines for clinical trial of herbal drugs. *J Pharm Bioallied Sci* 2015, 7, 329–333.
9. Geneva, Switzerland: 2014. Convention on International Trade in Endangered Species of Wild Fauna and Flora [Internet]. [cited 2014 Apr 29]; Available from: http://www.cites.org/eng/disc/what.php .
10. World Health Organization, IARC monographs on the evaluation of carcinogenic risks to humans, 2002, IARC Press: Lyon, France.
11. https://alephindia.in/drug-licence.php
12. Malik V. *Law Relating to Drugs and Cosmetics*. Eastern Book Company: Lucknow, 2013.
13. https://www.setindiabiz.com/ayush-license
14. https://www.fda.gov/food/guidance-documents-regulatory-information-topic-food-and-dietary-supplements/dietary-supplements-guidance-documents-regulatory-information, 2003.

15. Health Canada. Natural Health Products—Drugs and Health Products: Ottawa. http://www.hc-sc.gc.ca/dhp-mps/prodnatur/index.eng.php.
16. https://www.canada.ca/en/health-canada/services/drugs-health-products/natural-non-prescription/applications-submissions/product-licensing.html
17. Official Journal of the European Union: Directive 2004/24/EC; 31st March. 2004 [Internet]. [cited 2014 Apr 29]; Available from: http://www.eur-lex.europa.eu/LexUriServ/LexUriServ.do?uri=OJ: L: 2004:136:0085:0090:en: PDF .
18. North Sydney: Therapeutic Goods Administration; 2014 [Internet]. [Last updated on 2014 Apr 09; cited 2014 Apr 29]; Australian Government Department of Health. Available from: https://www.tga.gov.au/
19. Saudi Food and Drug Authority. Kingdom of Saudi Arabia: Data requirements for herbal and health products submission: Contents of dossier, version 1. 2012 [Internet]. [cited 2014 Apr 29]; Available from: https://www.sfda.gov.sa/sites/default/files/2019-12/Data%20Requirement%20for%20Herbal%20%28Draft%29.pdf
20. Geneva: WHO Library Cataloguing-in-Publication Data, World Health Organization; 2005 [Internet]. [cited 2014 Apr 29]; Guidelines on the Registration of Traditionally used Herbal Products, Department of Health, Republic of Philippines, Report of a WHO Global Survey. Available from: http://www.apps.who.int/medicinedocs/pdf/s7916e/s7916e.pdf.
21. Ishak, R., & Mohamad, J. *Guidelines on Registration of Traditional and Health Supplement Products*. Revised ed. Version 1.0. Malaysian Biotechnology Corporation SDN BH: Kuala Lumpur, 2009.

CHAPTER 11

Future Trends and Conclusion

ANKITA WAL[1*], E. SELVAKUMARI[2], C. S. KANDASAMY[3], HIMANGI VIJ[1], BIRESH KUMAR SARKAR[5], ARPAN KUMAR TRIPATHI[6], SAMIKSHA PRASHANT WARKE[7], and MOHD MASIH UZZAMAN KHAN[8]

[1]PSIT—Pranveer Singh Institute of Technology (Pharmacy), Kanpur, Uttar Pradesh, India

[2]Department of Pharmacognosy, College of Pharmacy, Mother Theresa Post Graduate and Research Institute of Health Sciences, Puducherry, India

[3]Department of Pharmacognosy, Karpagam College of Pharmacy, Coimbatore, Tamil Nadu, India

[5]Department of Pharmacy, Central Ayurveda Research Institute, Central Council for Research in Ayurvedic Sciences, Kolkata, West Bengal, India

[6]KIPS, Shri Shankaracharya Professional University, Bhilai, Chhattisgarh, India

[7]Department of Pharmaceutics, KYDSCT College of Pharmacy, Jalgaon, Maharashtra, India

[8]Department of Pharmaceutical Chemistry & Pharmacognosy, Unaizah College of Pharmacy, Unaizah, Saudi Arabia

*Corresponding author

Herbal Drug Industry: From Cultivation to Innovation and Global Impact.
Abhishek Tiwari, Varsha Tiwari, and Ajay Sharma (Eds.)

DOI: 10.1201/9781779640994-11

ABSTRACT

In our nation, a range of officially recognized health systems, including Ayurveda, Yoga, Unani, Siddha, homeopathy, and naturopathy, prominently feature herbal medicaments. These herbal remedies are a blend of age-old practices from diverse indigenous medical traditions and the collective healing wisdom passed down through the decades. To fully unlock the potential of herbal medicines, it is crucial to establish standardized protocols and gather data on their safety and effectiveness. Numerous academic and research institutions have undertaken extensive studies, employing cutting-edge methodologies, to explore herbal remedies and their formulations. The herbal medicine industry is undergoing a notable transformation, driven by both domestic and global demands. Nutraceuticals, which include botanical ingredients, are experiencing rapid growth due to worldwide concerns about health and lifestyle. One substantial obstacle in promoting herbal remedy-based enterprises in less developed nations is the lack of awareness about the economic and societal benefits that can result from the industrial utilization of medicinal plants. Government ministries should step up their efforts to promote herbal remedies, both domestically and internationally, and facilitate exchanges between educational institutions offering AYUSH education. This comprehensive approach ensures the continuous growth and integration of herbal medicines into modern healthcare systems, benefiting individuals across the globe.

11.1 INTRODUCTION

The wider population is beginning to turn more and more toward herbal medicines since they are perceived as "alternative remedies" that are less harmful and more benign than synthetic ones. Furthermore, a plethora of scientific evidence backs the medical application of herbal remedies for a variety of illnesses [1]. In recent years, scientists have made significant investments in the investigation and creation of innovative methods for delivering herbal drugs [2]. In the field of pharmaceutical manufacturing innovation, science and technology have progressed to the point where phytodosage forms have evolved from basic mixes and tablets to extremely sophisticated technology-based pharmaceutical delivery techniques [3].

In addition to lowering presystemic metabolic rates and the possible harm from drug accumulation in nontargeted regions, the application of modern technology in the application of herbal remedies or plant-based products also improved active drugs' stability and increased patient compliance due to ease of administration and adequate dosage [4]. It is especially difficult to design unique medicine delivery strategies for herbal medicines because of the wide range of active components. Therefore, in order to protect the molecule from various physiological diversions, including acidic pH, the reticuloendothelial route, and metabolic activities, innovative drug distribution strategies are required to optimize drug bioavailability. Therefore, for better treatment outcomes, herbal remedies or natural substances should be incorporated into cutting-edge drug delivery systems [5].

Innovative herbal medicine delivery systems are being developed to overcome the limitations of the herbal dose forms that are now available because of the many advantages that herbal medicines bring to humanity. New herbal medicine delivery technologies can help attain site specificity. By increasing the medication's surface area, the novel drug delivery technique not only makes drugs more soluble and active, but it also makes nanoparticles (NPs) more permeable via the blood–brain barrier [6]. Pharmaceutical research has combined to create modern drug delivery methods, which have unique physicochemical properties including a huge surface area to mass ratio, highly sensitive, regulated, and ultrasmall dimensions, and a functional framework. Many of the main drawbacks of conventional therapies can be solved thanks to enhanced pharmacokinetic and pharmacological properties, in addition to the stability of NP through physiochemistry. Additionally, constant delivery of drugs made possible by NPs lowers the amount of drug administration [7].

The rising popularity of nanoformulation has shown some encouraging results in the development of novel phytochemical delivery systems. Modern herbal preparations such as liposomes, phytosomes, microspheres, nanocapsules, polymeric nanoparticles, nanoemulsions, transferosomes, and ethosomes have been made possible by the utilization of plant bioactive components [8].

Because nanogels have benefits over other formulations, they are primarily accessible on the marketplace despite alternative approaches. An NP incorporating hydrogel is called "nanogel" having a cross-linked polymer chain. Nanogels are contemporary medications that require special attention because of their good chemical and physical features, exceptional colloidal stability, strong cell internalization characteristics, and propensity to stay inert in the blood. Furthermore, nanogels can readily overcome the difficulties that herbal formulations currently face [9]. Following logical structure and practical design, a hydrogel is a type of adaptable platform with a variety of biomedical applications. It uses materials engineering to modify its physicochemical properties (such as rigidity, pore diameter, viscoelasticity, structure, biodegradability, ligand display, stimulus-responsive properties, etc.) and affect the fate and cascades of cell signaling [10, 11]. Numerous groundbreaking studies have been conducted in the last few decades to investigate the relationships between cells and hydrogel matrices and determine the mechanisms that underlie them, opening the door for the clinical application of hydrogel-based therapeutics from the lab to the clinic. A family of water-swollen three-dimensional polymer networks known as hydrogels has tunable physicochemical attributes that are required to meet specific criteria in various scenarios [12]. They are a category of exciting substances that have been widely used in the biomedical area for a variety of purposes, including tissue regeneration, illness therapeutics, and investigations of biological and pathological processes [13].

This chapter provides an additional synopsis of a number of contemporary developments in the composition of herbal drugs, as well as an outlook for the future.

11.2 HERBAL NANOFORMULATIONS

The application of nanotechnologies in the manufacturing of herbal remedies has demonstrated the therapeutic efficacy of the pharmacologically active ingredients carried by the aforementioned transport proteins toward a range of human ailments, resulting in their anti-inflammatory, antimicrobial, antioxidant, cancer prevention, and other properties [14]. Herbal-laden NPs were produced by using the procedure to help: first, the phytochemical components of the herbs needed to be extracted, followed by they needed to be transformed into phytocompounds loaded with nanomaterials, which in turn encouraged therapeutic action in their intended form. Rapid progress is being made in the development of target treatments to improve the physicochemical properties and specificity of medications. The range of nano-applicability formulations has expanded due to ongoing research and development. Both the combination of certain transporters and the development of medications based on transporters have demonstrated the benefits of nanoformulation. The adaptable biological and physicochemical efficiency of NPs has led to important breakthroughs in herbal nanotechnology, some of which are currently in use are described below [15].

11.2.1 PHYTOSOMES

"Some" suggests a cell, while "phyto" refers to a plant. Typically measuring between 50 and a few hundred micrometers, phytosomes are complexes based on phytolipids [16]. The distribution technique assisted by phytosomes presents a fresh possible solution for lipid-bonded herbal medicines (Figure 11.1). Phytosomes exhibit greater solubility and bioavailability than standard herbal formulations since they are exceptionally well soluble in water and contain a lipophilic external surface. Due to their enhanced ability to bypass lipid-rich membrane barriers and reach the source, phytosomes are far more accessible than conventional herbal medications. Phytosomes are intriguing therapeutics and dietary supplements due to their exceptional pharmacological and pharmacokinetic properties. In either biological or physical environments, the following factors affect phytosomes behavior: volume and purity of the raw ingredient; physical traits, the percentage of enclosed solutes, transparency of the membrane, and chemical characteristics. Phytosomes enhance absorption by protecting essential elements of botanical extracts from being dissolved by stomach acid and intestinal microorganisms. Additionally, it increases bile's receptivity to components found in herbs. As the major phytoconstituent's bioavailability increases, the dose required for its reduction. When used in the production of phytosomes, phosphatidylcholine functions as a hepatoprotective as well as a carrier, creating a synergistic effect [17].

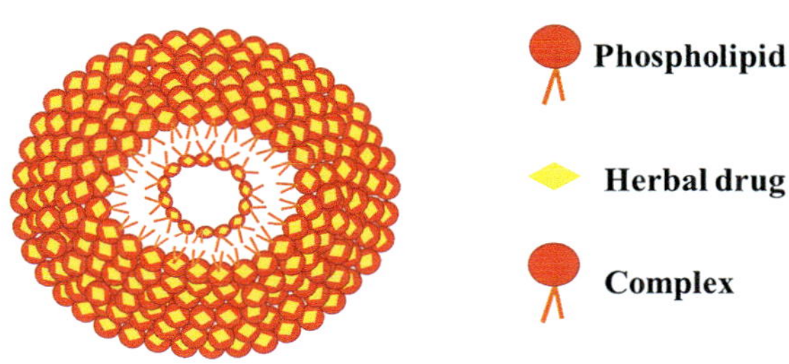

FIGURE 11.1 Phytosomes.

11.2.2 LIPOSOMES

"Lipos" denotes fat, but "Soma" implies the body. Drug firms commonly use liposomes, which are lipid-based liquid nanocrystals, due to their biocompatibility and ability to dissolve in cells when transferring encapsulated compounds. A small amount of the fluid is encased by two or more circular lipid bilayers, which disperse easily. Polar lipids, which include both hydrophobic as well as hydrophilic groups on one single molecule, are the building blocks of liposomes (Figure 11.2) [18]. Liposomes are advantageous due to their great biocompatibility, ease of manufacture, and chemical flexibility, which permits the loading of compounds that are lipid-soluble, amphiphilic, and polar solvents. Additionally, drug entrapment is significantly impacted by the particle number of bilayers. Because liposomes are biodegradable and can improve both paracellular and transcellular drug transport, they provide a great deal of potential as plant-based extract delivery vehicles [19].

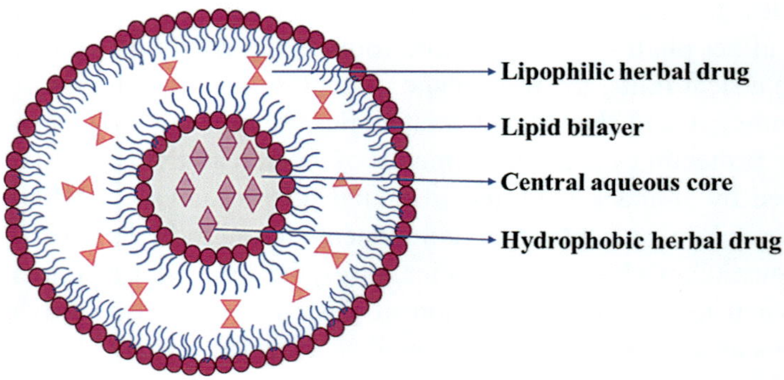

FIGURE 11.2 Liposome.

11.2.3 TRANSFEROSOMES

The term transferosomes means "body carrier." The Greek term "soma" that signifies "body," and the Latin phrase "transferee" that implies "to carry across," are the sources of the word "transferosome." One type of liposome is a transferosome, which is a type of liposome. A transferosome is a specialized type of liposome characterized by its high deformability and ability to penetrate the skin barrier. These formulations typically exhibit a broad range of pore sizes, with diameters ranging from approximately

20 to 400 nm. [20]. Transferosomes and liposomes have a fundamental structure; however, they differ from one another with regard to softness, ultradeformability, and the capacity to alter systemic membranes (Figure 11.3). One of transferosomes' most important characteristics is their ability to stick to and hold onto moisture. Due to the interdependence of their bilayer shape, the vesicle is able to regulate and optimize itself. This enables the transferosome to function as a pharmaceutical carrier for the noninvasive delivery of specific medications once it has easily navigated a variety of transportation hurdles. They are applied topically in a nonoccluded manner, and osmosis or wetness allows them to penetrate into the stratum corneum lipid lamellar regions. As drug transporters, it can transport a wide range of microscopic molecules, peptides, proteins, and herbal ingredients [21].

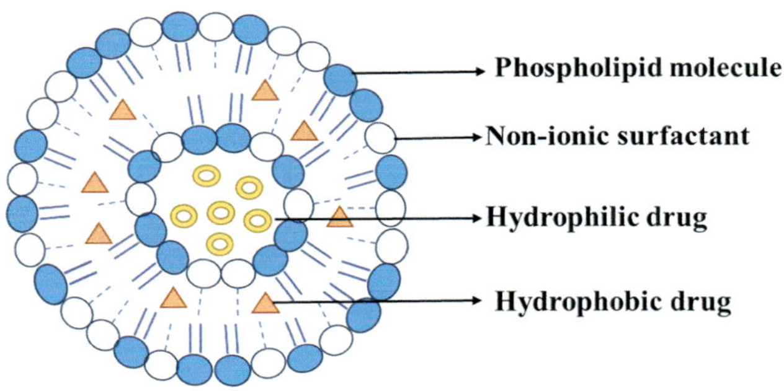

FIGURE 11.3 Transferosome.

11.2.4 ETHOSOMES

Ethosomes are a particular kind of adaptable liposome whereby the lipid bilayer is treated with alcohol to increase the molecule's flexibility. Hydrophilic, lipid-soluble, or amphiphilic medicines can be incorporated into ethosomes, which can penetrate the skin's layers and the blood vessels. Ethanol, water, and soy phosphatidylcholine comprise ethosomes complexes. They can form multilamellar coverings and have a high rate of entrapment for particles with different lipophilicities (Figure 11.4). Ethosomes' physiochemical properties allow for the legal passage of medication by the stratum corneum, inside the deep layer of skin, and maybe even into the bloodstream. This feature is essential as a transdermal distribution network and carrier of topical medications. Moreover, the ethosomes transporter has the potential to efficiently transport medications within cells that are lipid-soluble or hydrophilic [22]. Ethosomal delivery systems for drugs are employed extensively in the veterinary, cosmetic, and biopharmaceutical sectors. Patient compliance is good since the ethosomal medicine is supplied in a semisolid formulation. A recent development in vesicular studies for transdermal drug delivery systems is herbal ethosomes. Its future appears bright in the field of natural drugs. Modifications made to these medications have several advantages over synthetic pharmaceuticals and are thought to be harmless. Herbal ethosomes are ready for a noninvasive kind of transdermal medication administration [23].

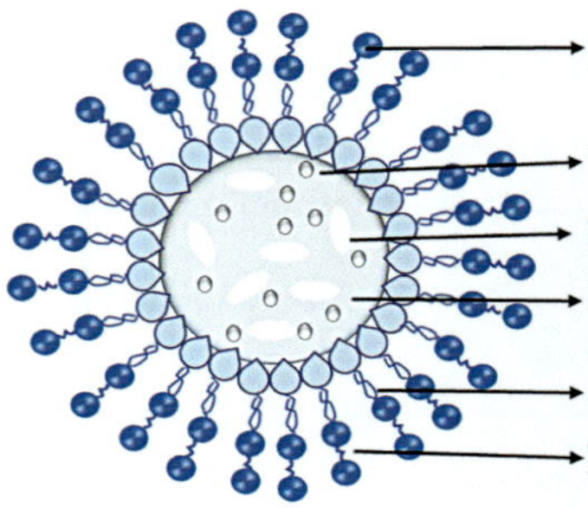

FIGURE 11.4 Ethosomes.

11.2.5 NIOSOMES

Niosomes are tiny lamellar aggregates which vary in dimension between 10 and 1000 nm. They are similar to liposomes in appearance, but because of their nonsurfactant bilayer, they are considerably more flexible. Pharmaceuticals that are both polar and nonpolar can be found in niosomes, and compared to liposomes, they are more chemically durable due to the presence of nonionic surfactants (Figure 11.5). Two major benefits of using niosomes are their ability to reduce systemic side effects by encapsulating therapeutic drugs and to minimize their excretion from the body's tissues through progressive drug release [24]. Compared to conventional oily formulations, they can enclose a significant amount of material in just a few inches of vesicles, leading to increased acceptance by patients, comfort, and effectiveness. Because of their special shape, niosomes may contain a broad range of substances, including drugs that are lipophilic, hydrophilic, and amphiphilic. Features such as structure, fluidity, and size of niosomes can be readily altered by altering their physical characteristics and production method. Niosomes can be applied topically, parenterally, or orally and come in a range of dosage forms, such as semisolids, powders, and solutions [25].

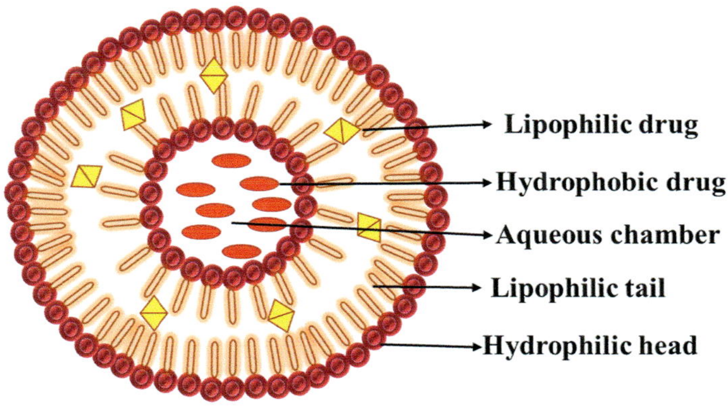

FIGURE 11.5 Niosome.

11.2.6 DENDRIMERS

Polymeric nanostructures called dendrimers have a globular or spherical form. They are branched-chain, monodispersed NPs that either ensnap the drug within their inner cores or stick to it at the edges (Figure 11.6). One distinctive feature of branching throughout the interior is that it significantly affects physicochemical qualities. The extremely small polydispersity of dendrimers adds to their utility as a technique for administering drugs. Due to their high penetration and inadequate drainage in the tumor vasculature, which causes macromolecule accumulation in the tumor, dendrimers are perfect for treating solid tumors. Additionally, targeted delivery reduces systemic toxicity by using less medicament. Additionally, pharmaceuticals can be continuously and carefully released. Reduced drug clearance due to altered drug distribution in organs at the site of localization and delivery, in addition to controlled and delayed drug release, results in improved effectiveness in therapy and fewer side effects. Its drug content is excessively high. Since pharmaceuticals can be incorporated into organisms without passing through any chemical processes, their action remains intact [26].

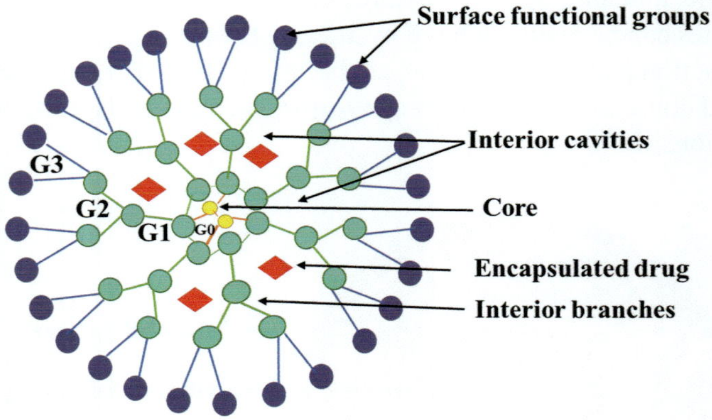

FIGURE 11.6 Dendrimers.

11.2.7 NANOSTRUCTURED LIPID CARRIERS

Nanostructured lipid carriers (NLCs) are a class of lipid-based delivery approaches that have many benefits, including improved absorption of the encapsulated bioactive, longevity, the ability to achieve a specific or controlled release, flexibility in encapsulation, highly hydrophilic and lipophilic pharmaceuticals, and high encapsulation efficacy. NLCs are submicron-sized colloidal carriers made up of an aqueous phase comprising a surfactant or combination of surfactants and a solid-lipid core made of a combination of solid lipids combined with a liquid lipid that creates an unstructured nanoscale matrix (Figure 11.7). Large packing capacities, long-lasting release profiles, and improved stability of the encapsulated bioactive are all made possible by the partly solid nanostructure. Because the lipid matrix is composed of biocompatible and biodegradable components, there is less chance of toxicity, either acute or chronic [27]. NLCs have the incredible ability to immobilize pharmaceuticals and prevent drug particle coalescence. NLCs offer benefits like better drug loading due to the increased solid matrix flaws and the liquid lipids available. The chemical stability of the medications covered by NLCs is also increased. Hydrophobic and hydrophilic pharmaceutical delivery by NLC was additionally investigated. NLC can be injected intravenously or given ingested into the brain. To be taken orally, NLC is exposed to pancreatic enzymes found in the duodenum, which breakdown fat into fatty acids and monoglycerides [28].

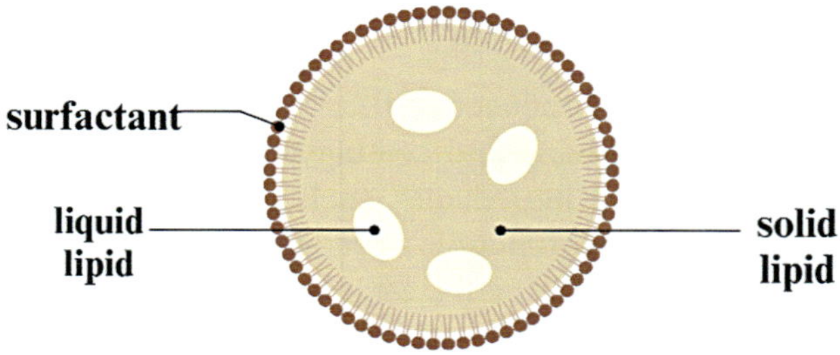

FIGURE 11.7 Nanostructured lipid carriers.

11.2.8 SOLID LIPID NANOPARTICLES

They are composed of lipids. In addition to the lipid, there is also water and an emulsifier. These submicron-sized particles serve as an extra-medication delivery mechanism for liposomes and emulsions. Phospholipids cover the water-resistant matrix of single-layer nanocarriers (Figure 11.8). Therefore, it is anticipated that these nanocarriers, as opposed to traditional liposomal nanocarriers, will prove superior in encasing hydrophobic medications in their matrix core. Advantages like location-specific targetability and being able to integrate solid lipid nanoparticles with certain moieties may make it more likely that target organs will be targeted [29].

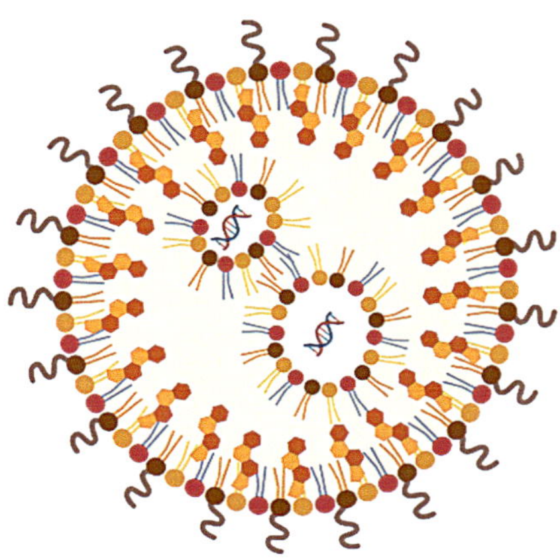

FIGURE 11.8 Solid lipid nanoparticles.

11.2.9 GREEN SYNTHESIS NANOPARTICLES

Green synthetic process-produced NPs are very productive, soluble, and long-lasting. By oxidizing and coating the freshly created particles, naturally occurring herbal ingredients, such as a range of both primary and secondary metabolites, function as reduction factors for silver ions. Biological techniques seem to be the easiest, fastest, safest, most reliable, and least harmful of all the synthetic methods available for producing silver nanoparticles (AgNPs). Under ideal conditions, these methods may produce established structural and dimensional features for conventional research. AgNPs are one of the more important and intriguing nanomaterials among the several metallic NPs employed in medical therapies [30]. Because they are able to be customized so easily, gold nanoparticles (AuNPs) provide an adaptable structure for nanobiological aggregates containing proteins, oligonucleotides, and antibodies. These days, AuNPs bioconjugates are thought to be suitable substitutes for producing novel biomaterials for use in medical research. In a typical green synthesis process, botanical extract and a metallic salt solution, which serves as the precursor for NPs, are combined. By giving them electrons, biomolecules such as polyphenols and terpenoids can lower metallic ions [31]. The reduced ions thus start to organize within a manner that mimics the crystalline structure's nucleus. The nuclei maintain the reduced ions, which will keep building up on their surface and enlarging the dimensions of the particles [32].

11.3 HYDROGEL

Hydrogels are a type of 3D polymer system that swells when moist and has adjustable physicochemical attributes that are required to meet certain demands in various environments. They are currently widely used in the biomedical industry as a sort of promising substance for anything from the regeneration of tissues and illness therapeutics to pathophysiological mechanism investigations. Hydrogels with great drug loading effectiveness have also drawn a lot of attention from researchers studying pharmaceutical formulation (Figure 11.9). Polymers, which might have natural or synthetic origins, are their main elements. Numerous characteristics, including origin, configuration, cross-linking, external appearance, and network electricity, are used to characterize hydrogels. The chemical makeup and origin of the polymeric material indicate whether the hydrogel is synthetic, organic, or hybrid. Hydrogels are classified as semicrystalline or amorphous based on their molecular structure, as either physical or chemical depending on cross-linking, as well as ionic or neutral depending on their electric charge [10].

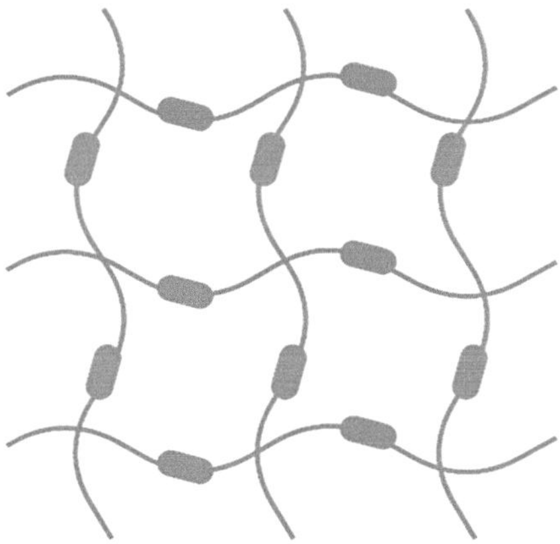

FIGURE 11.9 Hydrogel.

Alginate (Alg) is a significant natural polymer used in hydrogel manufacturing. It is an anionic polysaccharide made up of L-guluronic acid and D-mannuronic acid joined by a 1–4 bond. Alg may create bead, gel, microparticle, and nanosphere matrices when it gelates with simple divalent ions [33]. Collagen is a further kind of natural polymer and a key component of the connective tissues matrix of extra cells. Collagen has a very high mechanical strength. Hydrogels for the cornea and applications in tissue engineering have been created using it. In addition to natural polymers, a variety of synthetic polymers have been developed for hydrogel production thanks to advancements in the study of materials. In addition to natural polymers, a variety of synthetic polymers have been developed for hydrogel production owing to advancements in materials technology. Polymers made synthetically and derivatives of them often possess greater durability than natural polymers, but their overall toxicities and biodegradability have drawn more attention [34].

The great ability to absorb water of hydrogels sets them apart from other methods designed for the administration of medicinal herbs. This ability has made it easier to load herbal formulations, which are typically aqueous, into hydrogels. Certain hydrogels have also been reported to provide sustained and stimulus-controlled medication release thanks to advancements in the design of the material. An in-depth knowledge of the intricate and ever-changing relationship among cells and hydrogels is crucial for informing the sound engineering of hydrogels and easing their clinical application in the near future. This is because how they interact has an important effect on cells physiological, proliferation, emigration, differentiation, and pathological events like cell death, fibrosis, immune-mediated rejection, and so on [35, 36].

11.3.1 NATURAL POLYMER-BASED HYDROGEL FORMULATION

The goal of the biomaterial determines whether or not natural polymers are used in the hydrogel manufacturing process. For instance, biodegradable and harmless polymers are widely employed in hydrogels for regulated drug release since they meet these requirements. These polymers are frequently found in the environment; cellulose, the most prevalent polysaccharide, is one example [37].

11.3.1.1 HYALURONIC ACID

As a straight-chain copolymer of 2-acetamido-2-deoxy-D-glucose and D-glucoronic acid, hyaluronic acid (HA) exhibits significant electrostatic forces with various other substances due to its anionic attributes. Its fundamental structure can be made flexible through chemical changes caused by adding, condensation, or radical polymerization processes of volatile molecules. This makes it possible for HA to exist as hard hydrogels, fibers, sponges, sheets, networks, or nanoparticulate fluids. When applied, HA has been associated with certain therapeutic benefits such as angiogenesis, increased cell migration and proliferation, tissue repair, and regulation of the immune system's response [38].

11.3.1.2 CELLULOSE BASED

All cellulose-based compounds start with cellulose, a prevalent hydrophobic, recyclable polymer that may be found in plants and fibers from nature like linen and cotton. Chemical modifications to cellulose, including etherification or esterification involving its hydroxyl groups, result in the production of cellulosics, which are variants of cellulose. For instance, hydroxyl groups can be substituted for methyl or hydroxypropyl groups to create a hydrophilic polymer similar to methylcellulose with very little modification to the chemical makeup. Methylcellulose possesses an amount of replacement between 1.4 and 2.0 and is typically water soluble since this process weakens the bonds of hydrogen that are common in cellulose that are in charge of the polymer's high crystallinity. Aqueous cellulose ethers are cross-linked to create stable, irreversible gels or reversible gels, which is how all cellulose-based hydrogels are made [39]. By decreasing the pH of specific polymers in a solution of water having carboxyl groups, hydrogels bearing hydrogen bonds can be created. One such hydrogel is carboxymethylcellulose (CMC), a material with a network made by a dispersion of CMC in 0.1 M HCl. The process involves switching out the sodium atoms in the CMC solution for hydrogen atoms. It is through this replacement that hydrogen bonds are formed. These linkages cause CMC's solubility in water to decrease, which causes an elastic hydrogel to develop [40].

11.3.1.3 DEXTRAN BASED

One polymer of glucose, dextran, features a linear 1,6-glycosidic bond with some branching via 1,3-linkage. This polymer finds extensive application in the medical field, specifically as a blood viscosity-reducing and blood clot-preventing agent. Dextran exhibits breakdown and biological compatibility in a range of human organs. Glycidyl methacrylate, hydroxyethyl methacrylate dextran, and dextran hydroxyethyl methacrylate lactate are among the various kinds of dextran hydrogel. Although hydrogels were once considered as potential therapeutic media, their organized porosity has caused premature release of the entrapped medicines, which has limited their use as protein carriers [41].

11.3.1.4 ALGINATE BASED

Pseudomonas and *Azotobacter* are the two species of bacteria that create Alg, which is extracted from brown seaweed. Brine is used to dehydrate the algae in order to extract Alg from it. The copolymer of straight blocks, Alg polysaccharide, is composed of polyanionic blocks (1,4)-linked D-mannuronic (M unit) and a -L-guluronic acid (block G). In its raw form, this organic polymer is employed in clinical settings to treat arthritis and is also the foundation for hydrogel formulations [42]. Since Alg hydrogels are readily available, inexpensive, and biocompatible, they are particularly being explored for application in tissue engineering, drug administration, and wound healing purposes. Additionally, it has been extensively utilized as a thickening agent and emulsifier in the food business [43]. Alg gels are widely used as tissue engineering matrices, much like numerous other natural polymer hydrogels. It was discovered that the application of calcium sulfate cross-linking ($CaSO_4$) with Alg produced an uneven morphology, as it was explored to be utilized with carrier cells in tissue engineering. Therefore, researchers have hypothesized that adding calcium instead of additional metal ions during the Alg gelation process will enhance the hydrogels' physical makeup [44].

11.3.1.5 CHITOSAN BASED

Although chitosan is not commonly found in the natural world, it is readily extracted from the naturally occurring polymer chitin. Deacetylated chitin with a minimum of 60% D-glucosamine waste is referred to as chitosan. The procedure of chitin deacetylation can be carried out either by enzymatic hydrolysis with the help of certain enzymes, such as chitin deacetylase, or by chemical hydrolysis in an alkaline environment [45]. Chitosan and other organic polymers are extensively utilized because they are nontoxic, biocompatible, and biodegradable. In addition to these properties, chitosan has the ability to develop into a gel at low pH levels and is a mucoadhesive. Numerous studies have focused on the potential application of chitosan, a polymer made from natural materials, as a framework component in hydrogels because of its unique physicochemical and biological characteristics as well as its low toxicity and biodegradability. The main amine and hydroxyl groups on chitosan's backbone allow for chemical reactions that regulate the material's physical characteristics. New drug delivery methods that can release the pharmaceuticals incorporated inside them in response to a variety of outside stimuli have been created thanks to the sophisticated design of chitosan hydrogels [46].

Because of their favorable biological compatibility and adjustable physicochemical features, hydrogels are being extensively studied and used in clinical settings. The most common FDA-approved uses of hydrogels are in contact lenses, fillers, facial correction, and other applications.

These days, hydrogel materials are showing promise for treating diseases and regenerating different types of tissue.

11.4 NANOGEL

Among the numerous facets of nanomedicine, the nexus of nanotechnology, healthcare, and pharmaceuticals has been the development of nanogels as a viable method for providing and delivering drugs to consumers in the past few years. There was cross-linking in the polymeric nanogels. Networks with a nanoscale dimension and the capacity to absorb massive volumes of water. Hydrogels that are smaller than a nanometer are known as nanogels. A hydrogel is a polymer-based gel created by joining polymer chains to create a web of macromolecules (Figure 11.10). There are many techniques to make hydrogels, but they all start with the production of polymeric monomers, which need to be polymerized using useful cross-linker groups in order to generate a polymer framework that resembles a net [47]. The elements of the nanogel-forming mixture that are selected based on the biodegradability, as well as low immunogenicity, may also contain proteins and polysaccharides. A novel and exciting approach to drug shipment, nanogels have the promise of assisting in overcoming the obstacles associated with the chosen pharmaceuticals. By creating nanogels that protect the encapsulated pharmaceuticals from deterioration and provide regulated delivery over extended periods of time, the curative value of the loaded medication can be increased.

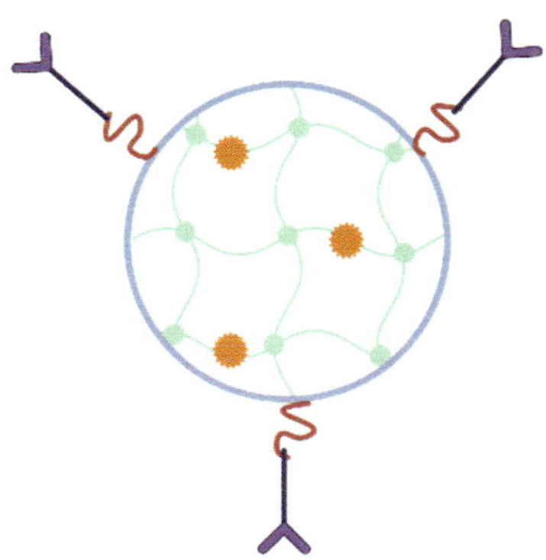

FIGURE 11.10 Nanogel.

It is possible for medications to enter the tiny spaces and thereafter pass through them. On the other side, hydrogels are basically what nanogels are, but on a 20,200 nm size. The vast majority of emulsion polymerization is made using most nanogels. Nanogels can be administered intraocularly, orally, pulmonary, nasally, or parentally. There are several ways that the drugs emerge through the nanogels, but one of the mechanisms involves activation by external stimulation, which modifies the internal features of the drug. The therapeutic payload is transported to the intended location as a result of this physical alteration, which makes the polymer network expands or contract [48].

A novel and exciting approach to drug shipment, nanogels have the promise of assisting in overcoming the obstacles associated with the chosen medications. By creating nanogels that protect the encapsulated pharmaceuticals from deterioration and provide regulated delivery over extended periods of time, the therapeutic index of the loaded medication can be increased. Biodegradable polymer-based nanogels are excellent choices for the delivery of drugs. Biopolymer-based nanogels perform better than synthetic ones with regard to biodegradability, biologically generated diversity in nature, and nontoxicity. The availability of numerous useful groups for later coupling with biomolecules is a further advantage [9].

In an attempt to increase the bioavailability of herbal medicines that are not very water soluble, nanotechnology modifies the release of these treatments. Nanogels are employed for both local as well as systemic effects of drugs due to their natural capacity to expand due to a chemical shift. This makes it possible for the medication to be delivered in the required dosage form. Nanogels can be used to create ionic delivery of medications, dermal patches, and biosensors. These microscopic structures can be distinguished based on the makeup of the polymer and lipids within them [49]. It is possible to enhance medication distribution from carbohydrate-based nanogels by using lectin activity. Nanogels consist of cross-linked chains of polymers that are nanoscale in size and have the capacity to absorb massive volumes of water, which sets them apart from other forms of nanoformulation. One of the most intriguing new drug delivery technologies currently available is nanoemulgel, which also presents the most promising options for managing and maintaining drug release systems. The ingredients of nanoemulgel are gel and nanoemulsion. In this case, the nanoemulsion and gel were produced independently. An o/w or w/o type nanoemulsion is possible. Last but not least, the nanoemulsion is distributed throughout the gel stages and is present in any herbal medicine's nanoemulgel composition. As a result, the aforementioned formulation promotes improved skin penetration and demonstrates a dual discharge control mechanism [50].

11.4.1 NANOGEL PREPARATION

Based on the size, polymerization technique, and nanometer scale, the methods utilized to produce nanogels fall into several types. The following part goes over the steps involved in making gels and managing their nanostructures.

11.4.1.1 PHYSICAL APPROACHES

Typical physical procedures for creating nanogels include inverse nanoprecipitation, microfluidics, and the mini-emulsion process. The mini-emulsion technique, which includes small fragments of oil-soluble surfactant found in a continuous organic phase, produces an oil-in-water emulsion. In the microfluidic technique, glass compartments or a silica capillary tube that replicates a polymer are utilized to produce droplets. The most methodical technique for creating aqueous nanogels is the last system, referred to as inverse nanoprecipitation, that consists of merely blending an aqueous polymer mixture with a miscible nonsolvent [51].

11.4.1.2 CROSS-LINKING TECHNIQUE

Among the most efficient methods of linking to form a gel matrix using a monomer containing a sensitive functional group with a lesser molecular weight is covalent linking. The extremely durable nanogels produced by covalent bonding through the cross-linking of the functional groups they contain were beneficial in the medication release and entrapment process when produced *in vitro*.

Chemical processes, including Schiff base response, free radical polymerization, and perhaps employed for this cross-linking. Cross-linking prepared polymers results in the formation of nanogels in surroundings with different colloidal states, like w/o microemulsions. The incorporation of biomacromolecules and small-molecule pharmaceuticals within nanogels is facilitated by this methodology. The quantity of polymer needed to achieve the required size is dependent on several factors, such as temperature, ionization constant, pH, and ionic strength. This approach's capacity ought to develop ellipsoid or disc-shaped NPs rather than spherical types in order to inhibit phagocytosis, which constitutes among its primary benefits. Because of current studies and manufactured items, the cross-linking process is used in conjunction with the microfluidic emulsification method to produce a homogeneous distribution of NPs. Given the strong relationship between particle size and bioavailability in medication delivery, particle size is a crucial factor to take into account [52].

11.4.1.3 NONCOVALENT LINKING

Structural cross-linking nanogels, which include weak van der Waal forces, hydrophobic and hydrophilic connections, and furthermore, are produced by interactions that are not covalent. Such forms are less secure, and the environment, cross-linking substance, the components all significantly affect the gel's sensitivity. It has been shown that using nanogels to create micelles can increase a medication's solubility by as much as 30,000 times when it comes to highly lipophilic drugs [53].

11.4.1.4 BIOCONJUGATION TECHNIQUE

One widely recognized and carefully regulated process for creating nanogels in a range of sizes and forms, notably core–shell nanogels, is using the free radical polymerization technique. Subinitiators in this biological conjugation process include functional impulses and micro initiators that prevent functions from being incorporated into the nanogel's interior, enabling multivalent biological conjugation. Because of the brittleness of the bonds that exist between polymer chains, hydrophobic, noncovalent, or hydrogen bonding physically cross-linked systems at reasonable environments are far more probable to develop weaknesses, brittle compared to their covalently cross-linked counterpart [54].

Due to their superior *in vivo* reaction, high drug loading ability, superior absorption, and cellular-like characteristics, nanogels have demonstrated great potential in the delivery of a variety of drugs to different bodily organs. Co-emulsifiers can enhance drug permeability and penetration, and research indicates that using nanogels in conjunction with co-emulsifiers enhances the properties of cutaneous release.

11.5 CONCLUSION

Biologically significant natural substances found in plants are known as herbal constituents. More than 10,000 plant-based substances and herbal medications have been used for a range of purposes, including sterility, aromatization, and the treatment of diseases like cancer, metabolic disorders, and infections. Organic compounds with therapeutic properties are frequently utilized and originate from common medicinal plants and herbs.

For the treatment of their ailments, the vast majority of people have turned to herbal remedies. A worldwide study has been conducted on herbal medications. The use of nanotechnology in the production of botanicals or phytonutrients is growing in acceptance. Particularly enhanced surface area is possessed by nanoformulations with a spectrum of biological purposes. Bioactive chemicals that are labile, insoluble, and not well absorbed can be effectively delivered with NP technologies. Bypassing the robust physiological obstacles and improving the bioavailability and lifetime of phytochemical components, nanoformulations are helping to address several issues.

Numerous methods of delivering herbal medicines based on nanotechnology are intriguing to investigators. Significant changes have occurred in drug delivery techniques, resulting in improved goods and new physicochemical characteristics. Effective herbal medication research is hampered by traditional drug delivery methods since oral or parenteral herbal formulations have been demonstrated to be ineffective due to numerous issues. Studies on natural plants have shown that novel nanodelivery systems for herbal medications offer several benefits, such as increased tissue dispersion, safer and less toxic side effects, greater therapeutic action, enhanced stability, and higher absorption and bioavailability. The present analysis provides a data set that researchers may use to support their future research on the production of AgNPs and AuNPs for biological applications, and it summarizes the already acknowledged potential to manufacture phytonanoparticles from. Because of its therapeutic uses, the AgNPs and AuNPs industry has already experienced tremendous growth and is expected to do so again in the coming years. If significant advancements in research are made, a sizable portion of this proportion will consist of plant-based AgNPs and AuNPs. To meet the standards that are frequently connected with NPs produced by chemical means, a great deal of research should be focused on the creation and growth of plant-based AgNPs and AuNPs synthesis.

Hydrogels have so far had a major effect on a wide range of biomedical domains, including cancer therapy, tissue engineering, drug screening, and aesthetic medicine. The in-depth and thorough knowledge of how cells behave and transmit signals as they react to the physicochemical and structural properties of the hydrogel matrix contributes to the continuous advancement of material techniques aimed at improving the regulation of the cell's biology and fate for desired purposes. Crucially, researchers concentrate on a wider range of hydrogel attributes and dimensions, such as 3D, hydrogel architecture, breakdown, and dynamic characteristics, so as to more fully recapitulate the complex native matrix. This helps to expand our knowledge regarding how hydrogel physiochemical, mechanical in nature, and structural cues control the phenotype, functioning, and destiny of tissue and cells.

When it comes to minimizing this delivery system's complexity and doing away with the drawbacks of earlier methods, nanogels have been shown to be more desirable. Multifunctional nanogels hold great potential as novel polymeric platforms for biomedicine. Their uses in pharmaceutical and gene transfer, innovative modalities of imaging, responsive materials, and multivalency as a therapeutic approach demonstrate this promise. Nanocarriers have changed and become more important in biomedicine as a result of recent advances in nanotechnology. Although nanomedicine is a vital weapon in the fight against new coronaviruses, significant challenges remain in the field of clinical practice, such as the toxicity of nanocarriers, *in vivo* behavior, and large-scale manufacture. Conventional chemotherapy drugs are transported by nanocarriers, which also serve as platforms for combination therapy and multifunction investigations.

KEYWORDS

- **herbal formulation**
- **nanoparticles**
- **phytosomes**
- **nanogels**
- **hydrogels**
- **green synthesis**

REFERENCES

1. Verma, M., Gupta, P. K., Varsha, B. P., & Purohit, A. P. Development of transdermal drug dosage formulation for the anti-rheumatic Ayurvedic medicinal plants. *Anc Sci Life* 2007, 1, 66–69.
2. Mandal, S. C., & Mandal, M. Current status and future prospects of new drug delivery system. *Pharm Times* 2010, 42, 13–16.
3. Chakrobarty, K., Shivakumar, A., & Ramachandran, S. Nanotechnology in herbal medicine. *Int J Herb Med* 2016, 4(3), 21–27.
4. Devi, V. K., Jain, N., & Valli, K. S. Importance of novel drug delivery systems in herbal medicines. *Pharmacog Rev* 2010, 4(7), 27.
5. Nalini, T., Kumari, S., & Basha, K. Novel nanosystems for herbal drug delivery. *World J Pharm Pharm Sci* 2017, 6(5), 1447–1463.
6. Bonifacio, B. V., da Silva, P. B., Ramos, M. A. D. S., Negri, K. M. S., Bauab, T. M., & Chorilli, M. Nanotechnology-based drug delivery systems and herbal medicines: A review. *Int J Nanomed* 2014, 9, 1–15.
7. Pravin, P., Adhikrao, Y., & Varsha, G. Different techniques for preparation of nanosuspension with reference to its characterisation and various applications-A review. *Asian J Res Pharm Sci* 2018, 8(4), 210–216.
8. Semalty, A., Semalty, M., & Rawat, M. S. M. The phyto-phospholipid complexes-phytosomes: A potential therapeutic approach for herbal hepatoprotective drug delivery. *Pharmacog Rev* 2007, 1, 369–374.
9. Chaudhari, P. M., & Paithankar, A. V. Herbal nanogel formulation: A novel approach. *Science and Technology* 2020, 5, 138–146.
10. Cao, H., Duan, L., Zhang, Y., Cao, J., & Zhang, K. Current hydrogel advances in physicochemical and biological response-driven biomedical application diversity. *Signal Transduct and Target Ther* 2021, 6, 426.
11. Ma, G., & Wu, C. Microneedle, bio-microneedle and bio-inspired microneedle: A review. *J Control Release* 2017, 251, 11–23.

12. Ning, X., Wiraja, C., Chew, W. T. S., Fan, C., & Xu, C. Transdermal delivery of Chinese herbal medicine extract using dissolvable microneedles for hypertrophic scar treatment. *Acta Pharmaceutica Sinica B* 2021, 11, 2937–2944.
13. Ventrelli, L., Marsilio Strambini, L., & Barillaro, G. Microneedles for transdermal biosensing: Current picture and future direction. *Adv Healthc Mater* 2015, 4, 2606–2640.
14. Singh, S., Sharma, B., Kanwar, S. S., & Kumar, A. Lead phytochemicals for anticancer drug development. *Front Plant Sci* 2016, 7, 1667.
15. Meng, J., Agrahari, V., & Youm, I. Advances in targeted drug delivery approaches for the central nervous system tumors: The inspiration of nanobiotechnology. *J Neuroimmune Pharmacol* 2017, 12, 84–98.
16. Khogta, S., Patel, J., Barve, K., & Londhe, V. Herbal nano-formulations for topical delivery. *J Herb Med* 2020, 20, 100300.
17. Sharma, G., Anabousi, S., Ehrhardt, C., & Ravi Kumar, M. N. V. Liposomes as targeted drug delivery systems in the treatment of breast cancer. *J drug target* 2006, 14(5), 301–310.
18. Ahmed, A., Shuaib, M., Shirsat, M. K., & Sharma, D. Herbal medicines and recent development on novel herbal drug delivery system. *Indonesian Journal of Pharmaceutical and Clinical Research* 2023, 6, 13–24.
19. Sogut, O., Sezer, U. A., & Sezer, S. Liposomal delivery systems for herbal extracts. *J Drug Deliv Sci Technol* 2021, 61, 102147.
20. Sakamoto, K., Lochhead, R. Y., Maibach, H. I., & Yamashita, Y. (Eds.). *Cosmetic Science and Technology: Theoretical Principles and Applications*. Elsevier, 2017.
21. Yanyu, X., Yunmei, S., Zhipeng, C., & Qineng, P. The preparation of silybin–phospholipid complex and the study on its pharmacokinetics in rats. *Int J Pharm* 2006, 307, 77–82.
22. El-Ridy, M. S., Badawi, A. A., Safar, M. M., & Mohsen, A. M. Niosomes as a novel pharmaceutical formulation encapsulating the hepatoprotective drug silymarin. *Int J Pharm Pharm Sci* 2012, 4, 549–59.
23. Fatima Grace, X., Rahul Raj, S., Reshma, I., Sandeep, T., Shanmuganathan, S., & Chamundeeswari, D. Herbal ethosomes—A novel approach in herbal drug technology. *Am J Ethnomed* 2014, 1, 226–230.
24. Yadav, D., Suri, S., Choudhary, A. A., Sikender, M., Hemant, B. N., & Beg, N. M. Novel approach: Herbal remedies and natural products in pharmaceutical science as nano drug delivery systems. *Int J Pharm Tech* 2011, 3, 3092–3116.
25. Bhokare, S. G., Dongaonkar, C. C., Lahane, S. V., Salunke, P. B., Sawale, V. S., & Thombare, M. S. Herbal novel drug delivery: A review. *World J Pharm Pharm Sci* 2016, 5, 593–611.
26. Bar-Zeev, M., Livney, Y. D., & Assaraf, Y. G. Targeted nanomedicine for cancer therapeutics: Towards precision medicine overcoming drug resistance. *Drug Res Updat* 2017, 31, 15–30.
27. Piazzini, V., Lemmi, B., D'Ambrosio, M., Cinci, L., Luceri, C., Bilia, A. R., & Bergonzi, M. C. Nanostructured lipid carriers as promising delivery systems for plant extracts: The case of Silymarin. *Appl Sci* 2018, 8, 1163.

28. Prasad, M., Lambe, U. P., Brar, B., Shah, I., Manimegalai, J., Ranjan, K., & Prasad, G. Nanotherapeutics: An insight into healthcare and multi-dimensional applications in medical sector of the modern world. *Biomed Pharmacother* 2018, 97, 1521–1537.
29. Tapeinos, C., Battaglini, M., & Ciofani, G. Advances in the design of solid lipid nanoparticles and nanostructured lipid carriers for targeting brain diseases. *J Control Release* 2017, 264, 306–332.
30. Karmous, I., Pandey, A., Haj, K. B., & Chaoui, A. Efficiency of the green synthesized nanoparticles as new tools in cancer therapy: Insights on plant-based bioengineered nanoparticles, biophysical properties, and anticancer roles. *Biol Trace Elem Res* 2020, 196, 330–342.
31. Singh, J., Dutta, T., Kim, K. H., Rawat, M., Samddar, P., & Kumar, P. 'Green' synthesis of metals and their oxide nanoparticles: Applications for environmental remediation. *J Nanobiotechnol* 2018, 16(1), 1–24.
32. Chugh, D., Viswamalya, V. S., & Das, B. Green synthesis of silver nanoparticles with algae and the importance of capping agents in the process. *J Genet Eng Biotechnol* 2021, 19, 1–21.
33. Bagre, A. P., Jain, K., & Jain, N. K. Alginate coated chitosan core shell nanoparticles for oral delivery of enoxaparin: In vitro and in vivo assessment. *Int J Pharm* 2013, 456, 31–40.
34. Das, D., Ghosh, P., Ghosh, A., Haldar, C., Dhara, S., Panda, A. B., & Pal, S. Stimulus-responsive, biodegradable, biocompatible, covalently cross-linked hydrogel based on dextrin and poly(n-isopropylacrylamide) for in vitro/in vivo controlled drug release. *ACS Appl. Mater. Interfaces* 2015, 7, 14338–14351.
35. Lin, Z., Gao, W., Hu, H., Ma, K., He, B., Dai, W., Wang, X., Wang, J., Zhang, X., & Zhang, Q. Novel thermo-sensitive hydrogel system with paclitaxel nanocrystals: High drug-loading, sustained drug release and extended local retention guaranteeing better efficacy and lower toxicity. *J Controlled Release* 2014, 174, 161–170.
36. Tang, W., Yang, J., Zhao, Z., Lian, Z. & Liang, G. Intracellular coassembly boosts the anti-inflammation capacity of dexamethasone. *Nanoscale* 2017, 9, 17717–17721.
37. Zu, Y., Zhang, Y., Zhao, X., Shan, C., Zu, S., Wang, K., & Ge, Y. Preparation and characterization of chitosan–polyvinyl alcohol blend hydrogels for the controlled release of nano-insulin. *Int J Biol Macromol* 2012, 50, 82–87.
38. Nolan, A., Badminton, J., Maguire, J., & Seymour, R. A. The efficacy of topical hyaluronic acid in the management of oral lichen planus. *J Oral Pathol Med* 2009, 38, 299–303.
39. Li, H., Niu, R., Yang, J., Nie, J., & Yang, D. Photocrosslinkable tissue adhesive based on dextran. *Carbohydr Polym* 2011, 86, 1578–1585.
40. Gulrez, S. K., Al-Assaf, S., & Phillips, G. O. Hydrogels: Methods of preparation, characterisation and applications. In: *Progress in Molecular and Environmental Bioengineering—From Analysis and Modeling to Technology Applications*, InTech, 2011, ISBN: 978-953-307-268-5.
41. Artzi, N., Shazly, T., Crespo, C., Ramos, A. B., Chenault, H. K., & Edelman, E. R. Characterization of star adhesive sealants based on PEG/dextran hydrogels. *Macromol Biosci* 2009, 9, 754–765.
42. Gasperini, L., Mano, J. F., & Reis, R. L. Natural polymers for the microencapsulation of cells. *J R Soc Interface* 2014, 11, 20140817.

43. Berger, J., Reist, M., Mayer, J. M., Felt, O., Peppas, N. A., & Gurny, R. J. E. J. O. P. Structure and interactions in covalently and ionically crosslinked chitosan hydrogels for biomedical applications. *Eur J Pharm Biopharm* 2004, 57, 19–34.
44. Zhao, W., Jin, X., Cong, Y., Liu, Y., & Fu, J. Degradable natural polymer hydrogels for articular cartilage tissue engineering. *J Chem Technol Biotechnol* 2013, 88, 327–339.
45. Ivanovska, J., Zehnder, T., Lennert, P., Sarker, B., Boccaccini, A. R., Hartmann, A., & Detsch, R. Biofabrication of 3D alginate-based hydrogel for cancer research: Comparison of cell spreading, viability, and adhesion characteristics of colorectal HCT116 tumor cells. *Tissue Eng Part C Methods* 2016, 22, 708–715.
46. Jiang, S., Liu, S., & Feng, W. PVA hydrogel properties for biomedical application. *J Mech Behav Biomed Mater* 2011, 4, 1228–1233.
47. Annabi, N., Mithieux, S. M., Zorlutuna, P., Camci-Unal, G., Weiss, A. S., & Khademhosseini, A. Engineered cell-laden human protein-based elastomer. *Biomaterials* 2013, 34, 5496–5505.
48. Sindhu, R. K., Gupta, R., Wadhera, G., & Kumar, P. Modern herbal nanogels: Formulation, delivery methods, and applications. *Gels* 2022, 8, 97.
49. Gupta, S., Gupta, J., Anand, A., & Ojha, S. Review on nanogel/emulgel formulations of traditional medicines. *Biol Sci* 2022, 2, 269–278.
50. Raut, B. P., Khan, S. A., Ubhate, A. A., & Ganjiwale, R. O. A review on herbal nanoemulgel for the treatment of acne vulgaris. *World J Pharm Res* 2021, 10, 487–497.
51. Mota, A. H., Sousa, A., Figueira, M., Amaral, M., Sousa, B., Rocha, J., & Reis, C. P. Natural-based consumer health nanoproducts: Medicines, cosmetics, and food supplements. In: *Handbook of Functionalized Nanomaterials for Industrial Applications*, Elsevier, 2020, pp. 527–578.
52. Basak, S., Khare, H. A., Roursgaard, M., Kempen, P. J., Lee, J. H., Bazban-Shotorbani, & Kamaly, N. Simultaneous cross-linking and cross-polymerization of enzyme responsive polyethylene glycol nanogels in confined aqueous droplets for reduction of low-density lipoprotein oxidation. *Biomacromolecules* 2020, 22, 386–398.
53. Yallapu, M. M., Jaggi, M., & Chauhan, S. C. Design and engineering of nanogels for cancer treatment. *Drug Discov Today* 2011, 16, 457–463.
54. Okay, O., & Lozinsky, V. I. Synthesis and structure–property relationships of cryogels. In: *Polymeric Cryogels: Macroporous Gels with Remarkable Properties*, 2014, pp. 103–157.

Index

Note: Page numbers followed by 'f' and 't' indicate figures and tables, respectively.

A

Access and Benefit-Sharing (ABS) provision, 275
Acid insoluble ash, 202
"Acute disease," 288–289
Adverse drug reaction (ADR) reporting, 294
Aegle marmelos, 193
Aesculus hippocastanum, 130
Aflatoxins, in natural products, 204
Agency for the Assessment and Application of Technology, 32
Alginate (Alg), 315
Alkaloids, 3
Alstonia boonei, 207
Alternative remedies, 304
American Botanical Council, 143
American Herbal Pharmacopeia (AHP), 164–167
  challenges and future directions, 167
  herbal industry, impact on, 166
  herbal research and education, contribution to, 166
  key features of, 165–166
  mission and objectives, 165
Analytical laboratories, 10
Anatomical therapeutic chemical (ATC) approach, 125
Andrographis paniculate, 186
Angelica dahurica, 198
Anti-inflammatory effects, 6
Antioxidant activity, 6
API. *See* Ayurvedic Pharmacopeia of India
Aristolochic acids (AAs), 117
Arnica montana, 130
Artemisia absinthium, 135
Artemisia annua (sweet wormwood), 3
ARTG. *See* Australian Register for Therapeutic Goods
Ash content, in natural products, 202
Ashwagandha *(Withania somnifera),* 101
AusPAT, 253*t*
Australian Register for Therapeutic Goods (ARTG), 122, 299
Ayurveda, Yoga and Naturopathy, Unani, Siddha and Homoeopathy (AYUSH), 119
Ayurvedic, Siddha, and Unani (ASU) medicines, 6, 47, 131–132
Ayurvedic HMPs, 40
Ayurvedic Pharmacopeia of India (API), 153–154
AYUSH. *See* Ayurveda, Yoga and Naturopathy, Unani, Siddha and Homoeopathy
Azadirachta indica, 101
Azotobacter, 317

B

Bacopa monnieri, 6
BFAD. *See* Bureau of Food and Drugs
BHP. *See* British Herbal Pharmacopoeia
Bioactive compounds, of herbal drugs, 3–4
Biodiversity Management Committees, 47
Biological Diversity Act of 2002, 46, 47, 232
"Biopiracy," 229
"Biopiracy-patents," 228
Blighia sapida, 207
Blood–brain barrier, 305
Botanical gardens and herbaria, 10
Botanical research, 9
Brahmi *(Bacopa monnieri),* 101
Bridelia ferruginea, 207
British Herbal Pharmacopoeia (BHP), 149–150, 167–169
  challenges and future directions, 169

global influence and collaboration, 150
herbal industry, impact on, 168
herbal research and education, contribution to, 168–169
historical pillars, 150
key features, 167–168
legal status and effectivity, 150
mission and objectives, 167
public health, role in, 150
Bureau of Food and Drugs (BFAD), 123–124

C

CAGR. *See* Compound annual growth rate
Canadian Patent Database (CPD), 253*t*
Capillary electrochromatography (CEC), 198–200, 199*f*
Capillary electrophoresis (CE), 183, 208
Capsules and tablets, 18
Cassia acutifolia, 130
Cassia sieberiana, 207
Catharanthus roseus, 187
CBD. *See* Convention on Biological Diversity
CE. *See* Capillary electrophoresis
Ceaning-in-place (CIP) systems, 63
Central Council of Indian Medicine, 47
Chamomile tea, 90
Charaka Samhita, 79
Citation analysis, 262
Clinical trial infrastructure, 10
Collaboration, 10
Committee on Herbal Medicinal Products (HMPC), 143, 146
Compound annual growth rate (CAGR), 115
Contaminants, in natural products, 200–207
aflatoxins, 204
ash content, 202
foreign organic matter, 201–202
fumigants, 206
heavy metals, 206, 206*t*
microbial contamination, 203–204
moisture content, 202–203
pesticides, 205, 205*t*
radioactive contamination, 206–207
Convention on Biological Diversity (CBD), 229, 274–275
Article 8(j) of, 230
major outcomes of, 230
relationship to traditional knowledge, 229–230
support plant patent law reform, 220
Convention on International Trade in Endangered Species of Wild Fauna and Flora, 284
Cordia linnaei, 197
Cosmetic herbs, 80
Cosmetics Act 1940, 47
COVID-19
declared as pandemic, 114
medications used in hospitals, 115
Croton membranaceus, 207
Culinary herbs, 80
Cuminum cyminum, 190
Curcuma longa, 101
Czech Republic Patent Database, 253*t*

D

DARE. *See* Department of Agricultural Research and Education
Daruharidra *(Berberis aristata),* 101
Demand and supply, 32, 55
Dendrimers, 311, 312*f*
DEPATIS, 253*t*
Dietary Supplement Health and Education Act of 1994, 5, 40, 134
Digitalis purpurea, 4
Digital Library of Traditional Knowledge (TKDL), 238
Directorate of Medicinal and Aromatic Plants Research (DMAPR), 50
Distillation, 91
DNA polymorphism, 44
Dosage forms, in herbal drugs, 17–19
capsules and tablets, 18
essential oils, 19
herbal extract sprays, 19
herbal teas (infusions and decoctions), 17
lozenges and pastilles, 19
poultices and compresses, 19
powders, 18

syrups, 18
tinctures, 17
topical preparations, 18
Drug license, 295–300
in Australia, 299
in Canada, 298
in European Union, 298–299
in India, 295–298
in Malaysia, 299
in Philippines, 299
in Saudi Arabia, 299
in United States of America, 298
Drug Regulatory Authorities (DRAs), 284, 295–300
Bureau of Food and Drugs, Philippines, 299
European Medicine Agency, 298–299
Food and Drug Administration, 298
Health Canada, 298
of India, 295–298
of Malaysia, 300
of Saudi Arabia, 299
Therapeutic Goods Administration, Australia, 299
Drugs and Cosmetics Act 1940 (India), 40, 119, 132, 295

E

EAE. *See* Enzyme-assisted extraction
EAPATIS, 254*t*
EAPO. *See* Eurasian Patent Organization
Eastern Mediterranean Region
adverse drug reaction reporting, 294
categorization of herbal medicines, 285–290
novel herbal medicines, 286–289
traditional herbal medicines, 285–286
herbal medicinal products registration requirements, 284–295
AYUSH license, documents required to apply for, 290*t*
drug license and minimum requirement, types of, 289*t*–290*t*
pharmacovigilance, 294
quality control, 291–294
approaches to quality assurance, 291
guidelines related to, 293–294
guidelines related to GACP and GMP, 292–293
of imported herbal drugs, 291–292
regulating promotion, 294–295
Echinacea purpurea, 130
Electrospray ionization-mass spectrometry (ESI-MS), 196
Enzyme-assisted extraction (EAE), 183, 188, 208
Equipment selection, 63
ESI-MS. *See* Electrospray ionization-mass spectrometry
Espacenet, 252*t*
Essential oils, 4, 19
Ethosomes, 309–310, 310*f*
Eugenia jambolana, 193
Eurasian Patent Organization (EAPO), 254*t*
European Medicine Agency, 121
European Patent Convention, 234
European Patent Office (EPO), 251
European Pharmacopoeia (EP), 151–152, 153, 161, 172
comprehensive quality control, 151
legal mandate, 151
scope of standards, 151
undertakings of Convention, 152
European Scientific Cooperative on Phytotherapy, 178
Expression, 91
Extraction techniques, 89–92
advantages and disadvantages of, 93*t*
distillation, 91
expression, 91
infusion, 90
maceration, 89–90
percolation, 90
Soxhlet extraction, 92
supercritical fluid extraction, 91–92

F

Finnish Patent and Registration Office, 254*t*
"First-to-document" (pharmaceutical company), 273
Flavonoids, 3
Food and Drug Administration (FDA), 5, 121

Foreign organic matter, in natural products, 201–202
Formulation development, 9
Fourier transform-infrared spectroscopy (FTIR), 183, 195
Freedom to operate (FTO) search, 250–251
FTIR. *See* Fourier transform-infrared spectroscopy
Fumigants, in natural products, 206

G

GACP. *See* Good Agricultural and Collection Practices
Gas chromatography (GC), 183
Gas chromatography-mass spectrometry (GC-MS), 86
Ginkgo biloba, 6, 130
Global market, of herbal drugs, 114–119
  CAGR, 116
  cosmetics industry, demand for natural ingredients, 115
  future perspectives of, 136–137
  market report, 116*f*
  regulatory requirements in safety and efficacy, 117–119
  value of, 116
Glycosides, 4
Glycyrrhiza glabra, 38
GMP-compliant manufacturing facilities, 125
Gold nanoparticles (AuNPs), 314
Good Agricultural and Collection Practices (GACP), 131, 137
Good manufacturing practices (GMPs), 9, 11, 32
  adherence to, 62, 66, 113–114, 284
  European Union, 114
  for quality of herbal medications, 53–54
Green synthesis nanoparticles, 314
Guidelines for Herbal ATC Classification, 125

H

Harmonization of Herbal Medicine, 124
Heavy metals, in natural products, 206, 206*t*
Heavy metal toxicity, 117–118
Heliotropium europaeum (garden heliotrope), 135
Herbal ATC Index, 125
Herbal drug evaluation, key parameters in, 162
Herbal drug production
  facilities
    construction guidelines for, 64
    state-of-the-art, 62
  plant design, 65–73
    construction challenges and considerations, 71–73
    equipment selection, 63, 68
    facility design, 66, 67*t*
    layout planning, 63, 68–70
    site selection, 62–63, 65–66
  quality control and assurance, 63–64
  rising significance of, 64–65
Herbal drugs or medicines, 283–284. *See also* Herbal products
  adaptation and innovation, 5
  bioactive compounds in, 3–4
  challenges, 7
  chemical structure of, 20*f*
  classification, 113
  clinical trials data on, 20, 20*f,* 21*t*
  community and identity, 5
  complexity of, 284
  connection to nature and land, 5
  cultural and traditional knowledge, 7–8
  cultural heritage, 4
  cultural significance, 4
  dosage forms in, 17–19
  in Eastern Mediterranean Region, 284–295
  future trends, 304–324
  holistic approach to health, 4
  infrastructure for. *See* Infrastructure, for herbal drugs
  limited scientific evidence, 7
  natural origin, 3
  overview, 2–3
  potential benefits, 6–7
    anti-inflammatory effects, 6
    antioxidant activity, 6
    cognitive enhancement, 6–7
    digestive health, 6
    immune support, 6
    stress reduction, 6

quality control and standardization, 7
regulatory frameworks for, 5–6
Canada, 5
China, 6
European Union, 5
India, 6
United States, 5
regulatory issues, 7
safety concerns, 7, 284
spiritual and ritualistic use, 4–5
traditional medicine systems, use in, 3
Herbal extract sprays, 19
Herbal formulations, 30–56
certification, 48
current trends in, 35–36, 36*t*
drawbacks of, 37–44
clinical trials, 40–42
formulations interactions, 39–40
regulatory control, absence of, 42–43
social misinformation, 44
toxicity, 37–39
entrepreneurship
development, 45–46
startup, 49–51
in India, 30–31
law and policy, 49
management of resources, 47–48
marketing, 48–49
modernization of, 44–45
overview, 33–35
parameters for, 52*f*
and poverty decline, 46–47
project selection and project reports, 51–52
quality and regulatory concerns, 53–54
Herbal medicine merchandise, 31
Herbal monograph. *See* Monographs
Herbal nanomedicines (HNMs), 35
Herbal products. *See also* Herbal drugs or medicines
challenges and issues, 133–136
clinical research, challenges associated with, 135–136
herbal-allopathic drug interaction, challenges associated with, 134
herbal drug safety, challenges related to, 134–135
status and safety, impact of regulatory guidelines, 133–134
classification, 80
commercialization of, 101–102
cosmetic herbs, 80
culinary herbs, 80
extraction techniques, 89–92
advantages and disadvantages of, 93*t*
distillation, 91
expression, 91
infusion, 90
maceration, 89–90
percolation, 90
Soxhlet extraction, 92
supercritical fluid extraction, 91–92
formulation, types of, 93–97
capsules, 96
decoctions, 94
glycerites, 95
herbal oils, 97
ointments and creams, 96–97
powdered herbal preparation, 97
tablets, 95
tinctures, 94–95
future perspectives and challenges, 103–104
identifying and authenticating herbs, methods of, 84–89
biological analysis, 88–89
chemical analysis, 86–88
DNA barcoding, 88
macroscopic analysis, 85
microscopic analysis, 85–86
standardization and quality control, methods for, 84*f*
Indian developed and commercialized, 101–102, 102*t*
manufacturing processes, 98–101, 98*f*
formulation stage, 99
grinding and milling, 99
raw material selection, 98–99
standardization, 100–101
medicinal herbs, 80
overview, 78–81
popularity, 79–80
recognition and acceptability, 80–81

regulatory requirements, lack of, 131–133
selection of herbs, 81–84
intended use, 82
potency, 83–84
quality, 83
safety, 82–83
stability issues of, 100*f*
Herbal teas (infusions and decoctions), 17
Herbal toxicity, 37–39, 54
High-performance liquid chromatography (HPLC), 87, 190–192, 208
High-performance thin-layer chromatography (HPTLC), 87
High-speed counter-current chromatography (HSCCC), 190
HMPC. *See* Committee on Herbal Medicinal Products
HNMs. *See* Herbal nanomedicines
Hot-water extraction (HWE), 187
HPLC. *See* High-performance liquid chromatography
HPTLC. *See* High-performance thin-layer chromatography
HSCCC. *See* High-speed counter-current chromatography
Hydrogels, 314–319, 315*f*, 324
alginate based, 315, 317–318
cellulose-based compounds, 316–317
chitosan-based, 318–319
dextran-based, 317
hyaluronic acid, 316
natural polymer-based formulation, 316–319
Hypericum perforatum, 130

I

IARC. *See* International Agency for Research on Cancer
ICAR. *See* Indian Council of Agricultural Research
ICAR-Directorate of Medicinal and Aromatic Plants Research (ICAR-DMAPR), 50
ICDRA. *See* International Conference of Drug Regulatory Authorities
India
government initiatives in, 153
harmonization efforts in, 163–164
herbal formulations, 30–31
Kani model of benefit sharing in, 277–278
medicinal herbs, 30
Ministry of AYUSH, 6
Ministry of Environment and Forests, 220
Pharmacopoeia Commission for Indian Medicine & Homoeopathy, 153
sale of traditional medicines in, 131
Indian Council of Agricultural Research (ICAR), 50
Indian Herbal Drugs Market, 116
Indian Medicine Central Council Act, 1970, 47
Indian Pharmacopoeia (IP), 133, 148–149, 153, 161–162, 172–173
historical roots, 149
legal authority and recognition, 148–149
postindependence developments, 149
standards and monographs, 149
Indigenous herbal remedies, 113
Industrial Property Office of Slovak Republic, 254*t*
Industry collaboration, 10
Infrastructure, for herbal drugs, 8–17
consumer awareness, 16–17
consumer information sources, 17
educational initiatives for, 17
healthcare professionals in, 16
regulatory bodies in, 16
cultivation, 8
distribution and marketing, 13–14
cultural acceptance and demand, 13
distribution channels, 14
marketing strategies, 13, 14
quality control and standardization, 14
regulatory frameworks, 13–14
supply chain management, 13
education and training, 12–13
academic programs, 12
continuing education, 13
public awareness and consumer education, 13
regulatory framework, 13
research collaboration, 12

research initiatives, 13
training programs, 12
equipment, 9
facilities, 9
farming practices, 8
harvesting, 8
international collaboration, 15–16
capacity building, 16
cultural and ethical considerations, 16
global standards, 15
public awareness and education, 16
regulatory harmonization, 15–16
research and development, 15
research exchange, 15
manufacturing facilities, 11–12
cultivation and sourcing, 12
extraction and processing equipment, 12
GMPs, 11
packaging and labeling, 12
quality control laboratories, 12
pharmacovigilance, 14–15
adverse event reporting systems, 15
monitoring programs, 15
quality control, 15
regulatory framework, 14
research and evaluation, 15
processing, 8–9
processing and extraction, 9
quality assurance, 9
quality control, 8–9
regulatory compliance, 10–11
product labeling and claims, 11
quality control and testing, 11
quality standards, 11
registration and licensing, 11
regulatory agencies, 11
safety monitoring, 11
research and development, 9–10
analytical laboratories, 10
botanical gardens and herbaria, 10
botanical research, 9
clinical trial infrastructure, 10
formulation development, 9
industry collaboration, 10
regulatory agencies, 10
research institutions, 10
traditional knowledge documentation, 10
storage facilities, 9
Infusion, 90
Innovative herbal medicine delivery systems, 305
INPAIRS, 253*t*
Instituto Nacional de Biodiversidad (INBio), 277
Intellectual property (IP), 223–224
claiming, 224
protection of, 33, 225
Intellectual property ownership, 223–224, 225
Intellectual property rights (IPR), 223–224, 239, 273
application of, 232
definition, 223
herbal industries, challenges faced by, 234–236
Indian herbal industries, role in, 225–226
over biological resources, 236
reform rich country, 278
TRIPS Agreement, 226
International Agency for Research on Cancer (IARC), 204
International Atomic Energy Agency, 207
International Conference of Drug Regulatory Authorities (ICDRA), 147, 178
International Cooperative Biodiversity Groups (ICBG) project, 276
International harmonization, 124–131
evaluation of efficacy and safety, 129–131
good manufacturing practice, 127–128
labeling of herbal drugs, 125–126
safety, 128–129
International Organization of Standards (ISO), 51
International Patent Classification (IPC), 256, 262
(In) Validity search, 252
IP.com, 255*t*
IP management, 269–279
ethical considerations and case studies, 273–279

protecting innovations in field, importance of, 270
relevant to herbal products, types of, 269–270
strategies, 270–272
collaboration agreements, strategic use of, 272
collaborative IP ventures, 271
customized IP policies, 271
defensive publishing, consideration of, 272
early assessment of patentability, 271
selective data sharing, 272
strategic filing of patents, 271
timely disclosures in patent applications, 272
trade secret protection, 271
IPONZ, 254*t*
IPOS Singapore, 254*t*
IPR. *See* Intellectual property rights
IPSum, 255*t*

J

Japanese Pharmacopoeia (JP), 172, 173
JplatPat, 252*t*

K

Kava kava, 130
Keyword analysis, 262
Khaya ivorensis, 207
KIPRIS. *See* Korean Intellectual Property Rights Information Service
Korean Intellectual Property Rights Information Service (KIPRIS), 254*t*

L

LC-NMR. *See* Liquid chromatography-nuclear magnetic resonance
Legal status examination, 262
Liposomes, 308, 308*f*
Lippia multiflora, 207
Liquid chromatography-nuclear magnetic resonance (LC-NMR), 196–197
Lisianthus seemanni, 197
Lozenges, 19

M

Maceration, 89–90
MAE. *See* Microwave-assisted extraction
MALDI. *See* Matrix-assisted laser desorption/ionization
MALDI-TOF mass spectrometry, 197–198
Mass spectrometry (MS), 183, 195–196
Matricaria chamomilla, 130
Matrix-assisted laser desorption/ionization (MALDI), 183
Medicinal herbs, 80
Medicines and Healthcare Products Regulatory Agency (MHRA), 53
Medi-Hub TBI, 49
Mekai leaf (*Pycnarrhena tumefacta* Miers), 203
MHRA. *See* Medicines and Healthcare Products Regulatory Agency
Microbial contamination, in natural products, 203–204
Microwave-assisted extraction (MAE), 183, 188, 208
Millingtonia hortensis, 191
Ministry of Agriculture and Farmers Welfare, Government of India, 50
Moisture content, in natural products, 202–203
Mondia whitei, 207
Monographs, 142–178
comparative study of, 148–163, 156*t*–160*t*
herbal drug evaluation, key parameters in, 162
herbal drug standards across major pharmacopoeias, comparison of, 163
introduction to other pharmacopeias, 153–162
types of pharmacopeias, overview of, 148–153
components of, 143–145
harmonization
challenges and need for, 147
efforts in India, 163–164
international pharmacopeias, 164–171

American Herbal Pharmacopeia, 164–167
British Herbal Pharmacopoeia, 167–169
national pharmacopeias *vs.*, 171–176
WHO guidelines, 169–171
parameters of, 142–143
regulatory context, 146–147
British Pharmacopoeia, 146
Committee on Herbal Medicinal Products, 146
European Medicines Agency, 146
International Conference of Drug Regulatory Authorities, 147
national pharmacopeias, 147
WHO, 146
WHO guidelines, role of, 143, 176–177
Monotes, 197

N

NAFDAC. *See* National Agency for Food and Drug Administration and Control
Nagoya Protocol, 275–279
Nanoformulation, 305–314. *See also* Nanogel
dendrimers, 311, 312*f*
ethosomes, 309–310, 310*f*
green synthesis nanoparticles, 314
liposomes, 308, 308*f*
nanostructured lipid carriers, 312, 313*f*
niosomes, 310–311, 311*f*
overview, 306–307
phytosomes, 307, 307*f*
rising popularity of, 305
solid lipid nanoparticles, 313, 313*f*
transferosomes, 308–309, 309*f*
Nanogel, 319–323, 319*f*. *See also* Nanoformulation
biopolymer-based, 329
preparation of, 321–323
Nanogels, 305–306
Nanoparticles (NPs), 305
Nanostructured lipid carriers (NLCs), 312, 313*f*
National Agency for Food and Drug Administration and Control (NAFDAC), 124
National Biodiversity Authority, 232
National Medicinal Plants Board (NMPB), 46, 47
Natural Health Product Directorate (NHPD), 122
Natural health products (NHPs), 5, 122, 284
Natural products, testing of, 182–208
characterization of, 184*f,* 192–200
capillary electrochromatography, 198–200, 199*f*
electrospray ionization-mass spectrometry, 196
Fourier transform-infrared spectroscopy, 195
HPLC-SPE-NMR system, 200
liquid chromatography-nuclear magnetic resonance, 196–197
MALDI-TOF mass spectrometry, 197–198
mass spectrometry, 195–196
NMR spectroscopy, 193, 195
UV–vis spectrometry, 192–193, 194*f*
collection and authentication of, 207*f*
contaminants in, 200–207
aflatoxins, 204
ash content, 202
fumigants, 206
heavy metals, 206, 206*t*
microbial contamination, 203–204
moisture content, 202–203
pesticides, 205, 205*t*
radioactive contamination, 206–207
extraction, 184*f,* 185–188, 189*f*
microscopic identification, 185
overview, 182–183, 184*f*
Niosomes, 310–311, 311*f*
NMPB. *See* National Medicinal Plants Board
Nuclear magnetic resonance (NMR), 193, 195, 208

O

Opposition search, 251
Over-the-counter (OTC) medications, 131

P

Pan American Network of Drug Regulatory Harmonization, 125
Panax ginseng, 130
Pastilles, 19
Patentable herbal medicine inventions, 236–237
Patent literature, for research, 258–269
  extracting information from patents, 259–262
    text mining techniques, 260–261
    visualization techniques, 261–262
  integrating patent findings into research, 262–264
    herbal product development, patented technologies for, 263–264
    patent literature influence on experimental design, 263
  potential pitfalls, 264–266
    addressing limitations and biases, 265–266
    keyword search, 264–265
    verifying and validating information obtained from patents, 266
  real-world examples, 267*t*–269*t*
Patent(s)
  analysis, 259*f*
  on Ayurvedic/herbal extracts, 267*t*–268*t*
  context and philosophy, 226–227
  distribution of, 225
  ethical and legal implications, 224
  granting, conditions for, 224
  identifying existing, 247–248
  inapplicability of current laws, 225
  Indian herbal industries, role of IPR, 225–226
  intellectual property ownership, need for modifications in, 225
  obstacles for, 225
  overlapping studies, 258
  overview, 220–224
  plagiarism and preservation, 227–239
    additional legal instruments, 231–232
    bilateral and multilateral agreements, significance of, 233
    "biopiracy-patents," 228
    CBD and TRIPs relationship to traditional knowledge, 229–230
    developing new medicines, costs of, 233
    equity considerations, 233
    European Patent Convention, 234
    exploitations of medicinal plants in underdeveloped nations, 233
    herbal industries in IPR protection, challenges faced by, 234–236
    IPR over biological resources, 236
    legislation and protection of traditional knowledge, 237
    major outcomes of CBD, 230
    new indication, 237
    patentable herbal medicine inventions, categories of, 236–237
    patents, role of, 233
    process patent in herbal medicines, 237
    process patents viewed as less valuable, 236
    protectable subject matters for pharmaceutical products, 234
    regulatory framework, 232
    strategies for safeguarding natural and herbal products, 237–239
    Sui generis systems, calls for, 232–233
    TRIPs Agreement, 231
    TRIPs in protection, role of, 231
  procedure for applying, 224
  systematic analyses, 258
  technology-specific research, 258
  on 30 medicinal plants in India, 268*t*–269*t*
  traditional herbal medicines granted with, 222*t*
  trends in, 258
  TRIPs Agreement, 226
  verifying and validating information from, 266
Patentscope, 252*t*
Patent searches
  conducting, 246–247
  decision models for, 250
  definition, 247
  introduction to, 247–248
  keywords and classification codes for, 255–257
  methods of conducting, 248–257

online patent databases, utilizing, 251, 252*t*–255*t*
strategies, 249
successful searches in herbal science, 257–258
literature review on patent search studies, 257–258
patent information retrieval, 257
types of, 249–251, 250*f*
freedom to operate (FTO) search, 250–251
(In) Validity search, 252
opposition search, 251
Prior Art/Novelty/Patentability search, 250
state-of-the-art search, 249–250
PatFT, 252*t*
PCIM&H. *See* Pharmacopoeia Commission for Indian Medicine & Homoeopathy
PEF. *See* Pulsed electric field extraction
Percolation, 90
Pesticides, in natural products, 205, 205*t*
PFE. *See* Pressurized fluid extraction
Pharmacopoeia, 123
Pharmacopoeia Commission for Indian Medicine & Homoeopathy (PCIM&H), 153
Phenolic compounds, 3
PHWE. *See* Pressured hot-water extraction
Phytochemicals, 112–113
Phytosomes, 307, 307*f*
Piper methysticum, 130
Plant design, 65–73
construction challenges and considerations, 71–73
compliance with regulatory standards, 72
hygienic design, 71
material selection, 71
project management, 72
utility and support systems, 71–72
validation and qualification, 72–73
equipment selection, 63, 68
facility design, 66, 67*t*
layout planning, 68–70
extraction and processing areas, 69
flexibility for expansion, 70
formulation and mixing, 69–70
quality control and assurance, 70
raw material handling, 69
safety protocols, 70
zoning, 68–69
site selection, 62–63, 65–66
PLE. *See* Pressurized liquid extraction
Poultices and compresses, 19
Powders, 18
Preparative high-pressure liquid chromatography (prep-HPLC), 183
Pressured hot-water extraction (PHWE), 187
Pressurized fluid extraction (PFE), 187
Pressurized liquid extraction (PLE), 183, 188, 208
Prior Art/Novelty/Patentability search, 250
Process patent
in herbal medicines, 237
viewed as less valuable, 236
Protection of Plant Varieties and Farmers' Rights Act, 2001, 231
Pseudomonas, 317
Pulsed electric field extraction (PEF), 183, 188, 208

Q

Quality control (QC), 32

R

Radioactive contamination, in natural products, 206–207
Regulatory agencies, for herbal drugs, 10, 11, 119–124, 120*t*
in Australia, 122
in Canada, 122
in European Union, 121–122
in India, 119
in Malaysia, 122–123
in Nigeria, 124
in Philippines, 123–124
research and development and, 10
in Saudi Arabia, 123
in United States of America, 121
Regulatory requirements
lack of, 131–133
status and safety of herbal drugs, impact on, 133–134

Research institutions, 10
Rhamnus purshiana, 130
Rhododendron latoucheae, 200
Rio de Janeiro Convention on Biodiversity, 1992, 230

S

Saponins, 4
Sarcostemma brevistigma, 195
SEP. *See* Sustainable entrepreneurship practices
Serenoa repens, 130
SFE. *See* Supercritical fluid extraction
Siddha and Unani Pharmacopeia, 154–155
Silver nanoparticles (AgNPs), 314
Silybium marianun, 130
SIPO (China), 253*t*
Slovenia Intellectual Property Office (SIPO), 255*t*
Small- and medium-sized enterprises (SMEs), 45–46
Small-scale business ideas, 50*f*
SMEs. *See* Small- and medium-sized enterprises
Social misinformation, 44
Society for Research and Initiatives for Sustainable Technology and Institutions (SRISTI), 276
Solid lipid nanoparticles, 313, 313*f*
Soxhlet extraction, 92
State Medicinal Plants Board, 46, 47
State-of-the-art search, 249–250
Sui generis systems, 232–233
Supercritical fluid extraction (SFE), 91–92, 183, 208
Sustainable entrepreneurship practices (SEP), 45
Swissreg, 255*t*
Synephrine, 43
Syrups, 18

T

Tanacetun parthenium, 130
Taxodium distichum, 187
Terpenoids, 3
Text mining techniques, 260–261
  neural networks-based technique, 261
  NLP-based techniques, 260
  property-function based techniques, 260
  rule-based techniques, 260–261
  semantic analysis-based techniques, 261
Therapeutic Goods Administration (Australia), 122
Thin-layer chromatography (TLC), 86–87, 183
THMPD. *See* Traditional Herbal Medicinal Products Directive
Tinctures, 17
Tinospora crispa, 186
TLC. *See* Thin layer chromatography; Thin-layer chromatography
Topical preparations, 18
Total ash, 202
Trade-Related Aspects of Intellectual Property Rights (TRIPs) Agreement, 226, 227
  foundation for WTO Agreements, 231
  intellectual property, protection of, 231
  relationship to traditional knowledge, 229–230
  support plant patent law reform, 220
Traditional Chinese medicine (TCM), 79, 114
Traditional Herbal Medicinal Products Directive (THMPD), 5
Traditional knowledge documentation, 10
Transferosomes, 308–309, 309*f*
TRIPs Agreement. *See* Trade-Related Aspects of Intellectual Property Rights Agreement
Tymus serpyllum L., 187

U

UAE. *See* Ultrasonic-assisted extraction
Ultrasonic-assisted extraction (UAE), 183, 186–187, 208
United States Food and Drug Administration (USFDA), 117
United States Patent and Trademark Office (USPTO), 251
United States Pharmacopeia (USP), 133, 155, 161, 172

global impact and utilization, 152
introduction, 152
three-tiered quality standards in USP-NF, 153
USP-National Formulary, 152
USFDA. *See* United States Food and Drug Administration
USP. *See* United States Pharmacopeia
USPTO. *See* United States Patent and Trademark Office
UV–vis spectrometry, 192–193, 194*f*

V

Valeriana officinalis, 130
Vijaysar *(Pterocarpus marsupium),* 101

W

Water soluble ash, 202
Western Pacific Regional Forum, 124
WIPO. *See* World Intellectual Property Organization
Withania somnifera, 193
World Bank, 46
World Health Organization (WHO), 32, 135, 178
adverse drug reaction database, 287
COVID-19 as pandemic, declared, 114
Drug Monitoring Programme, 176
Eastern Mediterranean Region, 285
Eastern Mediterranean Regional Office, 286, 288
Good Agricultural and Collection Practices, 131
guidelines for developing monographs, 143, 169–171, 176–177
Guidelines for the Assessment of Herbal Medicines, 129, 143
heavy metal limits as per, 206*t*
maximum residue limits for pesticides, 118
World Intellectual Property Organization (WIPO), 238, 251
World Trade Organization (WTO), 246

Z

Zoning regulations, 62